Tumors at a Glance

Vishal Jain
MD (Std)
All India Institute of Medical Sciences
New Delhi

PEEPEE
PUBLISHERS AND DISTRIBUTORS (P) LTD.®

Tumors at a Glance

Published by
Pawaninder P. Vij and Anupam Vij
Peepee Publishers and Distributors (P) Ltd.
Head Office: 160, Shakti Vihar, Pitam Pura
Delhi-110 034 (India)
Correspondence Address:
7/31, First Floor, Ansari Road, Daryaganj
New Delhi-110 002 (India)
Ph: 41512412, 23246245, 9811156083
e-mail: peepee160@yahoo.co.in
e-mail: peepee160@rediffmail.com
e-mail: peepee160@gmail.com
www.peepeepub.com

First Edition Reprint: **2018**

ISBN: 978-81-8886-716-5

This book is dedicated
to
my friend's mother
and
my beloved aunty,
Late Mrs Anjali Pal

This book is dedicated

to

my friend's mother

and

my beloved aunty

Late Mrs A[illegible] Pal

Preface

Compiling a book describing "TUMORS" is a mammoth task. As we all know that what all known about tumors in today's world may be proved, in near future, as tip of iceberg, with hidden mysteries lying underneath. Anyways, I have made a conscious effort to compile "TUMORS" in a concise yet comprehensive form. I have tried to include all the relevant and necessary information about the malignancies of the human body. A worth mentioning feature is the inclusion of " AIDS-RELATED MALIGNANCIES". My effort was to make a student-friendly compilation of oncology.

I hope you will appreciate my hardwork and will encourage me to improve on my further writings.

Vishal Jain

Contents

One

General Consideration

Cancer is a disease in which healthy cells stop functioning and maturing properly. As the normal cycle of cell creation and death is interrupted, these newly "mutated" cancer cells begin multiplying uncontrollably, no longer operating as an integrated and harmonious part of the body. They also become parasitic, and can develop their own network of blood vessels to siphon nourishment away from the body's blood supply. This process, if unchecked, will eventually lead to the formation of a cancerous tumor. As the abnormal cells circulate within the bloodstream, the cancer can also spread to other parts of the body. This can cause the formation of more tumors and further sap the body's energy supply, weakening and eventually poisoning the patient with toxic byproducts.

Cancer is almost always fatal if left untreated. With cancer claiming so many lives each year, the search for a cure has become a global industry. Yet, as enticing as the idea of a "magic bullet" for cancer may seem, because of the multiple factors related to the disease, conventional medicine may never be able to offer the same sort of protection against cancer that it has been able to offer, for example, against polio and tetanus.

CHARACTERISTICS OF CANCER

Despite the fact there are several hundred different types of cancer, it is still possible to list certain general characteristics. Cancer is a cellular disorder, and so these general characteristics pertain to cancer cells.

First, *cancer cells experience uncontrolled and disorganized growth.* Normal cells only divide about 50 (fifty) times before they die, but cancer cells enter the cycle of dividing and reproducing, over and over again and never differentiate. *In tissue cultures raised in labs, cancer cells lack the contact inhibition exhibited by normal healthy cells.* This means, normal healthy cells stop reproducing when they contact each other, or the sides of a culture bowl. Normal cells in a tissue culture grow in only one layer because they adhere to the glass bowl and stop dividing once they make contact with their neighbors. Cancer cells have lost all restraint and grow in multiple layers, most likely because of cell surface changes. In the body, a cancer cell divides to form a growth, or tumor, that invades and destroys neighboring healthy tissue. This new growth, termed *neoplasia*, is made up of cells that are disorganized, a condition termed *anaplasia*. The cells are disorganized because they don't differentiate into the tissue of the organ and they never fulfill the function of the organ. To support their growth, *cancer cells release a growth factor* that causes neighboring blood vessels to branch into the cancer tissue. *This phenomenon has been termed vascularization, and some modes of treatment are aimed at preventing vascularization from occurring.*

Second, Cancer cells detach from the tumor and spread around the body. To accomplish this, the cells often must make their way across a basement membrane and into a blood vessel or lymphatic vessel. It's been discovered that cancer cells have receptors that allow them to adhere to basement membranes; they also produce proteolytic enzymes that degrade the membrane and allow them to invade the underlying tissues. Cancer cells also tend to be motile. This may be associated with a disorganized internal cytoskeleton and their lack of intact microfilament bundles. After traveling through the blood or lymph system, cancer cells start new tumor elsewhere in the body. This process is called *metastasis*.

If the original tumor is found before metastasis has occurred, the chances of cure are greatly increased. This is the rationale for early detection of cancer. In fact, sometimes a person isn't even considered to have cancer unless metastasis has occurred. *Benign tumors are those that remain in one place; malignant tumors are those that metastasize.*

Most, if not all, cancer cells contain genetic damage that appears to be the responsible event leading to tumorigenesis. The genetic damage present in a parental tumorigenic cell is maintained (i.e. not correctable) such that it is a heritable trait of all cells of subsequent generations.

Genetic Damage Found in Cancer Cells is of Two Types

1. Dominant and the genes have been termed *proto-oncogenes*. The distinction between the terms proto-oncogene and oncogene relates to the activity of the protein product of the gene. A proto-oncogene is a gene whose protein product has the capacity to induce cellular transformation given it sustains some genetic insult. An oncogene is a gene that has sustained some genetic damage and, therefore, produces a protein capable of cellular transformation.

The process of activation of proto-oncogenes to oncogenes can include retroviral transduction or retroviral integration, point mutations, insertion mutations, gene amplification, chromosomal translocation and/or protein-protein interactions.

Proto-oncogenes can be classified into many different groups based upon their normal function within cells or based upon sequence homology to other known proteins. As predicted, proto-oncogenes have been identified at all levels of the various signal transduction cascades that control cell growth, proliferation and differentiation. The list of proto-oncogenes identified to date is too lengthy to include here, therefore, only those genes that have been highly characterized are described. Proto-oncogenes that were originally identified as resident in transforming retroviruses are designated as c- indicative of the cellular origin as opposed to v- to signify original identification in retroviruses.

Classifications of proto-oncogenes

Although there are numerous examples of each classification of proto-oncogene, the lists here are by no means exhaustive. New genes with tumor causing capabilitites are being isolated continuously.

1. *Growth factors:*

The c-Sis gene (the v-sis gene is the oncogene in simian sarcoma virus) encodes the PDGF B chain. The v-sis gene was the first oncogene to be identified as having homology to a known cellular gene. The int-2 gene (named for the fact that it is a common site of integration of mouse mammary tumor virus) encodes an FGF-related growth factor. The KGF (also called Hst) gene also encodes an FGF-related growth factor and was identified in gastric carcinoma and Kaposi's sarcoma cells.

2. *Receptor tyrosine kinases:*
The c-Fms (*fims*) gene encodes the colony stimulating factor-1 (CSF-1) receptor. and was first identified as a retroviral oncogene. The Flg (*flag*) gene (named because it has homology to the Fms [*fims*] gene, hence fms-like gene) encodes a form of the FGF receptor. The Neu (*new*) gene was identified as an EGF receptor-related gene in an ethylnitrosourea-induced neuroblastoma. The conversion of proto-oncogenic to oncogenic Neu requires only a single amino acid change in the transmembrane domain. The Trk (*track*) genes encodes the NGF receptor-like proteins. The first Trk gene was found in a pancreatic cancer. Subsequently, two additional Trk-related genes were identified. These three are now identified as TrkA, TrkB and TrkC. The Met gene encodes the hepatocyte growth factor (HGF)/scatter factor (SF) receptor. The c-Kit gene encodes the mast cell growth factor receptor.

3. *Membrane associated non-receptor tyrosine kinases:*
The v-src gene was the first identified oncogene. The c-Src gene is the archetypal protein tyrosine kinase. The Lck gene was isolated from a T cell tumor line (LYSTRA cell kinase) and has been shown to be associated with the CD4 and CD8 antigens of T cells.

4. *G-protein coupled receptors:*
The Mas gene was identified in a mammary carcinoma and has been shown to be the angiotensin receptor.

5. *Membrane associated G-proteins:*
There are three different homologs of the c-Ras gene, each of which was identified in a different type of tumor cell. The Ras gene is one of the most frequently disrupted genes in colorectal carcinomas.

6. *Serine/threonine kinases:*
The Raf gene is involved in the signaling pathway of most RTKs. It is likely responsible for threonine phosphorylation of MAP kinase following receptor activation.

7. *Nuclear DNA-binding/transcription factors:*
The Myc gene was originally identified in the avian myelocytomatosis virus. A disrupted human c-Myc gene has been found to be involved in numerous hematopoietic neoplasias. Disruption of c-Myc has been shown to be the result of retroviral integration and transduction as well as chromosomal rearrangements. The Fos gene was identified in the feline osteosarcoma virus. The protein interacts with a second proto-oncogenic protein, Jun to form a transcriptional regulatory complex. The p53 gene was originally identified as a major nuclear antigen in transformed cells. The p53 gene is the single most identified mutant protein in human tumors. Mutant forms of the p53 protein interfere with cell growth suppressor effects of wild-type p53 indicating that the p53 gene product is actually a tumor suppressor gene.

2. Recessive and the genes variously termed tumor suppressors, growth suppressors, recessive oncogenes or anti-oncogenes.

Given the complexity of inducing and regulating cellular growth, proliferation and differentiation, it was suspected for many years that genetic damage to genes encoding growth factors, growth factor receptors and/or the proteins of the various signal transduction cascades would lead to cellular transformation. This suspicion has proven true with the identification of numerous genes, whose products function in cellular signaling, that are involved in some way in the genesis of the tumorigenic state. The majority of these proto-oncogenes were identified by either of two means: as the transforming genes (oncogenes) of transforming retroviruses or through transfection of DNA from tumor cell lines into non-transformed cell lines and screening for resultant tumorigenesis.

Viruses and Cancer

Tumor cells also can arise by non-genetic means through the actions of specific tumor viruses. Tumor viruses are of two distinct types. There are viruses with DNA genomes (e.g. papilloma and adenoviruses) and those with RNA genomes (termed retroviruses).

RNA tumor viruses are common in chickens, mice and cats but rare in humans. The only currently known human retroviruses are the human T-cell leukemia viruses (HTLVs) and the related retrovirus, human immunodeficiency virus (HIV).

Retroviruses can induce the transformed state within the cells they infect by two mechanisms. Both of these mechanisms are related to the life cycle of these viruses. When a retrovirus infects a cell its RNA genome is converted into DNA by the viral encoded RNA-dependent DNA polymerase (reverse transcriptase). The DNA then integrates into the genome of the host cell where it can remain being copied as the host genome is duplicated during the process of cellular division. Contained within the sequences at the ends of the retroviral genome are powerful transcriptional promoter sequences termed long terminal repeats (LTRs). The LTRs promote the transcription of the viral DNA leading to the production of new virus particles.

At some frequency the integration process leads to rearrangement of the viral genome and the consequent incorporation of a portion of the host genome into the viral genome. This process is termed transduction. Occasionally this transduction process leads to the virus acquiring a gene from the host that is normally involved in cellular growth control. Because of the alteration of the host gene during the transduction process as well as the gene being transcribed at a higher rate due to its association with the retroviral LTRs the transduced gene confers a growth advantage to the infected cell. The end result of this process is unrestricted cellular proliferation leading to tumorigenesis. The transduced genes are termed oncogenes. The normal cellular gene in its unmodified, non-transduced form is termed a proto-oncogene since it has the capacity to transform cells if altered in some way or expressed in an uncontrolled manner. Numerous oncogenes have been discovered in the genomes of transforming retroviruses.

The second mechanism by which retroviruses can transform cells relates to the powerful transcription promoting effect of the LTRs. When a retrovirus genome integrates into a host genome it does so randomly. At some frequency this integration process leads to the placement of the LTRs close to a gene that encodes a growth regulating protein. If the protein is expressed at an abnormally elevated level it can result in cellular transformation. This is termed retroviral integration induced transformation. It has recently been shown that HIV induces certain forms of cancers in infected individuals by this integration induced transformation process.

Cellular transformation by DNA tumor viruses, in most cases, has been shown to be the result of protein-protein interaction. Proteins encoded by the DNA tumor viruses, termed tumor antigens or T antigens, can interact with cellular proteins. This interaction effectively sequesters the cellular proteins away from their normal functional locations within the cell. The predominant types of proteins that are sequestered by viral T antigens have been shown to be of the tumor suppressor type. It is the loss of their normal suppressor functions that results in cellular transformation.

Hereditary Cancer Syndromes

See Table 1.1.

Table 1.1: Hereditary cancer syndromes

Syndrome	*Cloned gene*	*Function*	*Chromosomal location*	*Tumor Types*
Li-Fraumeni Syndrome	P53	Cell cycle regulation, apoptosis	17p13	Brain tumors, sarcomas, leukemia, breast cancer
Familial Retinoblastoma	RB1	Cell cycle regulation	13q14	Retinoblastoma, osteogenic sarcoma
Wilms Tumor	WT1	Transcriptional regulation	11p13	Pediatric kidney cancer
Neurofibromatosis Type 1	NF1 protein=neuro-fibromin 1	Catalysis of RAS inactivation	17q11.2	Neurofibromas, sarcomas, gliomas
Neurofibromatosis Type 2	NF2	Linkage of cell membrane to cyto-skeleton	22q12.2	Schwann cell tumors, astrocytomas, meningiomas, ependynomas
Familial Adenomatous Polyposis	APC	Signaling through adhesion mole-cules to nucleus	5q21	Colon cancer
Tuberous sclerosis 1	TSC1 protein=hamartin		9q34	Facial angiofibromas
Tuberous sclerosis 2	TSC2 protein=tuberin	GTPase activation	16	Benign growths (hamartomas) in many tissues, astrocytomas, rhabdomyosarcomas
Deleted in Pancreatic Carcinoma 4	DPC4 also known as Smad4	Regulation of TGF-b/BMP signal transduction	18q21.1	Pancreatic carcinoma, colon cancer
Familial Breast Cancer	BRCA1	Repair of double strand breaks by association with Rad51 protein	17q21	Breast and ovarian cancer
Familial Breast Cancer	BRCA2	Similar to BRCA1?	13q12.3	Breast and ovarian cancer
Hereditary Nonpolyposis Colorectal Cancer	MSH2	DNA mismatch repair	2p16	Colorectal cancer
Hereditary Nonpolyposis Colorectal Cancer	MLH1	DNA mismatch repair	3p21	Colorectal cancer
von Hippel-Lindau syn-drome	VHL	Regulation of transcription elon-gation	3p26-p25	Renal cancers, hemangioblastomas, pheo-chromocytoma
Familial Melanoma	CDKN2A protein= cyclindependent kinase inhibitor 2A	Cell-cycle regulation	9p21	Melanoma, pancreatic cancer, others

Contd...

Contd...

Syndrome	*Cloned gene*	*Function*	*Chromosomal location*	*Tumor Types*
Gorlin Syndrome: Nevoid basal cell carcinoma syndrome (NBCCS)	PTCH protein=patched	Transmembrane receptor for *hedgehog* signaling protein	9q22.3	Basal cell skin cancer
Multiple Endocrine Neoplasia Type 1	MEN1	Unknown	11q13	Parathyroid and pituitary adenomas, islet cell tumors, carcinoid
Multiple Endocrine Neoplasia Type 2	RET, MEN2	transmembrane receptor tyrosine kinase for glial-derived neurotrophic factor (GDNF)	10q11.2	Medullary thyroid cancer, type 2A pheochromocytoma, mucosal hartoma
Beckwith-Wiedmann Syndrome	p57, KIP2	Cell cycle regulator	11p15.5	Wilms tumor, adrenocortical cancer, hepatoblastoma
Hereditary papillary renal cancer (HPRC)	MET	Transmembrane receptor for hepatocyte growth factor (HGF)	7q31	Renal papillary cancer
Cowden diseas	PTEN similar to tensin	Dual-specificity phosphatase,	10q23.3	Brest cancer, thyroid cancer, intestinal hamartomous polyps
Hereditary prostate cancer (HPC)	Unknown	Unknown	1q24-q25	Prostate cancer
Ataxia telangiectasia (AT)	ATM	DNA repair	11q22.3	Lymphoma, cerebellar ataxia, immunodeficiency
Bloom syndrome	BLM	DNA helicase?	15q26.1	Solid tumors, immunodeficiency
Xeroderma pigmentosum (XP)	Several complimentation groups: XPA, XPC, XPD, XPE, XPF	DNA repair helicases, nucleotide excision repair	XPA = 9q22.3 XPC = 3p25 XPD=19q13.2-q13.3 XPE=11p12-p11 XPF=16p13.3-p13.13	Skin cancer
Fanconi's anemia	FAC			

TUMOR VACCINES

How to destroy cancer cells without damaging the normal cells? How to make conventional methods of systemic cancer treatment that predominantly comprise cytotoxic drugs more selective and prevent the development of drug resistance? There is an abundance of such questions that do not have simple answers. If, a few years ago, unselective cytotoxic drugs were the method of choice for the treatment of cancer, in the last 25 years we are witnessing the rapid transition of mmunotherapy from the laboratories to the clinics. Among the most attractive and promising immunotherapies for cancer, a special place s reserved for tumor vaccines. Exploiting the latest knowledge in immunology, tumor physiology, as well as in molecular biology, many outstanding approaches for the creation of tumor vaccines have been developed.

Tumor vaccination strategies have been increased over the past years. This increase began with the identification of tumor antigens recognized by the immune system. Better understanding of the immune system and increasing knowledge about the antigen presentation process and the role of dendritic cells have opened new therapeutic possibilities. DNA vaccines, already successfully used against viral antigens and covering a broad repertoire of epitopes, might also be of advantage in tumor immunotherapy. Design and selection of vectors are of considerable importance for the vaccination. There are three major types of DNA-based recombinant cancer vaccines: DNA from tumor antigens can be used 1) to modify dendritic cells, 2) as 'naked' DNA-vaccine or 3) to construct recombinant viral vaccines.

The development of vaccines against disease has been one of medicine's high-water marks. And now a new era in vaccinology which includes customized vaccines made from tumors and traditionally prepared cells which stimulate immune response (antigens). Tumors vaccinations can be subdivided into two different areas.

In the first one, a vaccine is developed which is biochemically specific for the tumor. The limitations here are that direct tumor samples (meaning the need for an active tumor from which fresh cells can be produced) may be unattainable, so patients in remission or those seeking the vaccines for cancer prevention are not candidates. Such vaccines work better with the help of other cancer therapies, nutrition, supplementation and detoxification, so they are not ideal "magic bullets" to treat an active tumor.

In the second strategy are "non-specific" vaccines which prevent, manage and control tumors. This form of therapy is useful from the earliest-stage cases right on through remission. By lengthening and enhancing tumor control through human immune/defense systems while remaining completely free of side effects over long periods of use, they are the most nature-similar ways of controlling malignant growths. Innovative immunological programs in which such vaccines play a central role are becoming increasingly important in the prevention and control of cancer.

Humans normally produce cancer cells throughout their lives. Malignant cells exposed to a healthy, active immune system will either be attacked and destroyed (phagocytosis) or genetically programmed for self-destruction (apoptosis). These mechanisms help rid the body of cancer cells throughout life. On closer examination, science has shown that cells derived from the specialized white blood cells called lymphocytes and monocytes produce tentacle-like elongations which trap tumors cells and expose them to the immune system for destruction. They are called denditric cells (DC's). Many factors in modern life may affect the maturation process of denditric cells, rendering the body more susceptible to the growth, maturation and proliferation of tumor cells. Since the relatively recent discovery of DC's, the challenge to medicine in an area of cancer therapy which until now has been essentially ignored was haw to make DC's functional and active. It was learned that denditric cells can in fact pick up normal cells and will migrate with them to lymph nodes where they will be exposed to a high concentration of immune system cells. DC's can stimulate a response in which the immune system increases the activity of such "fighter" units as T-cells. In experimental models this exposure to tumor-derived proteins resulted in dramatic protective immunity. The procedure involves drawing from the patient blood containing mature and immature DC's and tumor cells. A bio-chemist induces the maturation and activation of DC's in the presence of proteins derived from the patient's tumor.

At this point a weapon has been created which, when administered to the patient, will act as a cellular vaccine-a "smart-bomb" in modern defence parlance-which will actively seek out, entrap and expose to the immune system tumor cells developed at every stage of malignancy.

The vaccine, being non-toxic, sterile and customized from the patient's own blood, is thus a safe and effective form of therapy.

Therapeutic Vaccines Targeted at HPV-associated Tumors

Therapeutic vaccines are designed to treat preexisting HPV infection cases. The potential vaccines focus on E6 and E7, the HPV oncoproteins. Since both of these are required to maintain the transformed states of HPV-induced neoplastic cells, they are the prime targets for therapeutic vaccine intervention.

Emphasis in Developing Vaccines have been Placed on

- Minimizing presentation of E6 and E7 to the inductive arm of the immune response
- Introducing cytokine-encoding genes into *ex vivo* to induce tumor-specific CTL response
- Vaccinating with autologous tumor cells which have been engineered to create cytokines
- Eliciting Th1—which induces IgG2a antibody— to confer antibody-dependent lymphocyte activated killer (LAK)

Tumors have Evasion Mechanisms, which Result From

- Point mutations in genes encoding CTL epitopes within HPV proteins
- Down-regulation of endogenous peptide processing machinery (TAP), required for antigen stimulated CTL response

Experiments in animal models have shown the ability of E6 and E7 to prevent tumor formation. BPV4 E7 has been shown to be a successful target for BPV4-induced papillomas, and areas of homology in the conserved regions of BPV4 E7 and HPV16 E7 suggests that HPV16 E7 may be successful target in humans.

THERAPEUTIC VACCINE TRIALS IN HUMANS

Cervical Cancer

One Phase I trial underway uses peptides containing proven immunogenic HPV16 E7 CTL epitopes restricted by HLA A* 0201 in cervical carcinoma patients expressing this haplotype. The peptide is administered in adjuvant known to predispose to Th1 response.

A trial of HPV16 E7 as bacterial fusion protein administered in alum demonstrated Th2-type immunogenicity and lack of toxicity.

Issues which require special attention for cervical cancer trials:

- For peptide vaccines adjuvants should be optimized to elicit Th1 rather than Th2 response.
- Therapeutic vaccines must establish specific CTL memory, and should avoid need for repeated immunization.

ANOGENITAL WARTS

There are no prospective therapeutic vaccines against genital warts in clinical trials. There are many treatments for HPV associated genital warts, though none are universally effective. One non-vaccine possibility is a topical ointment called imiquimod that acts to reduce wart infection by stimulating the host's Th1 immune response, notably INFg. Since HPV type 6 and 11 are responsible for anogenital warts, a prospective therapeutic vaccine must be type specific. Researchers are investigating the possibility of combined therapies using a vaccine along with topical and/or surgical therapies.

Many of the gene therapies involving cancer represent a form of cancer vaccines. The ability to introduce genes into cells is known as gene transfer. Investigators have used these techniques to introduce genes into tumor cells to make them more reactive to the patient's immune system. These genes contain the building blocks for immune hormones (ie., interferon, interleukin-2 (IL-2), granulocyte-macrophage colony-stimulatine factor (GM-CSF), etc.) or other stimulatory proteins which have been found to enhance the effectiveness of these vaccines in animal studies.

Cancer vaccines are only available in clinical trials and are not considered a primary form of therapy. Researchers have conducted melanoma and renal cell (kidney) cancer vaccine studies on humans for several years. Cancer vaccines used to treat malignant brain tumors and breast tumors are also being developed. Another cancer vaccine is under development to treat sarcomas in children and young adults that relapse after chemotherapy.

TUMOR MARKERS

Tumor markers are substances that can be detected in higher than normal amounts in the blood, urine, or body tissues of some people with certain types of cancer. A tumor marker may be produced by the tumor itself, or by the body in response to a cancer presence. When diagnosing cancer, blood and pieces of tumor tissue are tested, These tests help to determine the characteristics of the tumor (aggressiveness, rate of growth, and degree of abnormality). Tests for tumor markers may be used with other tests or X-rays to detect and diagnose some cancers.

Tumor markers may be proteins, antigens, or hormones. Tumor markers tests are not used alone in diagnosis because most markers can be found in elevated levels in people who have benign conditions, and because no tumor marker is specific to a particular cancer. Not every tumor will cause an elevation in the tumor marker test, especially in the early stages of cancer. Physicians can use changes in tumor marker levels to follow the course of the disease, to measure the effect of treatment, and to check for recurrence.

Tumor markers can be used for one of four purposes: (1) screening a healthy population or a high risk population for the presence of cancer; (2) making a diagnosis of cancer or of a specific type of cancer; (3) determining the prognosis in

Table 1.2: Common tumor makers currently in use

Tumor markers	*Cancers*	*Other conditions*	*Clinical importance*	*Sample*
AFP (Alpha-feto protein)	Liver, germ cell cancer of ovaries or testes	Also elevated during pregnancy	Help diagnose, monitor treatment, and determine recurrence	Blood
CA 15-3 (Cancer antigen 15-3)	Breast and others including lung, ovarian	Also elevated in benign breast conditions; doctor can use CA 15-3 or CA 27.29 (two different assays for same marker)	Stage disease, monitor treatment, and determine recurrence	Blood
CA 19-9 (Cancer antigen 19-9)	Pancreatic, sometimes colorectal and bile ducts	Also elevated in pancreatitis and inflammatory bowel disease	Stage disease, monitor treatment, and determine recurrence	Blood
CA-125 (Cancer antigen 125)	Ovarian	Also elevated with endometriosis, some other diseases and benign conditions; not recommended as a general screen	Help diagnose, monitor treatment, and determine recurrence	Blood
CEA (Carcino-embryonic antigen)	Colorectal, lung, breast, thyroid, pancreatic, liver, cervix, and bladder	Elevated in other conditions such as hepatitis, cirrhosis, inflamatory bowel disease, chronic lung disease, pancreatitis, and in cigarette smokers	Monitor treatment and determine recurrence	Blood
Estrogen receptors	Breast	Increased in hormone-dependent cancer	Determine prognosis and guide treatment	Tissue
HCG (Human chorionic gonadotropin)	Testicular and trophoblastic	Elevated in pregnancy, testicular failure	Help diagnose, monitor treatment, and determine recurrence	Blood, urine
Her-2/neu	Breast	Oncogene that is present in multiple copies in 20-30% of invasive breast cancer	Determine prognosis and guide treatment	Tissue
Monoclonal immunoglobulins	Multiple myeloma and Waldenstrom's macroglobulinemia	Overproduction of an immunoglobulin or antibody, usually detected by protein electrophoresis	Help diagnose, monitor treatment, and determine recurrence	Blood, urine
Progesterone receptors	Breast	Increased in hormone-dependent cancer	Determine prognosis and guide treatment	Tissue
PSA (Prostate specific antigen), total and free	Prostate	Elevated in benign prostatic hypertrophy, prostatitis and with age	Screen for and help diagnose, monitor treatment, and determine recurrence	Blood

a patient; (4) monitoring the course in a patient in remission or while receiving surgery, radiation, or chemotherapy.

No test meets all of those requirements. Specifically, no marker has been established as a pratical cancer screening tool either in a general healthy population or in most high risk poulations. The reason for this is the relative lack of sensitivity and specificity of the available tests, given the low prevalence of cancers in most population groups. Given the low prevalence of cancer in general, even tests that are highly sensitive and specific may have low predictive values.

Tumor markers include many substances that are not readily systematically organized. Those discussed here are generally products or the cancer cell, although none is unique to cancer cells; they represent aberrant tumor production of a normal element. Some markers are produced by the organism in response to the cancers presence.

TUMOR ANTIGENS

Include markers defined by both monoclonal antibodies and polyclonal antisera, often the so called oncofetal antigens. The oncofetal substances, present in embryo or fetus, diminish to low levels in the adult but reappear in the tumor.

Common Tumor Markers Currently in Use

See Table 1.2.

Neuron Specific Enolase

Neuron specific enolase is an isozyme of the glycolytic pathway that is found only in brain and neuroendocrine tissue. Its an immunohistochemical marker for tumors of the central nervous system, neuroblastomas, and APUD tumors.

Use of NSE has been evaluated in lung cancer and neuroblastoma.

Galactosyl Transferase II

Galactosyl Transferase II, an isozyme of galactosyl transferase, has been shown to be elevated in a variety of malignancies, predominantly gastrointestinal. In colon cancer its level correlated with the extent of disease and disease progression; in pancreatic cancer it was more sensitive and specific in distinguishing benign from malignant disease than CEA and other tests.

The following table illustrates some of the pitfalls in ordering tumor marker tests Table 1.3.

Table 1.3: ....

Tumor markers	*Cancers*	*What else?*	*When/How Used*	*Sample*
B2M (Beta-2 microglobulin)	Multiple myeloma and lymphomas	Present in many other conditions, including Crohn's disease and hepatitis; often used to determine cause of renal failure	Determine prognosis	Blood
BTA (Bladder tumor antigen)	Bladder	Gaining acceptance	Help diagnose and determine recurrence	Urine
CA 72-4 (Cancer antigen 72-4)	Ovarian	No evidence that it is better than CA-125 but may be useful when combined with it	Help diagnose	Blood
Calcitonin	Thyroid medullary carcinoma	Also elevated in pernicious anemia and thyroiditis	Help diagnose, monitor treatment, and determine recurrence	Blood

Contd...

Contd...

Tumor markers	*Cancers*	*What else?*	*When/How Used*	*Sample*
NSE (Neuronspecific enolase)	Neuroblastoma, small cell lung cancer	May be better than CEA for following this particular kind of lung cancer	Monitor treatment	Blood
NMP22	Bladder	Not widely used	Help diagnose and determine recurrence	Urine
Prostate-specific membrane antigen (PSMA)	*Prostate*	Not widely used, levels increase normally with age	Help diagnose	Blood
Prostatic acid phosphatase (PAP)	Metastatic prostate cancer, myeloma, lung cancer	Not widely used anymore, elevated in prostatitis and other conditions	Help diagnose	Blood
S-100	Metastatic melanoma	Not widely used	Help diagnose	Blood
TA-90	Metastatic melanoma	Not widely used, being studied	Help diagnose	Blood
Thyroglobulin	Thyroid	Used after thyroid is removed to	Determine recurrence evaluate treatment	Blood

RECOMMENDATIONS

1. Never rely on the result of a single test .
2. When ordering serial testing, be certain to order every test from the same laboratory using the same assay kit.
3. Be certain that the tumor marker selected for monitoring recurrence was elevated in the patient prior to surgery.
4. Consider the half-life of the tumor marker when interpreting the test result.
5. Consider how the tumor marker is removed or metabolized from the blood circulation.
6. Consider ordering multiple markers to improve both the sensitivity and the specificity for diagnosis.
7. Order the nonspecific markers for cost-saving and for their high sensitivity.
8. Be aware of the possibility of a hook effect.
9. Be aware of the presence of ectopic tumor markers.

Two

Cancer Chemotherapy

Cancer cells have the following general properties. They proliferate in a disregulated manner. They invade surrounding tissues probably through secretion of certain proteolytic enzymes. They metastasize or spread to secondary sites throughout the body. Cancer cells arise from normal tissue-renewal STEM CELLS. Cancer cells also fail to differentiate normally. Cancer cells also show alterations of cell surface components such as antigens, enzymes and oncogenes. Some of these may be shed into the blood and are detectable by immunologic techniques as tumor markers.

In general there are few unique or specific differences between normal and cancer cells. Any beneficial effect of cancer chemotherapy is due to quantitative differences and not qualitative differences.

Cancers growing in the body also occupy space and crowd out normal cells. They can invade through tissues and cause hemorrhage and infection. They metastasize to distant organs (e.g., liver, brain, lungs, bone) and destroy these tissues. They produce nutritional deficits and weight loss due to their high metabolic rate. Cancer cells also decrease host defense mechanisms against infection.

TYPES OF EFFECTIVE TREATMENT OF CANCERS

Surgery is the most effective treatment of cancer but it is ineffective for metastasized or disseminated tumors

Radiation is the next most effective treatment after surgery. Rapidly dividing cells are the most sensitive. It is useful primarily in cancers that are not widely disseminated. It is often combined with surgery and chemotherapy.

Immunotherapy and Biological Response Modifiers (BRMs) is effective against small number of tumor cells. Its most important role is in combination with other agents. Immunotherapy has been becoming more and more important in recent years due to improved knowledge as to how they work and through molecular biologic techniques their is a greater availability of agents that play a role in anticancer activity.

Chemotherapy is useful mostly for disseminated cancers and is often used in combination with other types of therapy such as surgery, radiation or immunotherapy.

Survival from cancer depends on the tumor stage at time of diagnosis. Tumors that have progressed to a greater degree are usually more slow growing and thus are more difficult to treat.

Thus the chances of survival are less than with the smaller more rapidly growing tumors. Also the longer a tumor has been growing the more likelihood of metastasis. Since metastases are more disseminated than the primary tumors they are difficult to treat without inducing much toxicity to normal tissues. Thus the chances of survival are less.

DETERMINANTS OF DRUG RESPONSE

Growth fraction: is the proportion of dividing cells in a tumor or normal tissue. It is the fraction of cells that are actively dividing with respect to the entire population of viable cells.

The mass doubling time: is the time it takes for the tumor to double in size.

Tumors with a high growth fraction are more susceptible to the cytotoxic effects of anticancer drugs than those with a high percentage of dormant cells. Usually, it is the dividing cell that is drug sensitive. Thus, those tumors with shorter mass doubling times are more amenable to treatment with drugs. As tumors get larger, the mass doubling time increases and the growth fraction decreases. Unfortunately, normal tissues with high growth fractions *(Bone Marrow, Oral and Intestinal Mucosa, Hair Follicles)* are also damaged by anticancer drugs, and treatment with many of these drugs may produce bone marrow depression (leukocytopenia and infection, thrombocytopenia and bleeding), stomatitis, GI tract ulceration, and alopecia.

Total tumor burden: In general, large bulky tumors are not curable with drugs. Tumor size is another limiting factor to successful chemotherapy in malignant disease. Drugs may not be able to penetrate into a solid tumor in amounts sufficient to kill the cells. Also, most cells in a bulky tumor may be in a nonproliferative stage at the time of treatment and thus survive to reestablish the tumor mass. Also the longer a tumor has been present the greater likelihood that it has already metastasized.

In general, tumor cell kill after drug treatment follows first order kinetics, i.e., each treatment results in killing of a constant proportion, rather than a constant number of tumor cells. The data deviate from first order kinetics at the two ends of the response curve. After initial treatment, the rate of cell kill may change because the growth fraction and mass doubling time change as the tumor mass decreases from a large, bulky tumor to a smaller tumor (this is called *"Recuitment"*). The slope of the response curve is also different for the residual cells because they are likely to be less sensitive to the drug or present in sites where drug does not penetrate as well. Treatment must continue even in the face of clinical remission until the tumor is totally eradicated. Cure is considered achieved when the *Disease-free survival Plateau* is reached. This time is different for different tumors (e.g., Burkitts' lymphoma-8 months; testicular cancer-1 year). NOTE: There is no clear survival plateau for certain cancers (e.g., breast cancer).

Tumor heterogeneity: Tumors are heterogeneous populations of cells. Some of these cells are proliferating, some can proliferate but are dormant and others are dying. The fact that tumors are not uniform must be considered. For any tumor therapy to be completely effective the most invasive metastatic cells must be killed.

Cell cycle phase: The response to certain cell phase-specific drugs depends on the percent of cells in a sensitive phase during the time of exposure to pharmacologically effective concentrations of drug. In general, for cycle phase specific agents such exposure should be for at least two cell cycle times. Cells in the G0 phase are, for the most part, refractory to chemotherapy. These cells may reenter the cell cycle and result in disease recurrence. Most anticancer drugs are effective against cells in one particular phase of the cycle (e.g., vincristine during M; cytarabine during S, etc.). Most drugs have their greatest activity during S phase when cells are undergoing DNA synthesis.

Drug resistance: This is one of the most important problems with cancer chemotherapy. As many as 40-45% of patients' cancers may have or may develop resistance to anticancer drugs. There are several different biochemical Mechanisms by Which Tumor cells Develop Resistance to Anticancer Drugs. These include:

1. Decreased intracellular drug levels. This could result from increased drug efflux or decreased inward transport. Among the drugs which become resistant by this mechanism are the anthracyclines, dactinomycin, vinca alkaloids, and epidopodophyllotoxins.
2. Increased drug inactivation. Included in this group are the alkylating agents, antimetabolites and bleomycin.
3. Deceased conversion of drug to an active form. This mechanism is most common among the antimetabolites which must be converted to the nucleotide before they are active.
4. Altered amount of target enzyme or receptor (gene amplification)..methotrexate is a classic example here as often in methotrexate resistant tumors there is an amplification in the target enzyme dihydrofolate reductase.
5. Decreased affinity of target enzyme or receptor for drug. Examples, here are the antimetabolites and hydroxyurea.
6. Enhanced repair of the drug-induced defect. The alkylating agents typically show resistance by this mechanism although other mechanisms are also important with these drugs.
7. Decreased activity of an enzyme required for the killing effect (topoisomerase II). This is a newly recognized target but decreased activity is important for resistanced to doxorubicin, m-AMSA, and the epipodophyllotoxins. Multidrug Resistance (MDR) This is a phenomenon whereby tumors become resistant to several, often unrelated drugs, simultaneously. The multidrug Resistance (MDR1) gene encodes an ATP-dependent efflux pump, called p-glycoprotein, that may become amplified in drug-resistant tumors. MDR activity may be reversed by drugs such as calcium channel blockers (e.g., verapamil), cyclosporin, or tamoxifen. Multidrug resistance occurs between several different structurally unrelated antitumor agents that apparently have different mechanisms of action. This resistance is obtained through stepwise selection and it reflects the amplification of a gene that encodes a transmembrane protein that pumps the drugs out of the cell. Thus the resistant cell maintains a lower intracellular drug level than the drug-sensitive parental cells. Ling etal discovered that cell lines with a high level of resistance produced large amounts of a 170,000 dalton glycoprotein that they called P170 or Pglycoprotein. It is now clear that P170 is overproduced as a result of gene amplification. The degree of P-glycoprotein overproduction correlates well with the degree of drug resistance.

Host factors: Included among these are the general status of the patient. The Karnofsky patient "performance status" is a useful index to evaluate whether or not the disease is progressing both during and after therapy. In general, if the patient's performance status is below 40%, it is less likely that his or her clinical condition can be markedly improved with chemotherapy. The best chance for increasing survival time is when treatment begins early. Also important is the patient's immune status. The status of a patient's cell-mediated immunity (i.e., the effects initiated by activated macrophages, cytolytic T-lymphocytes, and natural killer cells) is the most important factor in the immune response to malignant cells. Antibody-dependent cell-mediated cytotoxicity (so-called ADCC reactions) also plays a role in tumor cell killing. Circulating antigen-antibody complexes ("blocking factors") may inhibit the cell-mediated killing of cancer cells. The blood supply and site of neoplasm is also important. If any drug is to be effective, it must be present in sufficient concentrations at the site of its action. In cancer chemotherapy, this means that tumor cells, even if very sensitive to the administered drug, cannot be destroyed unless they have a reasonable access to blood supply. Failure of drug therapy may occur when tumors metastasize into the pleural space or the CNS.

Finally there is the scheduling of the drug therapy. Effective chemotherapy requires that the tumor cells be exposed to pharmacologically active drug concentrations for a period of time sufficient to catch the maximal number of tumor cells in a sensitive phase of the cell cycle (the concentration × time factor).

Tumor markers: Tumor markers are quite useful in diagnosis and therapy follow-up in cancer. Examples: hCG-, alpha-fetoprotein (AFP), prostate specific antigen (PSA).

Common effects of anticancer drugs: Most of the anticancer drugs act by inhibiting DNA synthesis in one way or another. Some exceptions are vincristine, vinblastine, and L-asparaginase which affect the microtubules and protein synthesis respectively. Many of the anticancer drugs have bone marrow toxicity. Some drugs with low bone marrow toxicity are bleomycin, steroid hormones, and vincristine. These latter drugs are often used in combination chemotherapy with drugs that have high bone marrow toxicity. Many of these are mutagenic and some have been shown to be teratogenic and carcinogenic. These latter effects are often seen when these drugs are given for prolonged time periods. Most anticancer drugs exhibit a greater toxicity for tissues with high growth fractions such as the bone marrow, gastrointestinal epithelium, hair follicles, and gonadal tissue. Many of these drugs produce some nausea and vomiting. This is a problem especially with the alkylating agents and cisplatin. There is a important need for new drugs that will prevent or treat the nausea or vomiting as they significantly decrease the compliance with these drugs.

Combination chemotherapy: The use of combinations of drugs in cancer chemotherapy has been one of the major advances made in this field. Combination chemotherapy has several important advantages. They are that it usually results in a decreased incidence of resistance. Thus you frequently see combination chemotherapy being used in the treatment of cancer. Secondly, there is often a greater than additive or synergistic effect of the drugs. Finally, by using drugs with different types of toxic effects you can decrease the overall toxicity or at least the toxicity to any one organm system. There are three generally accepted guidelines to choosing drugs for combination chemotherapy. They are:Select drugs that are active against the tumor when used alone. Select drugs with different mechanisms of action (to avoid combined resistance) and select drugs with minimally overlapping toxicities.

Adjuvant chemotherapy and neoadjuvant chemotherapy: Adjuvant Chemotherapy is when surgery is followed by chemotherapy. This has the theoretical advantage of eliminating any residual or metastatic cells thus improving on survival of the patient. This is being used more and more as it is often quite effective. Neoadjuvant chemotherapy has been introduced relatively recently. It is also called primary or induction therapy. Here chemotherapy is given prior to the surgery in contrast to adjuvant therapy. This has several advantages including the ability to monitor drug sensitivity in the intact primary tumor and allowing one to determine what definitive local therapy could be used.

ALKALOIDS

Microtubule Inhibitors

Microtubules are protein polymers that are responsible for various aspects of cellular shape and movement. The major component of microtubules is the polymer tubulin, a protein containing two nonidentical subunits (alpha and beta). These drugs act by affecting the equilibrium between free tubulin dimers and assembled polymers.

Vinca Alkaloids

- Vincristine
- Vinblastine
- Vindesine

These are large complex molecules produced by the leaves of the periwinkle plant (vindesine is actually a synthetic vinca alkaloid). There are slight structural differences between the different vinca alkaloids but significant differences in therapeut ic uses and toxicity.

Mechanism of action The vinca alkaloids are cell specific agents and block cells in mitosis. Their biological activity is explained by their specific binding to tubulin. Upon binding to vinca alkaloids, tubulin dimers are u nable to aggregate to form microtubules. This effectively decreases the pool of free tubulin dimers available for microtubule assembly, resulting in a shift of the equilibrium toward disassembly. Formation of paracrystalline aggregates by vinca-bound tu bulin dimers shifts the equilibrium even further toward disassembly and microtubule shrinkage. They block mitosis with metaphase arrest.

Resistance Drug resistance is due primarily to decreased drug accumulation and results from overexpression of the P-glycoprotein. Note that this is one of the drug classes that may show MDR-mediated cross-resistance with mu ltiple other natural products. Resistance can also be due to alterations in tubulin structure resulting in changes in drug binding to the tubulin.

Pharmacology Their absorption is unpredictable and they usually are given by i.v. infusion. They are very irritating to tissues. Both are rapidly cleared from the plasma and excreted predominantly by the liver by a combin ation of hepatic metabolism and biliary excretion. Caution should be used with decreased hepatic function. Many vinca metabolites have been found in humans and animals. It is believed that a number of these are active cytotoxic agents and that the pharma cological effects of these drugs are still felt long after the parent drug is gone. Vincristine is eliminated much more slowly than the other two vinca alkaloids.

Therapeutic Uses Despite close similarity in structure the different vinca alkaloids have quite different therapeutic uses. Vincristine is used mainly in combination therapy for the induction of remission in childhood acute leukemias. Vincristine together with prednison is the main therapy for induction of acute lymphocytic leukemia. Complete remissions are obtained in 80 to 90% of patients. It is also used for the treatment of Hodgkin's and non-Hodgkin's lymphoma where it is part of several complex protocols. Here again vincristine therapy is very successful.

On the other hand the most important clinical use of vinblastine is in the therapy of metastatic testicular tumors where it is combined with bleomycin and cisplatin. Beneficial responses have also been obtained in the treatment of Hodgkin's and non-Hod gkin's lymphoma. In Hodgkins disease it has been used in place of vincristine providing similar antitumor activity with less neurotoxicity. Vindesine the newest of the vinca alkaloids has significant activity in the treatment of acute leukemia, blast cris is of chronic myelogenous leukemia and Hodgkins and non hodgkins lymphomas.

Toxicity Like the therapeutic uses the toxicities of these drugs is different. The dose limiting toxicity of vincristine is mainly peripheral neuropathy and other neurological toxicities. The most common symptom is a depres sed Achilles tendon reflex which is usually followed by paresthesias in the extremities. Autonomic neuropathy often occurs early in the course of therapy resulting in abdominal pain, constipation, paralytic ileus, urinary retention and orthostatic hypoten sion. Unlike most antineoplastic agents vincristine usually does not cause significant bone marrow supression therefore vincristine is often found in combination therapies with other drugs that are myelosuppressive. Gastointestinal symptoms also are comm on with this vinca alkaloid.

Unlike vincristine the other vinca alkaloids produce mainly bone marrow depression. Myelosuppression (primarily neutropenia) is the major toxicity of vinblastine while lymphopenia is the dose limiting toxicity of vindesine but neurotoxicity also occurs frequently.The neurotoxicity produced by these drugs is similar to vincristine but less common and less severe.

Paclitaxel (Taxol) and Docetaxel

Paclitaxel was first isolated from the from the bark of the Pacific Yew (Taxus brevifolia). Docetaxel is a more potent analog that is produced semisynthetically.

Mechanism of action: In contrast to other microtubule antagonists, taxol disrupts the equilibrium between free tubulin and mircrotubules by shifting it in the direction of assembly, rather than disassembly. As a result, tax ol treatment causes both the stabilization of microtubules and the formation of abnormal bundles of microtubules. Studies have shown that taxol binds to microtubules at a ratio of about one drug molecue per molecule of polymerized tubulin dimer. The bindi ng site for taxol is apparently distinct from the binding sites for colchicine, vinblastine, podophyllotoxin and GTP.

Resistance: Resistance to these drugs arises through mechanisms similar to how it arises to the vinca alkaloids. Those are multidrug resistance and mutation of the gene coding for one of the tubuline subunits.

Pharmacology It is usually given i.v.preferably in 24 hr infusions in order to prevent certain severe hypersensitivity reactions from occurring. Taxol binds extensively to plasma proteins. It undergoes significant P-450 med iated hepatic metabolism to hydroxylated metabolites and this is believed to be the major mechanism of elimination.

Therapeutic uses: It has significant activity against ovarian cancer, breast cancer, carcinoma of the lung and head and neck carcinoma. Response rates in these cancers is fairly high.

Toxicity: The major toxicity of these drugs is bone marrow depression with neutropenia the common dose limiting toxicity. Hypersensitivity reactions are also common. They are characterized by dyspnea, urticaria and hypotensi on. It is not clear at this time whether they are due to the vehicle in which taxol is given or the drug itself. Avoidance of bolus injections and short infusions can minimize this toxicity as can pretreatment with steroids or antihistamines. Mucositis is also common and is manifested as ulcerations of the mouth and throat. Taxol also causes some reversible neurotoxicities most often numbness and paresthesias in the hands and feet.

Chromatin Function Inhibitors

This class of drugs owe their antitumor effects to disruption of chromosomal dynamics. Chromosomes are complex structures which undergo many changes in conformation and intracellular position during the cell cycle. Drugs that interfere with the protein s responsible for these changes are selectively toxic to proliferating cells.

Topoisomerase Inhibitors
Epipodophyllotoxins

- Etoposide (VP-16)
- Teniposide (VM-26)

These drugs are semisynthetic glycosidic derivatives of podophyllotoxin a natural compound produced in the roots of the Mayapple plant. These derivatives are referred to as etoposide (VP-16-213) and teniposide (VM-26).

Mechanism of action: DNA in eukaryotic cells must be packed very efficiently to be able to fit into the n ucleus. As a result, chromosomal DNA is twisted extensively and the activities of enzymes called topoisomerases are ne eded to permit selected regions of DNA to become sufficiently untangled and relaxed to allow transcription, replication, and other essential functions to proceed. To do this topoisomerases have the ability to break DNA strands and then to reseal these bre aks after the topological changes have occurred. The clinically useful drugs in this class are inhibitors of topoisomerase II as they break both strands of DNA. Several inhibitors of the type I enzyme are in early clinical trials but look promising as an ticancer agents.

The two drugs work similarly although teniposide is taken up by cells more rapidly and retained to a greater extent than etoposide. This may be because teniposide is more lipophilic than etoposide. These drugs form complexes with the topoisomerase II enzyme. This complex produces inhibition of the enzyme along with production of double stranded breaks in the DNA. Removal of the drug results in a rapid return of normal topoisomerase function. Arrest of cells occurs during the G2 phase of the cell cyc le. Early studies with these drugs led investigators to believe that their action was due to inhibition of microtubules. Although these drugs bind to tubulin they have no effect on microtubular function or structure at therapeutic concentrations.

Resistance: Resistance to these two drugs is commonly accompanied by cross resistance to several drugs. Resistant cells demonstrate overexpression of the MDR gene that the encodes the p-glycoprotein drug efflux transporter. In addition an "atypical " multidrug resistant phenotype has been identified in which cells that are resistant to topoisomerase-II inhibitors retain normal drug transport characteristics. These cells have altered or decreased topoisomerase activity.

Pharmacology: They are usually given i.v. as oral administration usually results in variable absorption. Approximately 30-50% of etoposide is recovered as unchanged drug. Almost all of this is found in the urine with a sm all amount excreted in the bile. As much as 20% is recovered as metabolites. Both drugs are extensively bound to plasma proteins.

Clinical uses Etoposide has shown activity against a variety of tumor types. Its greatest effectiveness is in the treatment of testicular tumors where it is effective against tumors resistant to treatment of other drugs. It is most effective when combined with bleomycin and cisplatin. Etoposide also has an important role in the treatment of small cell lung carcinomas where it is often combined with cisplatin. Teniposide has been studied clinically much less than etoposi de. It appears to be effective for the treament of acute lymphoblastic leukemia and childhood neuroblastomas as well as brain tumors in adults.

Toxicity: The principal dose-limiting toxicity of these drugs is *Bone marrow depression* primarily leukopenia and thrombocytopenia. Nausea and diarrhea are common but not severe. Mucositis can be severe at higher doses. Other toxic effects seen include fever, chills, erythema. Allergic reactions have been noted in some patients.

Camptothecin

The camptotecins are a new class of chemotherapeutic agents with a novel mechanism of action targeting the nuclear enzyme topoisomerase I. This compound was isolated from the bark of a Chinese tree. This drug and its derivatives are inhibitors of topoi somerase I. Camptothecin itself is poorly soluble and causes significant toxicity. Several more soluble and less toxic derivatives are now available. One derivative with a lot of promise is irinotecan (CPT-11). It is one of the most active compounds a vailable for the treatment of non small cell lung cancer. Leukopenia and diarrhea were the most severe toxicities seen. Nausea and vomiting were common but manageable.

COVALENT DNA-BINDING DRUGS (ALKYLATING AGENTS)

Nitrogen Mustards

Mechanism of action All of the alkylating agents form strong electrophiles through the formation of carbonium ion intermediates. This results in the formation of covalent linkages by alykylation of various nucleophiles moi eties. The chemotherapeutic and cytotoxic effects are directly related to the alkylation of DNA mainly through the 7 nitrogen atom of guanine although other moieties are also alkylated. The formation of one covalent bond with nucleophiles can result in mu tagenesis or teratogenesis but the formation of two of these bonds through cross linking can produce cytotoxicity. Bifunctional alkylating agents (those containing two reactive chloroethyl side chains) can undergo a second cyclization of the second side cahin and form acovalent bond with another nucleophilic group. The second group could be a 7-nitrogen of another guanine or some other nucleophilic moiety. These bifunctional alkylating agents such as nitrogen mustard react with another nucleophilic moiety resulting in the cross-linking of two nucleic acid chains or the linking of a nucleic acid to a protein. This type of alteration could cause a major disruption in nucleic acid function. Cytotoxicity of bifunctional alkylators correlates very closely with interstrand cross-linkage of DNA. The ultimate cause of cell death related to DNA damage in not known. Some of the cellular responses produced include cell-cycle arrest, DNA repair and apoptosis or programmed cell death. The nucleophilic groups of prote ins, RNA and many other molecules can also be subject to attack by the alkylating agents.although the exact result of these interactions is not known.

The alkylating agents are generally considered to be cell-cycle-phase nonspecific. They also are known to be most cytotoxic to rapidly proliferating cells. Thus although DNA alkylation can occur anytime in the cell cycle, the biological consequences are most severe when this interaction during DNA synthesis. This is because cells exposed to the alkylating agents earlier such as in G1 would have enough time to repair some of the DNA damage before the next DNA synthesis phase. Nonproliferating cells w ould have an even greater period for DNA repair to occur before irreversible damage occurs. Thus the alkyating agents are proliferation dependent but cell-cycle phase nonspecific.

Resistance Cross-resistance between different alkylating agents often occurs. Resistance may represent the summation of a series of changes, none of which by itself confers significant resistance. Several biochemical mechan isms have been implicated as a cause of resistance to these drugs including decreased permeability of the drug into the cells, increased production of nucleophiles such as glutathione and increased repair of DNA. Two mechanisms of resistance that are prob ably of clincal importance are increased drug inactivation and decreased drug uptake.

Pharmacology All of the *nitrogen mustards* are chemically unstable but they vary greatly in their degree of instability ranging from the highly unstable mechlorethamine to the highly stable chlorambucil and cyclophosphamide. The latter two compounds can be given orally and cyclophosphamide requires biochemical activation by liver microsomal enzymes before it becomes active as an anticancer compound. The original alkylating agents such as mechlorethamine were very unstable and had to be administered rapidly to avoid breakdown. This, mechlorethamine must be given into a running i.v. infusion.

Most of the clinically useful alkylating agents have structural modifications that have produced stable compounds that can be given orally as well as parenterally. For example, *cyclophosphamide* can be administered orally or parenterally. However, cyclo phosphamide is unique in that it must be converted to an active form by liver microsomal enzymes. Cyclophosphamide was originally designed so that it would be preferentially activated in tumor tissue which is believed to contain high levels of enzymes tth at would convert it to an active form. Although selectivity is now known not to be achieved the drug undergoes metabolic activation in the liver catalyzed by the cytochrome P-450 microsomal enzymes. One of the metabolites formed is believed to be active as a cytotoxic agent while another metabolite, acrolein, is believed responsible for the cystitis produced by cyclophosphamide. Ifosphamide is a recently developed structural analog of cyclophosphamide. It is metabolized by the cytochrome P-450 system an d it undergoes the same metabolic conversions as does cyclophosphamide. However, a smaller proportion of ifosphamide is converted to cytotoxic compounds and larger doses are used clinically as compared to cyclophosphamide.

Therapeutic uses: The nitrogen mustards can be used for treatment of a variety of tumors ranging from leukemias to solid tumors. Mechlorethamine is used mainly to treat Hodgkin's disease and other lymphomas (MOPP regimen). It is also used in the treatment of other lyphomas but the results have been less predictable. Chlorambucil is used almost exclusively in the treatment of chronic lymphocytic leukemia. Occasionally it has been used to treat certain lyphomas. Melphalan has been used principally to treat multiple myeloma. The most commonly used alkylating agent is cyclophosphamide. It is an extremely versatile alkylating agent. It is used in Hodgkin's disease and other lymphomas but in addtion is useful to treat acute lymphocytic leukemia and a variety of solid tumors. It can be given in a variety of ways and dosages unlike many of the other nitrogen mustards. Ifosphamide is an alkylating agent closely related to cyclophosphamide. The indications for the use of ifosphami de are similar to that of cyclophosphamide. It is used almost exclusively with mesna a compound that inactivates the alkylating activity and helps prevent the cystitis associated with this drug.

Toxicity: The dose limiting toxicity of all the nitrogen mustards is bone marrow depression. This is usually of a delayed nature. It is important to monitor leukocyte and platelet counts carefully during therapy with these d rugs. All of the nitrogen mustards produce an acute nausea and vomiting, and with some such as mechlorethamine the effect is quite severe. There are now a variety of drugs available on the market that will lessen or help prevent these effects. In addition cyclophosphamide can cause alopecia and an hemorhaggic cystitis. As discussed above this cystitis is attributed to formation of acrolein during the metabolism of cyclophosphamide. Its incidence can be reduced by ensuring good fluid intake and frequent vo iding and can be prevented coadministration of the sulfhydryl scavenging compounds such as N-acetylcysteine or MESNA. As with ifosphamide patients who take high dose cyclophosphamide should be treated with mesna.

Mechlorethamine but not the other nitrogen mustards will produce a severe necrosis if extravasated on the skin during administration and phlebitis. If extravasation occurs the area should be infiltrated with isotonic sodium thiosulfite which reacts wit h the electrophilic drug dervatives. Busulfan (Myleran)

Busulfan has few pharmacological effects other than myelosuppression. This property is important in both its therapeutic use and toxicity.Busulfan is an atypical alkylating agent, although it is converted to a bifunctional alkylator.

Therapeutic uses: Its action is limited mainly to the myeloid cells. It is useful for the treatment of chronic myelocytic leukemia (CML). It is effective during the chronic phase of this disease. At therapeutic doses is has little if any effect on lymphoid tissue.

Toxicity: Its toxicity is mainly on the bone marrow where it is toxic mainly to the granulocytes. At high doses it does effect platelets and red blood cells and in some patient a severe pancytopenia will result. Also at high doses toxicities such as pulmonary fibrosis occur.

Nitrosoureas

This class of alkylating agents appear to function as bifunctional alkylating agents but differ in both pharmacological and toxicological properties from the other alkylating agents. The nitrosoureas are converted nonenzmatically into a carbonium ion a nd an isothiocyanate molecule. The carbonium ion acts as a typical alkylating agent and is probably responsible for the cytotoxic action of the nitrosoureas. The isothiocyanate may interact with proteins and account for some of the toxic effects of these drugs.

Pharmacology *Carmustine* must be administered parenterally while *lomustine* and semustine can be given orally. All of them have short plasma half-lives. All of the nitrosoureas are very lipophilic and have very good penetrat ion into brain tissue. This allows them good therapeutic utility in various CNS neoplasms.

Therapeutic uses: The nitrosoureas are used mainly for the treatment of Hodgkin's disease and meningeal leukemia and brain tumors. Occasionally they are used in the treatment of solid tumors such as (lung, carcinoma, G.I. and breast carcinomas in combination with other anticancer agents.

Toxicity: The usual dose limiting toxicity of the nitrosoureas is a delayed bone marrow toxicity. They also produce an acute nausea and vomiting. Carmustine also produces an unusual interstitial pulmonary fibrosis.

Other Alkylating Agents

Several other alkylating agents have been available over the years. Most of them are quite toxic and have been used only in special circumstances. Included among them are dacarbazine, hydroxymethylmelamine, thiotepa and mitocycin C.

Dacarbazine is probably the most widely used of the miscellaneous agents. It functions as a methylating agent after metabolic activation in the liver. It is employed in combination regimens for the treatment of malignant melanomas, Hodgkins disease and adult sarcomas.

NONCOVALENT DNA-BINDING DRUGS (ANTITUMOR ANTIBIOTICS)

General properties These drugs interact with DNA in a variety of different ways including intercalation, DNA strand breakage and inibition with the enzyme topoisomerase II. Most of these compounds have been isolated from na tural sources and antibiotics. However, they lack the specificity of the antimicrobial antibiotics and thus produce significant toxicity.

Dactinomycin (Actinomycin D)

Dactinomycin is the only actinomycin used clincically. This compound contains a phenoxasone ring and two cyclic pentapeptides as part of its structure. The phenoxasone ring is the chromophore mo iety which imparts a red color to the drug.

Mechanism of action: At low concentrations dactinomycin inhibits DNA directed RNA synthesis and at higher concentrations DNA synthesis is also inhibited. All types of RNA are affected, but ribosomal RNA is more sensitive. Da ctinomycin binds to double stranded DNA, permitting RNA chain initiation but blocking chain elongation. Binding to the DNA depends on the presence of guanine. The binding of the drug to DNA has been demonstrated by spectroscopy, by DNA density and meltin g experiments and by kinetic studies. It appears that the phenoxasone chromphore region of the drug intercalates between bases in the DNA and that the 2-amino group of the guanine is important in the formation of a stable drug-DNA complex. X-ray crystall ography studies show that in the dactinomycin-DNA complex the phenoxasone ring lies between two deoxyguanosine molecules and strong hydrogen bonds connect the 2-amino group of guanine and the threonine residues in the polypeptide side chains of the drug. There is a very tight binding of the drug with the DNA and thus a very slow dissociation. This apparently relflects the intermolecular hydrogen bonds. Apparently the tight binding of the dactinomycin prevents unwinding of the DNA to facilitate its intera ction with RNA polymerase. This prevents the synthesis of RNA by the DNA dependent RNA polymerase and this blockade is responsible for the cytotoxic effect. The exact mechanism of the cytotoxicity is not clear but in some cells apoptosis is initiated. Da ctinomycin is cytotoxic to cells in any phase of the cell cycle and it is probably equally toxic to exponentially growing cells and stationary cells.

Resistance: Resistance results mainly from decreased retention of the drug in the cancer cell. Cells resistant to dactinomycin show cross-resistance to anthracyclines and vinca alkaloids as a result of amplification of the gene for P-glycoprotein. In addition resistance can be reversed by competition with verapamil and a variety of other lipophilic compounds. Thus dactinomycin is one of several drugs considered part of the multidrug resistant (MDR) complex.

Pharmacology Actinomycin D is usually given i.v. and can cause severe local necrosis if extravasation occurs. Therefore, it should be administered into the tubing of a rapidly flowing i.v. infusion. The Plasma half-life i s very short, but tissue half-life is long (48 hrs) due to DNA binding. Only a small amount of the drug is known to be metabolized. Urinary and fecal excretion of the drug is prolonged. In humans it does not appear to enter into the central nervous system.

Therapeutic uses: Actinomycin is used mainly in the treatment of pediatric solid tumors (e.g. Wilm's tumor, rhabdomyosarcoma). It also is an alternative drug used to treat choriocarcinoma when methotrexate can't be used bec ause of resistance. The treatment of several solid tumors utilizes combination therapy with actinomycin and radiotherapy. There seems to be an improved antitumor effect when the two are used in combination.

Toxicity: The primary and dose limiting toxicity of actinomycin is bone marrow depression. The leukocyte count and usually the platelet count are depressed with a low after one to two weeks. Also nausea, vomiting, malaise, ulceration of the oral mucosa and gastointestinal tract and acneiform eruptions of the skin occur. The nausea, vomiting and malaise begin several hours after treatment and last for as long as a day. As mentioned above it is sometimes used in patients who also are receiving X irradiation. If given to a patient who has had radiation, a "recall" effect may be observed (i.e., when actinomycin D is administered, the patient may develop a reaction in normal appearing tissue that was included in the field of r adiation).

Anthracycline Antibiotics

- Daunorubicin [Daunomycin, Cerubidine]
- Doxorubicin [Adriamycin]
- Idarubicin [Idamycin]

The anthracyclines are among the most important antitumor drugs available. Doxorubicineis widely used for the treatment of several solid tumors while daunorubicin and idarubicin are used exclusively for the treatment of leukemias. They all contain a f our membered anthracycline nucleus attached to a sugar molecule. Daunorubicin and doxorubicin are identical except for the presence of a hydrogen or hydroxyl at the 14 position of the anthracycline ring. Idarubicin is a recently introduced member of this group. It is 4-demethoxy-daunorubicin. This minor structural modification at position 4 of the chromophore ring makes the drug more lipophilic giving it a longer half-life.

Mechanism of action: The anthracyclines all bind to DNA and their cytotoxicity largely results from this binding.They bind to double stranded DNA. In human chromosome preparations treated with anthracyclines the bound drug is observed as well-defined, orange-red fluorescent bands. This interaction with DNA is by intercalation and has been identified as such by several methods. If the structure of the anthracyclines is modified so that the binding to DNA is altered their is usually a decrease or loss of antitumor activity. Thus, DNA binding seems to be critical for the anticancer activity of these drugs. However, the pathway leading to cytotoxicity is not all that clear. Inhibition of DNA and RNA synthesis is not though to be critical for cytotoxicity as it only occurs at high drug concentration.

These agents have a number of important effects any one or all of which have a role in the cytotoxic actions of these drugs. First of all they can intercalate with DNA affecting many functions of the DNA including DNA and RNA synthesis. Breakage of the DNA strand can also occur. This is believed to mediated either by the enzyme DNA Topoisomerase II or by the formation of free radicals. Inhibition of the enzyme topoisomerase II, for example, can lead to a series of reactions leading to double strand bre aks in the DNA.

Temporary double-strand breaks are induced by topoisomerase II in the course of its normal catalytic cycle, by formation of a cleavable complex. Disruption of this complex, which results in a permanent double-strand break, occurs infrequently in the absence of drugs. Inhibitors of topoisomerase II cause the cleavable complex to persist, thereby increasing the probability that the cleavable complex will be converted to an irreversible double-strand break.

Anthracyclines can also cause the formation of active oxygen species that then cause predominantly single-strand breakage. The anthracycline chromophore contains a hydroxyquinone, which is a well-described iron chelating structure. The drug-Fe-DNA co mplex catalyzes the transfer of electrons from glutathione to oxygen, resulting in the formation of active oxygen species.

Resistance: The most common mechanism of resistance to the anthracyclines is increased drug efflux due to amplification of the gene for P-glycoprotein, the multidrug transporter. Anthracyclines show cross-resistance with ot her drugs that are acted upon by the p-glycoprotein transporter such as dactinomycin and the vinca alkaloids. However, two other mechanisms of resistance have been reported. These are decreased topoisomerase II activity and increased glutathione peroxidase activity. The latter is consistent with free radical formation being important in the mechanism of action of these drugs.

Pharmacology: All three anthracyclines are administered i.v. since the glycosidic bond would be split in the gastrointestinal tract making these drugs inactive if given orally. The anthracyclines are very irritating to tissue and should not be extravasated. Thus, they are usually given into the tubing of a rapidly flowing i.v. infusion. These drugs are rapidly cleared from the plasma. The metabolic pathways of the anthracylines are very similar. They are eliminated by metabolic conversion to a variety of less active or inactive metabolites by liver enzymes. A major pathway is conversion to the alcohols daunorubicinol and doxorubicinol which also have cytotoxic activity like their parents. This reduction is catalyzed by cytoplasmic NADPH-dependent reductases. These enzymes probably play a major role in the pharmacokinetics of these drugs.

Daunorubicin is a better substrate for this enzyme than is doxorubicin, thus after a few hours the alcohol is the principal circulating form of this drug while with doxorubicin the parent drug is the principal circulating form. Glycosidases also act on the parent drugs as well as the metabolites. Since the Anthracyclines are detoxified in the liver patients with impaired hepatic function risk severe toxicity and the dosage must be reduced.

Therapeutic uses: Daunorubicin has limited clincal activity. It is very useful for the treatment of acute lymphocytic and especially acute myelocytic leukemia. Doxorubicin has a very broad range of clinical usefulness in contrast to daunorubicin. It is most active against solid tumors, particularly breast cancer. Other solid tumors against which it has good activity are ovary, bladder, and lung carcinomas. It is also active in the treatment of Non-Hodgkin's lymphoma and Hodgkin's disease. Idarubicin appears to be as effective as daunorubicin in combination treatment of acute myelogenous leukemia with perchaps more efficacy in patients less than 60 years old.

Toxicity: The toxic effects of all three anthracyclines are similar. They frequently cause nausea and vomiting and patients may experience anorexia and diarrhea. These drugs and their metabolites may color the urine red for one or two days after administration. Bone marrow depression is dose-limiting and occurs in 60-80% of patients. This is seen primarily as leukopenia which reaches a low point at approximately one to two weeks. Thrombocytopenia and anemia may also occur but is not as severe. Stomatitis is dose related and may be severe. Alopecia also occurs in most patients but reverses when therapy is stopped. The anthracyclines potentiate the effects of radiation and enhancement of radiation reactions and radiation recall effects on normal tissues have been seen.

Cardiac toxicity is a peculiar adverse effect observed with these agents in both adults and children. The total dose should not exceed 550 mg/m2 as the risk of cardiotoxicity increases markedly at that level. Two types of reactions are observed: (1) early, transient electrocardiographic changes, and (2) a delayed progressive cardiomyopathy. Acute changes int he electrocardiogram, including tachycardia, extrasystolic contractions, and ST-T wave alterations, may occur in the week following drug administration. Arrhythmias generally reverse within a few hours, and the S-T segment and T-wave abnormalities usually reverse in 1 or 2 weeks after a single dose. Pathological studies of patients who have died of congestive heart failure show a decrease in the number of cardiac muscle cells and signs of degeneration in the remaining cells. It is thought that the sarcoplasmic reticulum is the critical site of anthracycline induced damage within the myocardial cell. The cardiomyopathy is usually fatal.

There is now a great deal of evidence that the myocardial damage produced by these drugs is due to production of reactive oxygen species, in particular the hydroxyl radical (OH). These radicals are generated from redox cycling of the anthracycline quinone, which can undergo one electron reduction to the semiquinone or two electron reduction to the corresponding dihydroquinone derivative. The semiquinone reacts rapidly with oxygen to generate superoxide anion. Superoxide anion can dismutate to peroxide, which reacts with a number of species to produce OH. The heart may be especially prone to anthracycline toxicity because it contains lower levels of critical detoxifying enzymes (e.g. catalase and superoxide dismutase) than other organs such as the liver. It has been shown that doxorubicin administration leads to lipid peroxidation in cardiac tissue and that this process can be blocked by free radical scavenger such as alpha-tocopherol. However, free radical scavengers were found to be unsuccessful at controlling cardiac toxicity in humans. More successful in humans werer agents that acted as iron chelators. The rational being that anthracycline induced lipid peroxidation required iron. Dexrazoxane has recently been approved by the FDA to prevent anthracylcine induced cardiac toxicity.

Anthracenediones (Mitoxantrone)

These drugs are analogs of the anthracyclines. They lack the sugar moiety of the anthracyclines but retain the planar polycylic aromatic ring structure that permits intercalation into DNA. They have shown impressive clinical activity but appear to cau se less cardiac toxicity most likely because they cannot produce quinone type free radicals.

Mechanism of action: *Mitoxantrone* interacts with DNA by a high-affinity intercalation. It also produces a lower affinity binding as a result of electrostatic interactions. As discussed for the anthracyclines, intercalation of mitoxantrone into DNA interferes with the strand-reunion reaction of topoisomerase II, resulting in production of protein-linked double-strand DNA breaks. Although mitoxanthone is cytotoxic to cells throughout the cell cycle, cells in late S phase are more sensitive. Tumor cells resistant to mitoxanthone may show cross resistance to other natural products.

Pharmacology: Mitoxanthone is given by i.v. infusion. It undergoes extensive binding to several different tissues. The drug has been detected in tissues of patients who died several weeks to several months after receiving th e last dose.

Therapeutic uses: Mitoxanthone has a much narrower range of therapeutic activity that the anthracyclines. It is used mainly for treatment of the leukemias (mainly acute myelogenous leukemia) and lymphomas as well as advanced breast cancer.

Toxicity: Patients should be warned of a possible blue-green coloration of the sclerae and nails as well as the urine. The primary acute toxicity is nausea and vomiting which is mild to moderate and occurs in about 40% of patients.It causes less nausea and vomiting and alopecia than does doxorubicin. Its major toxicities are bone marrow depression and mucositis. The bone marrow depression is of a delayed nature with the lowest counts being seen at one to two weeks.

Bleomycin (Blenoxane)

The bleomycins are a group of antitumor agents isolated from Streptomyces vericillus. The drug employed clinically is a mixture of compounds of complex structure containing about 70% bleomycin A2. Bleomycin is a metal binding water soluble glycopeptide antibiotic. Bleomycins have attracted interest because of their significant anticancer activity against certain solid tumors as well as the fact that they are minimally toxic to the bone marrow unlike most other anticancer agents.

Mechanism of action: Bleomycin has been found to profoundly inhibit DNA synthesis while RNA and protein synthesis are much less affected. Bleomycin usually produces a block in the early G2 phase of the cell cycle. The cytotoxic activity results from their ability to cause fragmentation of DNA. Single strand breaks occur predominantly but double strand breaks occur also. Damage to the DNA correlates with the cytotoxic effect of the drug. Bleomycin has two major domains in its structure. One portion interacts with DNA and one binds iron. Both iron and oxygen are required for bleomycin to degrade DNA. The drug binds Fe^{++} and binds DNA by intercalation between GT or GC bases, and acts as a ferrous oxidase (Fe^{++} Fe^{+++}) resulting in production of oxygen free radicals that cleave DNA.

Resistance: Several mechanisms of resistance have been described. One of the most common is an increased degradation of bleomycin by certain amidase enzymes. Low levels of this enzyme are found in tumors sensitive to the drug and high levels in many tumors resistant to it. However, some studies have not been able to correlate tumor responsiveness with levels of degradative enzymes. Changes in transport have also found in some resistant tumors.

Pharmacology: Bleomycin is given parenterally most commonly i.v. or i.m. After administration there are relatively high concentrations of the drug found in the skin and lungs. These organs are major sites of bleomycin toxicity. The primary route of excretion of the drug is renal, thus *Renal failure increases risk of toxicity*. As much as two-thirds of the drug is excreted in the urine within 24 hrs. Bleomycin is rapidly inactivated by a tissue enzyme, bleomycin hydrolase, which cleaves the amide bond of the aminoalanine moiety. Its activity is higher in drug-resistant tumors. Particularly low levels of the drug inactivating enzyme are found in skin and lung, and consequently high levels of biologically active drug are found in these two tissues. Therapeutic uses Bleomycin is highly active against squamous cell tumors of the head, neck and lungs. It is also highly effective against germ cell tumors of the testis and ovary. It is often used to treat testicular carcinomas along with with cisplatin a nd vinblastine. It is also active against Hodgkin's disease and other lymphomas where it is often included in the ABVD regimen.

Toxicity Bleomycin is *Marrow sparing* and is *not immunosuppressive* and is therefore a useful compound to use in combination drug protocols. In the usual doses the gastrointestinal tract, liver, kidneys and CNS are also not affected. Despite these advantages bleomycin is quite toxic. The *most common toxicity involves the skin and mucous membranes*. Oral mucositis is dose related and common in the more aggressive regimens. Alopecia occurs in about 10-20% of patients. Toxic reactions of the skin include hyperpigmentation, sclerotic changes with collage infiltration, edema and erythema of the hands and feet. These cutaneous changes are reversible when the drug is discontinued. As mentioned above the skin contains very littl e if any of the bleomycin inactivating enzymes.

Pulmonary toxicity is the dose-limiting toxicity and most severe toxicity associated with use of bleomycin. Symptoms include dyspnea, tachypnea, and a nonproductive cough. Fine rales are heard at the base of the lungs and radiography often shows a pat chy basilar infiltrate and in some cases fibrosis. The overall incidence of pulmonary toxicity is about 10% with fatalities occurring in about 1% of patients. There is an increasing incidence when the total dose of bleomycin goes above 400 units. It oc curs more commonly in patients with compromised renal function and when the drug is used with cisplatin which is itself nephrotoxic. In general pulmonary function testing has not been very helpful in predicting the toxicity to bleomycin and patients sho uld be monitored by respiratory symptoms e.g. cough, dyspnea, physical examination and periodic chest X-ray. Extreme caution should be employed in anyone having preexisting pulmonary disease.

Other toxicities of bleomycin include nausea, vomiting, anorexia, drug-induced fever and chills are common. These effects are usually seen within the first few hours of bleomycin therapy. About 1% of lymphoma patients develop allergic reactions similar to anaphylaxis. For this reason, lymphoma patients are given 2 units or less for the first 2 doses. If no acute reactions occur, the regular dosage schedule may be followed.

Plicamycin (Mithramycin)

This drug is most commonly referred to as mithramycin. It is an antibiotic derived from Streptomyces plicatus. It is part of a group of drugs referred to as chromomycin antibiotics and is the only one of this group used clinically in the U.S. It is rar ely used in cancer chemotherapy because of its toxicity. A number of drug-related deaths have occurred from the use of mithramycin. Its use is now limited to the treatment of hypercalcemia associated with malignancy where it is used in lower dosage than that used for the treatment of tumors.

ANTIMETABOLITES

Antimetabolites are structural analogs of naturally occurring compounds. Antimetabolites interfere with the production of nucleic acids. They work through a variety of mechaninsms including competition for binding sites on enzymes and incorporation into into nucleic acids. Antimetabolites inhibit the growth of the most rapidly proliferating cells in the body (e.g., bone marrow, G.I. tract, etc.). Their are three categories of antimetabolites: antifolates, purine analogs and pyrimidine antimetabolites.

Antifolates-*Methotrexate* (Folex, Mexate). The importance of folates in tumor cell growth was demonstrated in 1948 by Farber and colleagues where they (aminopterin) were shown to produce remissions in leukemia. Antifolates produced both the first striking remissions in leukemia and the first cure of a solid tumor, choriocarcinama. Although aminopterin was the first clinically useful folate methotrexate was soon introduced in therapy and it has become the major folate used in cancer therapy.

Folic acid is an essential growth factor from which is derived a series of tetrahydrofolate cofactors that provide single carbon groups for the synthesis of RNA and DNA precursors such as thymidylate and purines. Folic acid must be reduced in two successive steps by dihydrofolate reductase before it can functiion as a coenzyme. The fully reduced form in the one that picks up and delivers single carbon units in various metabolic processes. The enzyme dihydrofolate reductase (DHFR) is the primary site of action of most folate analogs such as methotrexate. Inhibition of this enzyme leads to toxicity through partial depletion of cofactors required for the synthesis of purines and thymidylate. Methotrexate is a strong inhibitor of DHFR. It has a high affinity for the tumor cell enzyme blocking dihydrofolate reductase (DHFR) and formation of tetrahydrofolate needed for thymidylate and purine synthesis. Cell death probably results from inhibition of DNA synthesis. As with most antimetabolites methotrexate is only partially selective for tumor cells and is toxic to all rapidly dividing normal cells such as those of the gastrointestinal epithelium and and bone marrow.

Several factors influence the effectiveness of methotrexate treatment. Included among them are factors that concentrate the drug intracellularly such as transport and conversion to the higher molecular weight polyglutamates that are preferentially retained within the cell. Also important are changes in the amount and structure of dihydrofolate reductase. Changes in the latter will influence methotrexate binding and determine how well the drug is able to inhibit nucleotide synthesis.

Resistance: Several biochemical mechanisms of resistance have been demonstrated. The major mechanisms are decreased drug uptake, amplification of the dihydrofolate reductase gene and thus an increase in the target enzyme, mutations in the DHF gene, and decreased ability to form methotrexate polyglutamate inside cells. In the clinic there are now several documented cases where there is a lack of response to methotrexate and a correlation to amplified DHFR genes in tumor cells.

Pharmacology: Methotrexate can be administered by several different routes including chronic oral, intermittent oral or i.v.high-dose intravenous and intrathecal. Its absorption from the gastrointestinal tract depends on the dose, with large doses being only partially absorbed while low doses are efficiently absorbed. These differences are most likely due to dependence on a saturable folate carrier. At high doses methotrexate is most likely taken up by passive diffusion. Only a small percentage crosses the into the CSF thus necessitatating intrathecal administration for the treatment of tumor cells in the CNS. Approximately 50% of the methotrexate is bound to plasma proteins thus there is the distinct possibility of drug interactions with drugs that also are significantly bound to plasma proteins. Metabolism is usually minimal although after administration in high dose therapy 7-hydroxymethotrexate is formed which is potentially nephrotoxic. Elimination is primarily renal and there is a clear relationship between serum levels of MTX and toxicity.

Therapeutic uses: Methotrexate is useful for the treatment of several different tumors. It is the drug of choice for gestational choriocarcinoma and related trophoblastic tumors of women where cures are obtained in a substantial number of women. In this cancer, it is usually used in combination with dactinomycin. Methotrexate is very useful for the treatment of acute lymphocytic leukemia in children where it is used for the maintenance of remissions. It is however of limited value for adult leukemias. It has also been used for the treatment and prevention of leukemic meningitis where it is given by intrethecal administration. Finally, high dose methotrexate along with leukovorin rescue is used for the treatment of osteogenic sarcoma and leukemias and lymphomas. Methotrexate is also used to treat several non-neoplastic diseases such as psoriasis and several immunological diseases such as rheumatoid arthritis, Wegener's granulomatosis and systemic lupus erythematosis.

Toxicity: The primary toxic effects are against the rapidly dividing cells of the bone marrow and gastrointestinal epithelium. The severity of the clinical effects depends largely on the duration of exposure to inhibitory levels of the drug. All of the stem-cell types of the marrow can be affected to produce leukopenia, thrombocytopenia and with long-term administration, anemia. Methotrexate therapy must therefore be modified according to the patients hematological status and leukocyte and platelet counts must be carefully monitored. Mucositis is one of the earliest signs of toxicity and its appearance indicates that the dose must be reduced or other serious toxicities will occur. If diarrhea and ulcerative stomatitis occur therapy with the drug must be stopped. Methotrexate causes kidney damage which is a frequent complication of high dose therapy. It is manifested by elevated serum creatinine and decreased creatinine clearance. Crystalline deposits of methotrexate and methotrexate derived material have been found in the renal tubules which seems to account for most of the nephrotoxicity. Alkalinizing the urine to increase the solubility and ensuring good urine flow minimizes most of the nephrotoxicity due to high-dose methotrexate. Both low and high dose therapy can cause hepatotoxicity. High dose therapy results in elevated liver enzymes and low dose therapy produces a different type of hepatotoxicity which includes cirrhosis. Methtrexate can cause a reversible pulmonary syndrome which has been observed primarily in children undergoing maintenance therapy. Intrathecal and high-dose administration is accompanied by several types of neurotoxicity. These range from acute manifestations to long-term delayed toxicity in the form of encephalopathy. Nausea and anorexia frequently occur as acute side effects of methotrexate therapy.

High dose MTX-rescue therapy Administration of high doses of methotrexate plus folinic acid (leucovorin) can be very beneficial in certain types of cancer. This therapy involves administration of methotrexate at high doses along with leucovorin to rescue host tissues from the effects of the intense methotrexate therapy. The leucovorin provides the normal tissues with the reduced folate leucovorin which circumvents the inhibition of DHFR. The protection seems to be selective in that it does not alter the antitumor effect of the methotrexate. Apparently only the host cells are able to utilize the leucovorin. A more recent explanation is that of differential reactivation of DHFR in host and tumor cells. Beneficial effects have been observed in patients with osteosarcoma as well acute leukemia.

Purine Antimetabolites

6-mercaptopurine (6-MP, Purinethol) and 6-thioguanine (6-TG). The two major anticancer drugs in this category are 6-mercaptopurine and *6-thioguanine*. These drugs are analogs of hypoxanthine and guanine, respectively. Several other purine analogs are also now commercially available. Among these compounds are not only anticancer drugs but immunosuppressives (azathioprine) and antiviral compounds (acyclovir, ganciclovir etc.). The antipurines can both inhibit nucleotide and nucleic acid synthesis and be incorporated into nucleic acid and sometimes they can do both.

Mechanism of action: Most studies indicate that the thiopurines work at multiple sites and that their mechanism of action is a result of combined effects at these different sites. The thiopurines must first be converted into the nucleotide form in order to be active. This conversion is catalyzed by phosphoribosyltransferase enzymes. The nucleotide forms inhibit the first committed step in the de novo purine synthesis pathway (PRPP amidotransferase) and the key step in guanine nucleotide biosynthesis, IMP dehydrogenase. This latter site is the branch point where IMP is channeled towards either guanine nucleotide synthesis or adenine nucleotide synthesis. The mononucleotide derivatives are ultimately converted to triphosphates which can be incorporated into RNA and DNA.

6-MP is an analog of hypoxanthine and thus can't be incorporated directly into DNA but must first be converted into a TG analog (thio-IMP to thio-GMP). Both drugs are thus incorporated as the same form. Although RNA incorporation can be significant most studies indicate that the biological effects of the drugs are due to incorporation into DNA. Exactly why these compounds are toxic to tumor cells is not known but it may result from multiple effects buy it is well known that these compounds exhibit significant antitumor activity.

Resistance to the thiopurines For these antipurines to work efficient generation and maintenance of the nucleotide forms is necessary. In experimental tumors, lack of an altered phosphoribosyltransferase enzyme is the most commonly encountered mechanism of resistance. This enzyme is primarily responsible for forming the nucleotide. A different pattern is seen in humans receiving thiopurine therapy where increased alkaline phosphatase activity seems to be a major cause of resistance. This enzyme catalyzes the breakdown of the nucleotide form and could protect tumor cells by antagoning the accumulation of thiopurine nucleotides. As would be expected there is cross resistance between these two purine analogs.

Pharmacology

6-Mercaptopurine (Purinethol) After oral ingestion, absorption is incomplete and variable, but it is still routinely given this way. 6-MP is widely distributed in the body with the exception of the CNS where little drug is found. As far as metabolism 6-mercaptopurine is methylated on the sulfhydryl group with subsequent oxidation of the methylated derivatives. In addition 6-mercaptopurine is oxidized to thiouric acid by xanthine oxidase. This pathway is blocked by allopurinol. Therefore, if it used along with allopurinol the dosage of 6-MP must be reduced otherwise toxicity will be increased. 6-Thioguanine is also given orally but it is slowly absorbed after oral administration. Unlike mercaptopurine it is metabolized mainly to inorganic sulfate. There is no formation of thiouric acid with 6-thioguanin thus unlike 6-MP it can be used in combination with allopurinol without the dosage being reduced.

Therapeutic uses: Both drugs are used primarily in the treatment of leukemias. Response rates are higher in children than adults. 6-MP is used in the maintenance therapy of acute lymphocytic leukemia and 6-TG in the treatment of acute nonlymphocytic leukemia.

Toxicity: Bone marrow depression is dose limiting with both drugs. The maximum effect on the blood count may be delayed and it is important to discontinue these drugs temporarily if there is an abnormally large fall in the leukocyte count or abnormal depression in the bone marrow. Other major toxicities include nausea and vomiting and stomatitis. Hepatotoxicity is seen as jaundice in]about 33% of the patients treated with 6-MP. As mentioned above 6-MP is a substrate for xanthine oxidase which converts it to 6-thiouric acid by oxidation. This appears to be an important route for inactivation of the drug. Allopurinol, a drug used to prevent the hyperuricemia and uricosuria that often follow marked cell kill consequent to leukemia therapy, inhibits this conversion. When 6-MP and allopurinol are used together, the dose of 6-MP is usually lowered. 6-TG is not extensively deaminated and only a small amount is converted to 6-thiouric acid. Therefore, no reduction in dosage is necessary with allopurinol.

Chlorodeoxyadenosine and Pentostatin: These are two newly introduced purine analogs which have good activity against certain types of leukemia. The presence of a halogen in the adenine ring of several purine analogs led to a group of compounds which resisted metabolic degradation by deamination. 2-chlorodeoxy-adenosine (CdA) showed the greatest activity of these compounds. It was found to be an inhibitor of ribonucleotide reductase and consequently DNA synthesis. It also inhibited DNA strand elongation after incorporation into the DNA. This drug was found to cause extensive DNA damage. It has been found to be very useful in the treatment of indolent B-cell lymphocytic leukemias such as hairy cell leukemia and chronic lymphocytic leukemia. Many of these have been resistant to other therapies. Additional studies have shown that this drug may be promising in lymphomas, and acute and chronic granulocytic leukemias also. The dose limiting toxicity is mild bone marrow depression.

Pentostatin (2'-deoxycoformycin) is a natural product isolated from bacteria. It binds tightly to and inhibits the enzyme adenosine deaminase. Lack of this enzyme has been implicated in some immunodeficiency syndromes. It has significant activity in patients with B-cell chronic lymphocytic leukemias. Toxicities are varied and somewhat unpredictable. Lymphopenia is often encountered leading to infectiions. Acute renal failure and neurological toxicities are less common but have been seen to be life threatening.

Pyrimidine Antagonists

There are several different compounds in this group but the principal members used in the treatment of cancer include the fluoropyrimidines and cytosine arabinoside. Pyrimidine analogs have also been used in the treatment of diseases as diverse as cancer, psoriasis, fungal infections and viral infections. The best characterized agents in this class are the halogenated pyrimidines.

Fluoropyrimidines

5-fluorouracil (Adrucil), 5-fluorodeoxyuridine (FdUrd) (Floxuridine) The most important members of this group are *5-fluorouracil (5-FU)* and 5-fluorodeoxyuridine (FdUrd).

Mechanism of action: Members of this group are direct inhibitors of thymidylate synthetase the key enzyme in thymidylate synthesis. Methotrexate in contrast is an indirect inhibitor of this enzyme through inhibition of dihydrofolate reductase. These agents produce multiple biochemical lesions as a result any one of which has the potential to be cytotoxic. 5-FU must first be converted to the nucleotide form to be active as a cytotoxic agent. The nucleotide (5'-FUMP) can be formed by several different pathways. FUMP can be incorporated into RNA and also can be converted to the deoxynucleotide(F-dUMP). This latter reaction is crucial to the cytotoxic effects of 5-FU. FdUMP may also be formed by the direct conversion of FdURD by thymidine kinase. FdUMP inhibits the enzyme thymidylate synthetase which leads to deletion of TTP, a necessary constituent of DNA. Ordinarily, thymidylate synthetase catalyzed the methylation of dUMP in a multistep process. When FdUMP is utilized the process becomes inhibited at an intermediate step. A complex between the enzyme, the pseudosubstrate and the folate cofactor is formed. The complex dissociates very slowly and is sufficiently stable so that the enzyme no longer can catalyze the reaction. DNA synthesis is inhibited until the drug is removed and new enzyme synthesis occurs. Since FdUrd is converted to FdUMP directly in one step it is a more potent inhibitor of TMP synthetase than is 5-FU. It is often effective in the low nanomolar concentration range. On the other hand 5-FU will require micromolar concentrations to be effective and at such concentrations other active metabolites are formed such as FUTP which can become incorporated into RNA in place of UTP. Incorporation into RNA has resulted in observed effects on the function of both rRNA and mRNA. Although incorporation into RNA is much higher than incorporation into DNA recent studies have shown this to occur also. The biological consequences of this are not known, however. An important question that is always asked is whether the effects on RNA or on those on DNA are important for the cytotoxic action of these compounds. There are many conflicting studies on this point. It is most probable that the cytotoxic action of these drugs is not the same in all cell lines and that this heterogeneity is the basis for the wide variability in response to FU.

Resistance: A number of biochemical mechanisms have been identified that are associated with resistance to 5-FU and FudR. The major ones include decreased conversion to the nucleotide form and increased breakdown of the nucleotide. For each of these mechanisms changes in several different enzymes might account for resistance.

Pharmacology: The oral absorption of fluorouracil is erratic, so it is usually given parenterally either by bolus (intravenous) or by continuous infusion (intravenous or arterial). Administration by continuous infusion overcomes the problem of rapid disappearance of FU from the circulation. Since these drugs work best if they are present during the S phase of the cell cycle their short time in the circulation would ordinarily present a problem as the plasma levels would greatly fluctuate. Protocols using continuous infusion were developed to overcome this potential problem. Metabolic degradation occurs particularly in the liver. 5-FU readily enters the CSF.

Therapeutic uses: Fluorouracil is used to treat several common solid tumors. It produces partial responses in up to about 1/3 of patients with metastatic carcinomas of the breast and the gastrointestinal tract. Topically it has been used for the treatment of basal cell carcinomas and premalignant skin keratoses. FU is used in many different combinations in order to enhance its activity. Some involve combination with other cytotoxic agents like methotrexate while others involve combination with agents that by themselves lack toxicity but modulate the cytotoxic effects of FU. Combination with leucovorin has been very successful as the leucovorin enhances formation of the ternary complex. FudR is primarily used by continuous infusion into the hepatic artery for treatment of metastatic colon cancer.

Toxicity: The toxicities of these two drugs are similar and somewhat dependent on the mode of administration. Anorexia and nausea are among the earliest toxicities seen. These are followed by stomatitis and diarrhea which are indicative of a sufficient dose being given. The frequency of effects varies with the treatment schedule employed. Stomatitis and diarrhea are the most common dose-limiting toxicities when continuous infusions are used. The major toxicity resulting from a bolus dose is bone marrow depression. This is manifested by leukopenia and somewhat less often by thrombocytopenia and anemia. The lowest blood counts occur at one to two weeks. Skin toxicity manifested by alopecia, thinning of the skin, nail changes, dermatitis and photosensitivity can also occur. FU also produces an acute cerebellar syndrome in less than 1% of patients. This includes ataxia, nystagmus, slurred speech and dizziness.

Cytosine Arabinoside (Cytosar; ara-C): This is an analog of 2'-deoxycytidine with the 2'-hydroxyl in a position trans to the 3'-hydroxyl of the sugar. The bases of polyarabinsides cannot stack normally as do the bases of polydeoxynucleotides.

Mechanism of action: Ara-C is first converted to the monophosphate nucleotide (AraCMP) by deoxycytidine kinase. The monophosphate can then react with appropriate kinases to form the di and triphosphate nucleotides. AraCTP is believed to be the key active component. Its accumulation causes potent inhibition of DNA synthesis in many cells. This nucleotide is a competitive inhibitor of DNA polymerases. Also, the triphosphate is a substrate for DNA polymerases and it is incorporated into the DNA. It apparently causes inhibition of DNA chain elongation when ara-C in incorporated at the terminal position of a growing DNA chain. Unlike most of the antimetabolites the effects of ara-C are directed almost exclusively towards DNA and it has little or no effect on RNA synthesis or function. The relative biological impact of DNA synthesis inhibition versus incorporation into DNA has been studied for several years now. The evidence indicates that synthesis inhibition is secondary to analog incorporation. However, the precise cause of cellular death by ara-C is not known.

Resistance: The overall balance between the anabolic (kinases) and catabolic enzymes (deaminases) involved in the metabolism of ara-C determine the amount of araCTP and thus the sensitivity or resistance of cells to araC. For example, in patients with refractory acute leukemia, who received high doses of ara-C upon relapse there was a significant correlation between the area under the curve and clinical response rate. The same relationship in newly diagnosed acute leukemias does not seem as well established.

Pharmacology: Cytarabine is very poorly absorbed after oral administration in humans. It is routinely given i.v. by continuous infusion sometimes in high dose regimens. Intrathecal administration is also used for meningeal leukemia and lymphoma. Ara-C reaches the CNS reasonable well with CSF levels as high as 40% of the plasma levels. It has a very short plasma half-life due to cytidine deaminase activity in liver and elsewhere, and its metabolites are renally excreted. Metabolism accounts for 70-90% of the Ara-C eliminated with most of the drug being excreted as ara-U.

Therapeutic uses: AraC is an important antimetabolite used primarily for the treatment of acute myelocytic leukemia due to its potent myelosuppressive action. It is the single most effective agent for induction of remission in this disease and it is used primarily in combination with daunorubicin. It has occasionally been used to treat acute lymphocytic leukemia and in high doses it has been used for non-Hodgkins lymphoma and chronic myelocytic leukemia. It is not active against solid tumors.

Toxicity: The principal toxicity is bone marrow depression manifested as granulocytopenia and thrombocytopenia. Other toxicities include oral ulceration, nausea, vomiting and diarrhea, and peripheral neurotoxicity with high doses. *Use caution with decreased hepatic function* since the liver is a major site of deamination.

Fludarabine: A new nucleoside analog that has modifications in both the base and sugar moieties. Like ara-C it is metabolized to the nucleotide triphosphate by sequential action of several kinases. It then interferes with DNA synthesis by DNA polymerase inhibition and by incorporation into nascent DNA. Unlike ara-C this compound is much more likely to act as a chain terminator. It also apparently acts as an inhibitor of the proofreading exonuclease activity of DNA polymerase epsilon. Fludarabine has been shown to be very effective against chronic lymphocytic leukemia. It gives a response rate exceeding 80% in previously untreated patients. Moderate to severe myelosuppression occurs at therapeutic doses, while neurologic toxicity occurs especially at higher doses.

ENZYMES

L-Asparaginase

This drug was developed after it was noted that guinea pig serum suppressed the growth of lymphosarcomas in mice. The active serum component was found to be *L-asparaginase,* an enzyme that hydrolyzes L-asparagine to L-aspartate. The enzyme is effective because a few neoplastic cells have low levels of asparagine synthetase activity and require L-asparagine for growth. The use of L-asparaginase in cancer chemotherapy is limited to acute lymphocytic leukemia to induce remission. Resistance rapidly develops to in most cancer cells.

Hydroxyurea

Hydroxyurea inhibits DNA synthesis without inhibiting the incorporation or precursors into RNA or protein. Specifically, it inhibits ribonucleotide reductase to block deoxyribonucleotide formation and DNA synthesis. This enzyme is closely related to proliferative status in cancer cells. It is involved in the de novo synthesis of all the precursors used in DNA synthesis. It converts ribonucleotide diphosphates to deoxyribonucleotides. Hydroxyurea is an S phase specific drug. Resistance is due to c hanges in the ribonucleotide reductase.

The drug is well absorbed from the gastrointestinal tract and is routinely given orally. It is primarily eliminated through the kidney and should be used with caution in patients with compromised renal function. Hydroxyurea is used primarily in the treatment of myeloproliferative disorders including chronic granulocytic leukemia, polycythemia vera and essential thrombocytosis. It has also been used in a variety of solid tumors including carcinomas of the head and neck and those of the genitourinary systems.

Mild nausea and vomiting are experienced by most patients who receive hydroxyurea. The major dose-limiting toxicity is bone marrow depression mainly seen as leukopenia. This is reversible when the drug is discontinued. With large amounts of the drug stomatitis and gastrointestinal ulceration may occur.

ANTIESTROGENS

Tamoxifen

Mechanism of Action Tamoxifen is a competitive inhibitor of estradiol binding to the estrogen receptor.It acts as a complete antagonist in some systems and as an antagonist with partial agonist activity in other systems. By binding to the receptor it competes with the binding of endogenous estradiol and its major therapeutic effect reflects this antiestrogenic mechanism. It induces a change in the 3 dimensional shape of the receptor inhibiting its binding to the estrogen response element on DNA.

Pharmacology: Tamoxifen is administered orally. It is metabolized by the cytochrome P-450 system to at least 6 metabolites some of which possess estrogen binding activity. These metabolites are conjugated principally as glucuronides and excreted in the bile. The metabolites have very long half-lives because of extensive protein binding in the plasma and efficient reuptake from the intestinal tract.

Therapeutic uses: It is used in the treatment of metastatic breast cancer. It is used alone for palliation of advanced breast cancer in women with estrogen receptor-positive tumors, and it is used for adjuvant therapy in certain types of early stage disease depending on the patients age, receptor status of the tumor and degree of nodal involvement. It also may have benefit as a preventive agent for breast cancer especially in women with risk factors. However, at the present time this is very controversial because of the possibility of increased incidence of endometrial cancer.

Toxicity: Tamoxifen is very well tolerated. The most frequent side effect is acute nausea and vomiting. This usually disappears after a few weeks and it can be reduced by taking the drug with meals. More chronic side effects include hot flashes, transient and mild thrombocytopenia and leukopenia; vaginal bleeding; skin rashes; hypercalcemia; retinopathy and corneal opacities with high dose long-term therapy

NONSTEROIDAL ANTIANDROGENS

Flutamide

This is a nonsteroidal antiandrogen. It is used in combination with gonadotropin releasing hormone analogs in therapy for patients with cancer of the prostate

Toxicity: Occasional diarrhea, nausea, vomiting and reversible liver function abnormalities are the significant toxicities of this drug.

Aromatase Inhibitors

Anastrozole (Arimidex)

A selective nonsteroidal aromatase inhibitor. Aromatase is a P-450 enzyme that catalyzes various steps in the conversion of androgen to estrogen. It is used for the treatment of postmenopausal women with advanced breast cancer that has progressed during treatment with tamoxifen.

PLATINUM COMPOUNDS

Cisplatin is one of a number of platinum coordination complexes with antitumor activity. Recently carboplatin was put on the market. These are now the only two platinum compounds available clinically although a number of similar compounds have had acti vity in experimental systems.

Mechanism of action: The platinum compounds are DNA cross-linking agents similar to but not identical to the alkylating agents. The platinum compounds exchange chloride ions for nucleophilic groups of various kinds. Both the cis and trans isomers do this but the trans isomer is known to be bioligically inactive for reasons not completely understood. To possess antitumor activity a platinum compound must have two relatively labile cis-oriented leaving groups. The principal sites of reaction are the N7 atoms of guanine and adenine. The main interaction is formation of intrastrand cross links between the drug and neighboring guanines. Intrastrand cross linking has been shown to correlate with clinical response to cisplatin ther apy. DNA-protein cross linking also occurs but this does not correlate with cytotoxicity. Cross-resistance between the two groups of drugs is usually not seen indicating that the mechanisms of action are not identical. The types of cross linking with DNA may differ between the platinum compounds and the typical alkylating agents.

Resistance: No clear-cut dominant mechanism of resistance to cisplatin has been identified. Often, resistant cells have an increased ability to repair intrastrand adducts but in many cases this is insufficient to explain th e extent of resistance. Resistance is some cases has been shown to correlate with the increase in sulfhydryl compounds such as glutathione or the metal binding protein metallothionein. Thus, as with the alkylating agents multiple causes of resistance may occur.

Pharmacology: Both cisplatin and carboplatin must be given parenterally often by i.v. injection. Cisplatin is given i.v. and by local introduction into the bladder and into the peritoneal space. After i.v. infusion it has an plasma half-life of about a half hour. This is followed by a period of slow decline. Cisplatin binds extensively to plasma protein. Carboplatin generates a reactive species much more slowly than with cisplatin. Thus its pharmacokinetic and toxicologic characteristics are different. Its plasma half-life is several fold longer that cisplatin.

Therapeutic uses: Cisplatin is one of the most frequently used anticancer drugs. It is an effective component of several different combination drug protocols used to treat a variety of solid tumors. Carboplatin was introduce d in the hope that it could reduce the toxic potential of cisplatin. These drugs are used in the treatment of testicular cancer (with bleomycin and vinblastine),bladder cancer, head and neck cancer (with bleomycin and fluorouracil), ovarian cancer (with cyclophosphamide or doxorubicin) and lung cancer (with etoposide). Cisplatin has been found to be the most active single agent against most of these tumors.

Toxicity: The dose limiting toxicity with cisplatin is nephrotoxicity. This effect is dose related and is manifested by a decrease in creatinine clearance and electrolyte imbalances particularly hypomagnesemia. The nephrotoxicity is initiated by a decrease in proximal tubular function. Several studies in both humans and in animals have shown that several approaches can reduce the nephrotoxicity. This includes the use of diuretics and hydration. Thiol containing compounds such as thiosulfate have also been shown to prevent the nephrotoxicity and may allow increased dosage of the cisplatin. On the other hand concomitant therapy with other nephrotoxic drugs such as aminoglycosides can augment the nephrotoxicity of cisplatin.

Other toxic effects associated with this drug include bone marrow depression, severe nausea and vomiting, anaphylactic reactions and peripheral neuropathy. The degree of bone marrow depression is usually moderate. Nausea and vomiting occur in virtually all patients receiving cisplatin and this usually occurs within a short period of time. Cisplatin also causes a neurotoxicity that most commonly is seen as a peripheral neuropathy with sensations of numbness in the hands, feet, arms, and legs. In most cases stoppage of the drug allows the symptoms to disappear.

With carboplatin the dose limiting toxicity is bone marrow depression. Other toxic effects include moderate nausea and vomiting and a low potential for ototoxicity and peripheral neuropathy.

Biological Response Modifiers

These include agents e.g., interferons, interleukins that affect the patient's bioligical response to a neoplasm beneficially. Some of the agents in this category act directly on the tumor cells while most of them act indirectly by enhancing the hosts immunological response to the neoplastic cells. Recombinant DNA technology has greatly facilitated the production of these compounds. These agents include growth factors, agents increasing differentiation and the interferons and interleukins. The first two groups of compounds are discussed below in separate sections.

Interferons: These compounds were originally discovered as natural anti-viral compounds. Human interferons are classified into three groups: alpha, beta, and gamma. Interferon alpha is produced by leukocytes and lymphoblastoid cells stimulated by viruses and certain microbial cell components. Interferon beta is produced by fibroblasts and gamma or immune interferon is produced by T lymphocytes in response to antigenic or mitogenic stimulation. The antitumor effects of the interferons result from a combination of direct cytotoxicity to tumor cells and from stimulation of natural killer cells and macrophages. The only interferon presently used clinically for anticancer activity is alpha. The alpha interferons are members of a multigene family. They are acid stable polypeptides. IFNalpha has demonstrated activity in a broad range of malignant disorders. Its best activity has been in the treatment of hairy cell leukemia. In the treatment of other neoplasms it is still in the early stages of clinical development.

Interleukin-2: It was originally discovered in the growth medium of mitogen stimulated murine and human peripheral blood lymphocytes and shown to stimulate T-cell proliferation and maintenance in culture. Human IL-2 is a glycoprotein with a M.W. of 17.2 kD. It is now known to stimulate B lymphocytes also as well as having several other effects. It is being studied in the treatment of acute myelogenous leukemia where it has been shown to induce remission in relapsed patients. When used alone toxicity is related to the activation and expansion of lytic lymphocytes has occurred. This has produced inflammation and vascular leak as well as the secondary release of other cytokines. It also has been used in adoptive immunotherapy to stimulate clonal expansion of lymphokine-activated killer (LAK) cells and tumor infiltrative lymphocytes (TIL).

Adoptive Immunotherapy

This is an approach in which cells with antitumor activity are administered to a tumor bearing host and mediate either directly or indirectly the regression of established tumor. This has been approached in several ways. One idea is to take the person's own lymphocytes and activate them in vitro with appropriate activating factors and then inject them back into the patient. IN this approach lymphocytes are incubated with recombinant IL-2 which stimulates a population of lymphocytes that whebn activated can lyse fresh, noncultured, natural killer cell-resistant tumor cells but not normal cells.

Hematopoietic Growth Factors

Several growth factors have recently been found to be very useful in reducing some of the bone marrow toxicity associated with the use of the anticancer agents. These are a subset of regualtory polypeptides of the cytokine family that are involved in the proliferation and differentiation of granulocytes and monocyte/macrophages.The ones most commonly used are granulocyte-macrophage stimulating, and granulocyte stimulating factor. Both of these have been shown to replenish peripheral blood neutrophils after high dose chemotherapy followed by autologous bone-marrow transplantation. Positive benefits include decreasing the frequency of infections and shortening the stay in the hospital. Erythropoietin has been used to replenish red blood cells in aplastic anemia and after cancer chemotherapy.

Induction of Tumor Cell Differentiation

This therapy takes advantage of the ability to initiate the differentiation of certain kinds of cells into functioning cells rather than allow them to stay in their immature form. A recent increase in the amount of research on the mechanisms of cellular differentiation has resulted in the first widespread use of a differentiation agent for the treatment of leukemia as well as generating several promising new anti-cancer drugs. All-trans-retinoic acid is now in widespread clinical tests for treating acute promyelocytic leukemia

Gene Therapy

Alteration of a cell's gene dosage for specific genes could significantly affect the outcome of a malignant growth.. For example, if a tumor supressor gene could be delivered to leukemic cells the malignant process may be able to be stopped or reversed. On the other hand if the DNA coding for a particular gene were incorporated into the cells genetic apparatus a permanent reprogramming of the cell might be achieved. This might be achieved in cells removed from a patient or by a viral vector. It might also be achievd in vivo by injection of a viral vector targeted to the desired cell type.

Antisense Therapy

This is another approach to regulating gene expression in cancer cells. An antisense piece of DNA or RNA is introduced into the cancer cells. Most commonly this is done by introducing a small piece of DNA (oligonucleotide) into the cell. This oligo is complementary to the normal gene. Such an approach might be used to inhibit the expression of cancer associated genes if it could be directed towards cancer cells. This approach has worked well with in vitro cultured cancer cells. Recent studies have shown it is promising for in vivo systems also, although problems with specificity have to be worked out.

Tumor Vaccines

Vaccines may prevent the onset of cancer for those tumors initiated or promoted by infectious viruses. These vaccines would be derived from inactivated viruses or from a preparation of viral antigens. However, vaccination of patients who already have cancer would be much more difficult to accomplish successfully. Some studies have shown promising results but overall there has been limited success with these therapies.

Therapy Directed Against Tumor Metastases

Studies over the last several years have provided much information on the steps involved in tumor metastasis. This has provided the basis for the development of drugs that can inhibit this process. The area where the most progress has been made has been in developing inhibitors of proteolytic enzymes which are known to play an important role in the invasive and metastatic process. Batimistat is one such inhibitor which is now in phase II clinical trials.

Inhibitors of Angiogenesis

Angigenesis is important in the process of tumor growth and in metastasis. Angiogenesis involves the growth of new blood vessels. The identification of inhibitors of this process will be very important for inhibiting tumor growth. Despite some prominent setbacks in the field, the experimental angiogenesis inhibitor bevacizumab became the first of these agents to show a survival benefit in a phase 3 clinical trial.

Three

Cancer Pain

Goals of Cancer Pain Management

A. Overall Strategy
   1. Palliative care is active treatment, not passive
B. Approach
   1. Identify the cause of pain
   2. Prevent the pain from recurring
   3. Erase the memory of the pain
   4. Maintain a clear sensorium and normal affect

Pathophysiology of Cancer Pain

A. Address all components to achieve effective management
B. Components
   1. Physical (biological) component 25%
   2. Psychological (emotional) component 25%
   3. Social Component 25%
   4. Spiritual Component 25%

Non-Pharmacologic Therapies

A. Relaxation
B. Support Groups
C. Biofeedback
D. Mental Imagery
E. Physiotherapy
F. Transcutaneous electrical Nerve Stimulation (TENS)
G. *Physical Activity*
H. Individual, Family and Group Psychotherapy

Other Palliative Management

A. Palliative radiotherapy
   1. Metastatic bone pain
   2. Neuropathic pain
      a. Lumbosacral plexopathy and brachial plexopathy
B. Palliative surgery
C. Palliative *Chemotherapy*

Guidelines or Pearls for Management

A. Oral route for analgesics is preferred
B. Do not assume the pain is part of the malignancy
   1. Make specific anatomic, and pathologic diagnoses
C. Consider the patients feelings and listen to fears
   1. Pain threshold varies with mood and morale
   2. Less pain is experienced if patient can express fears
D. Administer around the clock scheduled dosing
   1. Scheduled dosing requires less overall analgesic need

2. Avoid as needed medication dosing as much as possible
   a. As needed dosing results in break-through pain

E. Prescribe adequate amounts of analgesics
   1. Titrate dosing to the patient's pain
   2. Do not limit dosing to book values

F. Start with *non-Narcotic* medications if possible

G. Do not be afraid of *Narcotic* use
   1. When *non-Narcotics* fail, move to *Narcotics* quickly
   2. Moderate to Severe pain will require *Narcotics*
   3. Addiction is rare when *Narcotics* are used for pain

H. Make use of non-pharmacologic therapies
   1. See *Cancer Pain* Management

I. Make use of consultants or colleagues

J. Provide support for the entire family
   1. Treat anticipatory grief for family
   2. Prevent isolation and loneliness
   3. Intervene quickly for crises

K. Maintain air of quiet confidence and cautious optimism
   1. Aim for small goals and graded relief
   2. Builds patient's trust and hope
   3. Exhibit determination to succeed

L. Maintain clear sensorium
   1. *Methylphenidate*
      a. Overcomes *Narcotic* associated confusion, drowsiness

■ General Pointers

A. Assess patient's pain with a self rating pain scale

B. Scale
   1. No pain: 0
   2. Mild pain: 1-4
   3. Moderate pain: 5-6
   4. Severe pain: 7-10

■ WHO Analgesic Ladder

A. Step 1: Mild Pain (pain score of 1 to 4)
   1. Adequate analgesia for 20-25% of cancer patients
   2. Acetaminophen
   3. Aspirin
   4. *NSAIDs* or *COX2* Inhibitors

B. Step 2: Moderate Pain (pain score of 5 to 6)
   1. *Acetaminophen with codeine (Tylenol #3)*
   2. *Acetaminophen* with Hydrocodone (Vicodin, Lorcet)
   3. *Tramadol (Ultram)*

C. Step 3: Severe Pain (pain score of 7 to 10)
   1. *Morphine Sulfate*
   2. Hydromorphone
   3. *Transdermal Fentanyl*
   4. Levorphanol
   5. *Methadone*
   6. Avoid *Meperidine (Demerol)*
      a. Too short acting, lower efficacy

■ Routes of Administration

A. Oral Route (90% of cancer cases, preferred route)

B. Subcutaneous (5% of cancer cases)
   1. Programmed Subcutaneous pump is first choice option

C. Rectal (5% of cancer cases)

D. Avoid regular Intramuscular dosing (no indication)

■ Management: Somatic Pain Including Bone Metastases

A. Pain Characteristics
   1. Aching or throbbing sensation
   2. Stabbing sensation
   3. Pressure sensation

B. Medications: General
   1. See *Cancer Pain Narcotics*

2. *COX2 Inhibitors* (e.g. *Vioxx* or *Celebrex*)
3. Nonsteroidal Antiinflammatory drugs *(NSAIDs)*
   a. Diclofenac (Voltaren)
   b. *Naprosyn*
4. Radioactive Strontium

C. Medications: Bone Metastases
1. *Pamidronate (Aredia)* 90 mg IV over 2-4 hours qMonth
2. Calcitonin
3. Corticosteroids
   a. Prednisone 30 to 60 mg/day PO
   b. *Dexamethasone* 16 mg/day PO
   c. *Methylprednisolone* 120 mg/day PO

■ *Management: Neuropathic Pain*

A. Type I: Chronic Lancinating Pain (Paroxysmal pain)
1. Characteristics
   a. Sudden sharp, stabbing or "Zinger" pain
   b. Sudden knifelike pain
2. Medications
   a. *Gabapentin (Neurontin)* 100 mg PO tid
   b. *Carbamazepine (Tegretol)* 200 mg PO bid
   c. *Valproic Acid (Depakote)* 10 mg/kg/day PO
   d. *Clonazepam (Klonopin)* 0.5 mg PO tid
   e. Lamotrigine *(Lamictal)* 50 mg PO qd
   f. Baclofen (Lioresal) 5 mg PO tid

B. Type II: Continuous Dysesthesias
1. Characteristics
   a. Continuous burning
   b. Continuous electrical sensations
2. Medications
   a. *Tricyclic Antidepressants*
      i. *Amitriptyline (Elavil)* 30 to 100 mg PO qhs
      ii. Doxepin (Sinequan) 50 to 75 mg PO qhs
      iii. *Imipramine (Tofranil)* 50 to 75 mg PO qhs
   b. Systemic Anesthetics
      i. Mexiletine (Mexitil) 200 mg PO q8 hours
      ii. Tocainide (Tonocard) 400 mg PO q8 hours
   c. Other medications for refractory pain
      i. *Gabapentin (Neurontin)* 300 mg PO tid
      ii. *Clonidine (Catapres)* 0.1 mg PO bid
      iii. Capsaicin *(Zostrix)* 0.025% AAA tid

■ *Management: Visceral Pain*

A. Capsule swelling (e.g. hepatic)
B. *Corticosteroids*

Four

Oncological Emergencies

These include:
- Superior vena cava obstruction
- Spinal cord compression
- Hypercalcaemia
- Hyponatraemia

SUPERIOR VENA CAVA OBSTRUCTION

Anatomy

The superior vena cava is formed proximally by the union of the right and left brachiocephalic veins within the superior mediastinum. This occurs at the level of the right first costal cartilage. From this point, the SVC runs for about 5-7 cm inferiorly, slightly medially and anteriorly. It ends at the superior vena caval orifice in continuity with the right atrium deep to the third right costal cartilage in the middle mediastinum. It becomes ensheathed by pericardium superior to this point. Posteriorly, at the level of the second costal cartilage, the azygous vein arches anteriorly over the root of the right lung to merge with the posterior surface of the SVC.

The relation of the SVC include:
- *Superoposterior and medially:* the trachea with the right vagus nerve passing inferiorly on its surface
- *Posteroinferiorly:* the right azygous vein arching superior to the right lung root
- *Laterally:* right phrenic nerve running inferiorly with mediastinal parietal pleura more laterally
- *Superomedially:* arch of aorta
- *Inferomedially:* pericardium separated by transverse sinus of heart from ascending aorta
- *Superiorly:* brachiocephalic veins
- *Inferiorly:* right atrium

Superior vena caval obstruction often results from pressure on the vessel from tumour masses in the superior mediastinum. It may also be due to tumour involvement of the vessel and formation of mural thrombus.

Aetiology

The most common cause is lymph node metastases from primary bronchial carcinoma.

Other causes include:
- lymphadenopathy due to lymphoma
- thymoma
- mediastinal tumour
- retrosternal goitre
- mediastinal fibrosis
- thoracic aortic aneurysm

In children the most important causes are:
- T cell leukaemia
- lymphoma

Clinical Features

Possible clinical features include:
- Dilated subcutaneous veins over the upper limbs, neck and chest

- If there is collateral inferior vena cava circulation then there may be dilatation of the subcutaneous veins of the abdomen
- Tissue oedema
- SVCO may be of rapid, often thrombotic, onset or gradual onset
- There may be development of stridor due to progressive obstruction to the main bronchi or trachea

SVC Obstruction Diagnosis and Tests

An examination may show dilated cutaneous (skin) veins of the face, neck, and upper chest. *Blood pressure* is often high in the arms and low in the legs.

A *bronchoscopy* may be performed if *lung cancer* is suspected.

Obstruction of the SVC may show on:

- *Chest X-ray*
- *MRI of chest* or *CT scan of the chest*
- *Coronary angiography*
- *Doppler ultrasound*
- *Radionuclide ventriculography*

Treatment: is based on treating the acute symptoms, and making the underlying diagnosis

- Dexamethasone may be useful in acute SVCO
- Biopsy may be important
- Radiotherapy or, if a sensitive tumour, then cytotoxic chemotherapy, are useful in the long term
- Note that there may be complete regression of signs of SVCO without complete regression of the mass

SVC Obstruction Complications

The throat could swell and block the airways

SPINAL CORD COMPRESSION

Spinal cord compression is characterised by a combination of a progressive history of neurological deficit and a sensory level on examination.

This is a lesion that causes lower motor neurone signs at the level of the lesion and upper motor neurone lesions below that level.

It is a neurological emergency because:

- The final events are ischaemic, so they are fast and irreversible
- The patient may be left in a wheelchair, incontinent of urine

  Note that the commonest cause of acute cord compression is metastatic disease

The causes of spinal cord and root compression can be divided into:

- Vertebral causes
- Extradural causes
- Intradural extramedullary causes
- Intramedullary causes

The causes of cord compression originating from disease within the spinal vertebrae includes:

- Congenital bone anomalies
- Trauma: fracture, dislocation
- Disc prolapse, spondylosis, spondylolisthesis and atlanto-axial subluxation in rheumatoid arthritis and Down's syndrome patients due to the transverse ligament being insufficient to restrain the odontoid peg
- Tumour:
  a. metastatic: breast, bronchus, prostate
  b. primary, e.g. plasmacytoma
- Infection: TB–Pott's disease, staphylococcal septicaemia
- Paget's disease of the spine–may be monostotic or polyostotic; most commonly compresses the cauda equina

The causes of spinal cord compression which arise within the vertebral canal but outside the dura include:

- Neoplasia: lymphoma, leukaemic infiltrate, metastases
- Extradural abscess: e.g. as part of a staphylococcal septicaemia causing acute vertebral osteitis and subsequent vertebral collapse
- Extradural cyst

Causes of spinal cord compression which arise from within the dura but outside the spinal medulla include:

- Tumours: usually, neurofibroma and meningioma, in equal proportions across a population
- Arachnoiditis
- Arachnoid cyst

Causes of spinal cord compression which arise from within the spinal medulla include:

- Tumours:
  a. primary–most common; usually, ependymoma, astrocytoma
  b. metastatic–less common; from bronchial primary tumour or seeding from malignant intracranial tumour
- Syringomyelia
- Cyst-from degeneration of intramedullary tumour
- Intramedullary haematoma–haematomyelia

The presentation of a spinal cord compression depends upon:

- Site of lesion-intramedullary lesions produce within spinal segmental damage only; others produce cord both root and segmental damage
- Extent of lesion-partial, e.g. Brown Sequard, or complete
- Level of lesion-roots only damaged below L1
- Speed of onset-rapidly progressive lesions usually produce permanent deficits 'spinal shock'–upper motor neurone disease-but with a flaccid paralysis, loss of The pertinent investigations for spinal cord and root compression are:
- General-FBC; U and E's-kidney function; LFT's-for liver metastasis
- chest X-ray
- Spinal X-ray:
  a. antero-posterior:
    § erosion of pedicles suggests malignant extradural tumour
    § thinning of pedicles with increased inter-pedicular distance suggests chronic intra-dural or intramedullary expansion
  b. lateral:
  c. 'acalloping' of posterior surface of the vertebral body suggests chronic intradural lesion
    § narrow disc space and canal, hypertrophic joints suggests osteoarthritis/spinal stenosis
    § collapse of vertebral body suggests osteoporosis or malignant infiltration
  d. oblique:
  e. expansion of intervertebral foramina suggests neurofibroma
- Myelography-identifies level of lesion and site, i.e. intra-dural or extra-dural.
- CSF-of limited benefit-increased protein suggests a complete block; leucocytosis suggests abscess or TB; a positive Queckenstedt's test suggests complete block
- CT-valuable once level of lesion is known; intrathecal contrast provides most information-degree of compression and extent
- MRI-investigation of choice if available; sagittal views most informative
- Reflexes, absent plantar reflexes

The Tobey Ayer test is for a block in the spinal canal.

Pressure is applied to the neck in order to compress the internal jugular veins; this reduces venous outflow from the cranium and raises the intracranial pressure. A spinal puncture will displace CSF into the spinal sac and cause the measured CSF pressure, e.g. by manometer, to rise rapidly. This is not seen if a spinal block to the flow of CSF is present, as in Froin's syndrome.

The test is very unreliable.

MANAGEMENT

Treatment is largely symptomatic:

- Dexamethasone 10-20 mg iv.

- Radiotherapy if diagnosis is known to be metastatic disease and tumour is radiosensitive.
- If diagnosis unknown, surgical intervention.

The prognosis of spinal cord compression is related to the severity of the neurological deficit at the time of presentation. *If paraplegia and sphincter involvement have occurred then recovery is uncommon.*

HYPERCALCEMIA

This is an abnormally high level of plasma calcium i.e. greater than 2.6 mmol per l.

The common causes of hypercalcaemia include:

- Malignancy accounts for 50% of cases and is frequently accompanied by hypoalbuminaemia:
  a. metastases with osteolytic deposits e.g. breast
  b. osteoclast activating factors e.g. multiple myeloma
  c. ectopic parathyroid hormone like peptide e.g. hypernephroma, ovarian tumour, bronchial carcinoma
- Primary hyperparathyroidism accounts for 20% of cases and is more important in the young

Rarer causes of hypercalcaemia include:

- Increased extrarenal synthesis of calcitriol in chronic granulomatous disease:
  a. sarcoidosis
  b. pulmonary tuberculosis
  c. berylliosis
- Addison's disease
- Paget's disease with bed rest
- Immobilisation-especially in adolescence when bone turnover is increased
- Vitamin A and/or D toxicity
- Drugs:
  a. thiazide diuretics
  b. lithium
- Thyrotoxicosis:
  a. usually mild and accompanied by hypercalciuria
  b. due to increased bone turnover
- Familial hypocalciuric hypercalcaemia
- Tertiary hyperparathyroidism

Features of hypercalcaemia may include:

- GIT problems:
  a. constipation
  b. nausea and vomiting
  c. peptic ulceration-due to increased gastrin secretion
  d. abdominal pain
- Psychological:
  a. depression is common
  b. dementia and psychoses occur infrequently
- Renal:
  a. polyuria due to a decreased sensitivity to antidiuretic hormone
  b. compensatory polydipsia
- General:
  a. lethargy
  b. weakness
  c. anorexia
  d. bone pains
- Calcification:
  a. cornea
  b. conjunctival flare
  c. urolithiasis, nephrolithiasis and nephrocalcinosis
  d. less commonly, chondrocalcinosis

In severe hypercalcaemia (total calcium > 3.5 mmol per l):

- Cardiac arrhythmias
- Renal tubular damage-hypokalaemia, dehydration, sodium loss; renal vasoconstriction; acute renal failure

Possible biochemical indicators of malignancy include low plasma albumin, low chloride, raised phosphate, raised alkaline phosphatase, alkalosis and hypokalaemia.

Possible biochemical indicators of hyperparathyroidism are normal or low albumin, a normal or reduced phosphate, a raised PTH (or inappropriately in the normal range), and a normal urea. PTH should be suppressed by high calcium concentration due to any other cause. The exception is familial benign hypercalcaemia where PTH may be normal or elevated but when, unlike other causes, the calcium excretion index (CEI) is low despite high plasma calcium. (CEI = [Ca] urine * [creat.] plasma/[creat.] urine)

Other biochemical indications:

- Raised albumin + raised urea-implies dehydration
- Raised albumin + normal urea-implies a cuffed sample
- Normal or low albumin + normal or raised phosphate:
  a. raised alkaline phosphatase-suggests bony metastases, sarcoidosis, or thyrotoxicosis
  b. normal alkaline phosphatase-myeloma (raised plasma protein), vitamin D excess, milk-alkali syndrome, thyrotoxicosis, sarcoidosis.

A ten day glucocorticoid suppression test may be diagnostically useful.

Hypercalcaemia Causes a Shortening of the QT Interval

The underlying cause of the condition must be treated.

Hypercalcaemia of greater than 3.5 mmol/l, or the presence of dangerous symptoms e.g. severe abdominal pain, clouding of consciousness, or pyrexia requires immediate treatment in order to correct hypercalcaemia and alleviate symptoms. Symptomatic hypercalcaemia is associated with high mortality.

- Adequate rehydration with 0.9% saline e.g. 3-6 litres in 24 hr period as necessary with potassium supplements, as indicated be serum monitoring
- Loop diuretics help induce calcium excretion, but should only be given when needed to prevent heart failure (1). Never administer thiazide diuretics-decrease Ca^{++} excretion
- Haemodialysis may be required if in renal failure
- Correction of hypokalaemia and hypomagnesaemia using IV supplements
- Monitor plasma sodium, potassium, magnesium, urea, CVP
- In hypercalcaemia of malignancy IV diphosphonates are probably the treatment of choice e.g. pamidronate, clodronate, etridonate. Pamidronate is the most potent.
- Mithramycin inhibits bone resorption-effective if due to hyperparathyroidism or malignancy-but toxic to liver, kidneys and platelets
- Calcitonin has an acute but very short-lived hypocalcaemic effect. Used only in severe hypercalcaemia
- Oral steroids are an effective intervention in patients with multiple myeloma, sarcoidosis, and vitamin D overdose
- Beta blocker therapy e.g. propranolol may protect against adverse cardiac effects

HYPONATREMIA

Hyponatraemia is a low plasma sodium, defined as sodium less than 135 mmol/l.

The causes of hyponatraemia may be categorised into:

- Hypervolaemic with increased total body sodium and body water
- Normovolaemic with normal total body sodium and slightly increased body water
- Hypovolaemic with greatly reduced total body sodium and reduced body water

Hyponatraemia is usually asymptomatic when plasma sodium is above 125 mmol per litre. Features become evident if plasma sodium falls rapidly towards this level or falls below about 120 mmol per litre; the rate of decrease may be as important as the absolute value in determining severity.

Features of moderately severe hyponatraemia i.e. plasma sodium less than 120 mmol/l):

- Headache, nausea, vomiting
- Malaise, irritability, depression, personality change
- Cramps, muscle weakness

Features of severe hyponatraemia i.e. plasma sodium less than 110 mmol/l):

- Confusion, drowsiness, convulsions
- Diminished reflexes, extensor plantar response
- Coma, death

Patients with a plasma sodium concentration *greater than 125 mmol/l* rarely need specific therapy for hyponatraemia.

Otherwise the principles of management include:

- Restriction of fluid intake to 500 ml per day to raise plasma sodium to 130 mM
- Frequent measurements of plasma osmolality and sodium
- Monitoring of body weight
- Demeclocycline hydrochloride:
  a. may be given if water restriction is poorly tolerated or ineffective
- In very rare circumstances hypertonic saline and frusemide may be administered but must be done with extreme caution

Excessively rapid correction of hyponatraemia may cause central pontine myelinolysis.

Five

Paraneoplastic Syndromes

The paraneoplastic syndromes represent a diverse group of conditions that affect virtually every organ system. By definition, they reflect the remote effects of cancer rather than direct effects caused by tumor growth and invasion, complications of therapy, nutritional deficiencies, or ischemic complications.

The recognition of these syndromes is important, because they frequently herald the presence of a tumor, and recognition can lead to earlier detection of tumor and earlier treatment. The signs and symptoms of paraneoplastic syndromes are the results of peptide hormone production, stimulation of autoantibody production, and, possibly, increased susceptibility to viral infections.

More recent data suggest a role for tumor-derived growth factors. The paraneoplastic syndromes pose diagnostic challenges; direct complications of cancer or its treatment must be excluded before making a definitive diagnosis.

PARANEOPLASTIC DISORDERS OF THE NERVOUS SYSTEM

See Table 5.1.

PARANEOPLASTIC CUTANEOUS SYNDROMES

These skin changes may coexist with or precede the diagnosis of cancer. The differentiation of these changes from similar dermatologic changes in patients with nonmalignant conditions can be a diagnostic challenge. The incidence of underlying malignancy varies, depending on the specific dermatologic disorder; therefore, the aggressiveness with which a tumor work-up is pursued should reflect this variation.

In general, the onset of symptoms in paraneoplastic cutaneous lesions is more rapid than when associated with benign conditions. The appearance of skin lesions in patients with occult or obvious malignancy may be valuable in the detection and management of the cancer, because the skin is readily accessible to examination and biopsy. The causes of cutaneous lesions in most instances are unknown. However, because many cutaneous paraneoplastic syndromes are proliferative, tumor-derived growth factors may play a pathogenic role. Autoantibodies also may be involved.

Acanthosis nigricans: is characterized by a hyperpigmented, gray-brown, velvety soft thickening of the skin. The most common sites of involvement are the nape of the neck, axilla, palms, soles, perineum, antecubital fossae, and intertriginous areas. Most cases of acanthosis nigricans are not tumor-related and are associated with obesity and endocrine abnormalities. When associated with a malignancy, acanthosis

Table 5.1: Paraneoplastic neurologic syndromes

Paraneoplastic neurologic syndrome	*Cause or associated antibodies*	*Clinical manifestations*	*Associated malignancy*	*Treatment*
Cerebellar degeneration	Anti-Yo (most commonly in breast or gynecologic cancer) Anti-Ma	Acute or subacute onset of ataxia, dysarthria, vertigo, and nystagmus	Small cell lung cancer, gynecologic tumors, breast cancer, Hodgkin's disease	Treatment of tumor usually not effective, except in Hodgkin's disease
Encephalomyelitis	Anti-Hu (especially in small cell lung cancer) Anti-Ta (in testicular cancer)	Cerebellar signs, brain stem dysfunction, encephalopathy, myelopathy, autonomic dysfunction	Small cell lung cancer, breast cancer, gynecologic tumors, gastrointestinal tumors, Hodgkin's disease, testicular cancer	Treatment of tumor in rare cases helpful; immunosuppression may be effective
Opsoclonus-myoclonus ataxia	Anti-Ri (present in some cases)	Rapid irregular and uncontrollable movement of eyes and postural shaking of body	Neuroblastoma in children; lung, breast, and ovarian tumors in adults	May respond to corticosteroids and intravenous immune globulin
Lambert-Eaton myasthenic syndrome	Antibodies to presynaptic calcium channels impair acetylcholine release; proven to be causal	Proximal muscle weakness, dry mouth, ptosis, blurred vision, autonomic dysfunction	Small cell lung cancer	Plasmapheresis, immunosuppression, 3,4-diaminopyridine
Myasthenia gravis	Antibodies to postsynaptic acetylcholine receptors	Muscle fatigue (especially ocular) and ptosis	Thymoma	Thymectomy, acetylcholinesterase inhibitors, steroids, azathioprine
Necrotizing myelopathy	Unknown	Subacute onset of progressive ascending or descending spinal cord deficits; pain is rare	Lung, breast, kidney tumors; lymphoma	None
Sensory neuropathy	Anti-Hu (more commonly in small cell lung cancer) Anti-CV2	Subacute onset, pain, paresthesias, gait disturbance, numbness in distal limbs; can be associated with paraneoplastic encephalomyelitis	Small cell lung cancer usually; also, non-small cell lung cancer and breast cancer	Treatment of underlying tumor may lead to some improvement
Retinopathy	Anti-recoverin antibodies	Subacute onset of progressive visual loss	Small cell lung cancer, gynecologic tumors	May respond to corticosteroids and intravenous immune globulin

nigricans is seen in patients with adenocarcinoma, of which 50 to 60% is gastric carcinoma. Other primary sites include the lung, liver, uterus, breast, and ovary. In nonobese adults, the appearance of this cutaneous eruption should raise the clinician's suspicion of an underlying malignancy. Evaluation should include a physical examination, a complete blood count (CBC), and consideration of upper gastrointestinal endoscopy. Successful treatment of the underlying malignancy often leads to improvement.

The *Leser-Trélat sign* is the sudden and rapid appearance of pigmented, pruritic, seborrheic keratoses in patients with an underlying malignancy. Not only do new lesions appear, but preexisting keratoses increase in size over several days. These lesions most commonly appear on the trunk, followed by the extremities, face, abdomen, and neck. Again, this sign most is often associated with tumors of the gastrointestinal tract; it also has been associated with non-Hodgkin's lymphoma

Sweet's syndrome: is an acute, febrile, neutrophilic dermatosis characterized by fever, leukocytosis, and painful erythematous plaques or nodules that primarily occur on the face, limbs, and neck. Sweet's syndrome has been associated with hematologic malignancies, most commonly acute myelocytic leukemia; therefore, a careful physical examination and CBC should be sufficient screening. Generally, a rapid response to corticosteroid therapy is seen, regardless of the presence of malignancy.

Paraneoplastic acrokeratosis of Bazex: symmetrically affects the hands, scalp, feet, ears, and nose with violaceous, psoriasiform scales. Nail changes are common and consist of subungual hyperkeratosis with onychodystrophy and a white, flaking nail surface. This syndrome is associated with head and neck cancer, gastrointestinal tract cancers, and lung cancer. Virtually all patients with this syndrome have an underlying malignancy; therefore, a thorough evaluation for an internal neoplasm is warranted. This dermatosis generally improves with treatment of the underlying malignancy, and has been shown to reappear with recurrence of the malignancy.

Dermatomyositis: is a cutaneous, muscle disease of adults that has been associated with malignancy. Classic clinical manifestations include a purplish (heliotrope) rash of the eyelids and cheeks with periorbital edema, erythematous or violaceous papules over the knuckles (Gottron's papules), poikiloderma, and a photosensitive rash. The muscle disease, similar to polymyositis, is characterized by proximal muscle weakness. Approximately 25% of patients over 40 years of age with dermatomyositis have an underlying malignancy-most often lung, but also breast, ovarian, cervical, and gastrointestinal. Polymyositis also is associated with an underlying malignancy, but to a lesser degree than dermatomyositis

Once the diagnosis of dermatomyositis is made, work-up should include history and physical examination, CBC, chest radiograph, and stool sample for occult blood testing. If these tests have normal results, the value of a more extensive work-up is unclear. Dermatomyositis has been reported to precede diagnosis of a neoplasm for up to 5 years; therefore, continued surveillance for malignancy should be considered. The pathogenesis of this disorder remains unknown, but accumulating data suggest that it is a humoral autoimmune disorder. Treatment with corticosteroids results in improvement of skin rash, improvement of muscle strength, and normalization of serum muscle enzyme levels. Azathioprine and cyclosporine also have been effective in some patients.

Hypertrichosis lanuginosa acquisita: describes an abrupt, progressive development of fine lanugo hair in the adult. The long, downy, nonpigmented hair initially covers the face and ears, rapidly spreading to cover all hair-bearing skin and sparing the genital regions. The development of "malignant down" is quite rare, and usually is associated with occult malignancies. The most common neoplasms are tumors of the lung, colon, and uterus, as well as lymphoma

Erythema gyratum repens: is a rare, bizarre eruption characterized by erythematous bands that form a gyrate pattern moving in waves over the body. This condition almost always is associated with an underlying malignancy, most commonly lung cancer, breast cancer, and gastrointestinal cancer.

Necrolytic migratory erythema: is associated with glucagon-producing islet-cell tumors of the pancreas. Skin lesions include erythematous vesicles, pustules, and bullae, which typically involve the perineum and intertriginous areas of the skin. The cutaneous lesions can be confused with seborrheic dermatitis or candidiasis. Removal of the tumor or effective chemotherapy clearly improves the skin eruption.

Erythroderma: a diffuse erythema of the skin, most commonly is associated with hematologic malignancies, including leukemias and lymphomas (most frequently T-cell type, as in Sézary syndrome and mycosis fungoides). Facial and upper body flushing is primarily seen in patients with a carcinoid neoplasm and is caused by secretion of serotonin and other vasoactive peptides.

Several *vesiculobullous disorders* are associated with malignancy.

Pemphigus vulgaris: is associated with lymphoma and chronic lymphocytic leukemia. More than 50% of the time, the dermatologic findings precede the malignancy.

Paraneoplastic pemphigus: is a recently described form of pemphigus, which, as its name implies, always is associated with cancer. Patients have blistering mucocutaneous lesions. The disorder has been associated with lymphoma, chronic lymphocytic leukemia (CLL), sarcoma, squamous cell carcinoma, and thymoma. Unlike other forms of pemphigus, it usually does not respond to steroids, plasmapheresis, or immunosuppressive agents.

Papulosquamous disorders: also have been associated with malignancy.

Acquired ichthyosis: most often associated with Hodgkin's disease, should prompt a workup, including history and physical examination, CBC, chest radiograph, and potentially an abdominal CT scan. Pruritus of unknown origin is associated with Hodgkin's disease.

Numerous *inherited dermatoses* have been associated with the development of a wide range of malignancies

PARANEOPLASTIC RHEUMATIC SYNDROMES

Malignant neoplasms are associated with many paraneoplastic rheumatic syndromes. The most common of these are *hypertrophic osteoarthropathy*, *carcinoma polyarthritis*, and *paraneoplastic vasculitis*. Less frequently seen are such entities as fasciitis, panniculitis, erythema nodosum, Raynaud's syndrome, digital gangrene, erythromelalgia, and lupus-like syndromes.

Like the cutaneous syndromes, musculoskeletal manifestations of malignancy may precede, coincide with, or follow the diagnosis of cancer. Hematologic malignancies, including lymphomas and leukemia, most often are associated with paraneoplastic rheumatic diseases, although solid tumors, such as lung, breast, and ovarian cancers, also have been implicated.

The clinical course generally parallels that of the primary disease, with treatment of the underlying malignancy often resulting in regression of the rheumatic disorder. Rheumatic manifestations that suggest an occult malignancy include rapid onset of an unusual inflammatory arthritis, clubbing, or diffuse bone pains in a patient >/=50 years, chronic unexplained vasculitis, refractory fasciitis, Raynaud's syndrome unresponsive to vasodilator therapy, or rapidly progressive digital gangrene.

Treatment considerations include control of the underlying cancer and symptomatic management of the rheumatic syndrome with nonsteroidal anti-inflammatory drugs (NSAIDs) or corticosteroids

Paraneoplastic endocrine syndromes: the most interesting of the paraneoplastic syndromes, result from cancer-produced peptide hormones (ectopic hormone production). Recent advances in protein chemistry assays and sensitive methods of measuring hormone levels have helped to delineate the paraneoplastic endocrine syndromes. It is important to recognize these syndromes because they cause significant morbidity, which may be worse than the tumor growth and spread, and because the initial diagnostic clue to the cancer may be its hormone excess syndrome.

Ectopic Adrenocorticotropic Hormone (ACTH) Syndrome

Small cell lung cancer is the most common tumor associated with *ACTH* production.

Seventy percent of associated cancers arise in the lung, pancreas, and thymus, which suggest an embryologic relationship among tumors of these tissues. Elevated levels of ACTH can be found in both blood and tumor extracts. The classic clinical features of hypercortisolism-centripetal obesity, striae, buffalo hump, and moon facies-occur infrequently in patients with ectopic ACTH production.

Patients usually present with polyuria and polydipsia (from elevated blood glucose levels), edema, muscle wasting, fatigue, hypertension and hypokalemia. Laboratory evaluations reveal excessive cortisol production (e.g., elevated 24-hour urine-free cortisol) and lack of dexamethasone suppression of morning cortisol levels. Plasma ACTH levels >200 pg/mL suggest ectopic ACTH production and warrant a search for an underlying malignancy, especially a primary lung or pancreatic tumor.

Specific treatment is directed at the underlying tumor. Excessive hormone levels can be reduced by drugs that inhibit adrenal cortisol production, including aminoglutethimide, metyrapone, or mitotane. These agents must be used with caution, require careful monitoring, and require that treated patients receive supplementary steroids.

Hypercalcemia

Humoral hypercalcemia of malignancy (HHM) is most common in patients with squamous cell cancers. While squamous cell lung cancers are often associated with this syndrome, HHM has also been observed in squamous cell cancers of the head and neck, esophagus, cervix, and skin. Rarely, adenocarcinomas of the breast, ovary, kidney, and GI tract can produce HHM.

The presence of bony metastases is not necessary for the clinical syndrome; rather, HHM is caused by the production of circulating humoral factors leading to hypercalcemia. Since the identification of a *parathyroid hormone-related peptide (PTHrP),* most cases of HHM appear to be related to production of this factor. PTHrP shares homology with PTH at the amino terminus, allowing it to interact with PTH receptors in the bone and kidney.

Other humoral factors, such as interleukin-1 and TNF have also been implicated in hypercalcemia. The presence of bony metastases in any malignancy can induce hypercalcemia secondary to bone resorption. Multiple myeloma, for example, often presents with elevated serum calcium levels.

Treatment of HHM focuses on reversal of the hypercalcemic state.Acutely, intravenous fluid hydration and loop diuretics can help stabilize the patient. Calcitonin works most quickly to inhibit the effects of PTHrP in the kidney, and decrease serum calcium levels.

Bisphosphonates are the mainstay of therapy for hypercalcemia. Medications such as pamidronate and zoledronate are potent inhibitors of bone resorption. Given intravenously, these agents have a high affinity for bone mineral and prevent osteoclastic activity. Bisphosphonates are also effective at reducing skeletal complications from malignancy and can prevent formation of new bone metastases.

Hypoglycemia

Extrapancreatic tumors that reportedly induce hypoglycemia include mesotheliomas (most common cause), soft-tissue sarcoma, leiomyosarcoma and fibrosarcoma, hepatoma, and adrenal cortical carcinoma.

Tumors in hypoglycemic patients are often extremely large and often extensively involve the liver. Although the mechanism for cancer-induced hypoglycemia is not fully understood, two families of peptides (distinct from insulin), somatomedins and insulin-like growth factors, have been postulated to be responsible.

Both cancer-and noncancer-related causes of hypoglycemia have the same symptoms and signs. They frequently follow fasting or physical exertion. Neurologic symptoms may clinically mimic CNS metastases; therefore, hypoglycemia should be considered when evaluating a cancer patient with neurologic symptoms.

The acute treatment of hypoglycemia includes parenteral glucose administration. Chronic management, which is difficult, initially is directed at treatment of the underlying cancer; however, this approach is not often possible. Frequent small meals can reduce symptoms of hypoglycemia, but continuous parenteral glucose is sometimes required. Long-acting glucagon or high-dose corticosteroid therapy may be effective.

Syndrome of Inappropriate Antidiuretic Hormone Secretion

The *syndrome of inappropriate antidiuretic hormone secretion* (SIADH) has numerous causes, including CNS disorders, pulmonary infections, drug toxicities, and idiopathic causes.

SIADH should be suspected in patients presenting with hyponatremia. Various neoplasms, usually small cell lung carcinoma (or, less frequently, non-small cell lung cancer), have been associated with SIADH. In the patient with idiopathic SIADH, an extensive search for an occult lung cancer is recommended and should include a chest CT scan and bronchoscopy, even if the chest radiograph is normal. The pathogenesis of SIADH is tumor production of arginine vasopressin.

Successful treatment of the underlying tumor is the best therapeutic approach. Fluid restriction will slowly increase plasma osmolality. More serious hyponatremia requires treatment with hypertonic saline and furosemide. Occasionally, therapy must be directed at inhibition of arginine vasopressin activity. Demeclocycline (150 to 300 mg orally 4 times daily) is the most potent inhibitor of arginine vasopressin.

RENAL MANIFESTATIONS OF MALIGNANCY

Protein-losing nephropathy is relatively uncommon in patients with malignancies; it often precedes the diagnosis of cancer.

As many as 10% of all patients have some form of glomerulonephritis during the course of their malignancy. The most common cancers associated with nephrotic syndrome are Hodgkin's disease and lung, colon, ovarian, breast, and gastric cancers.

The most common glomerular lesion in paraneoplastic nephrotic syndrome is *membranous glomerulonephritis*, seen in 60 to 70% of patients. Other glomerular lesions include *membranoproliferative glomerulonephritis* and *minimal change disease*.

Most patients with malignancy-associated minimal change disease have Hodgkin's disease; less frequently, they have lung or gastrointestinal tract tumors. Although the glomerulonephropathy is theoretically related to immune complex deposition, specific antigens have not been identified. These antigens may be tumor-related, not tumor-related, or perhaps viral antigens. Both treatment of the underlying cancer and corticosteroid therapy improve malignancy-associated nephropathy.

HEMATOLOGIC PARANEOPLASTIC SYNDROMES

Hematologic abnormalities are among the most common paraneoplastic syndromes. During the past decade, significant advances were made in understanding both the regulation of normal hematopoiesis and the pathophysiology of paraneoplastic hematologic syndromes.

Anemia: is one of the most frequently encountered clinical findings in patients with malignant disease. It has numerous causes, including bone marrow involvement with underlying cancer, blood loss, chemotherapy, radiation therapy, infections, nutritional deficiencies, and myelofibrosis.

Chronic anemia of malignancy: is caused by a poorly understood defect in the production of erythrocytes. The erythrocytes in this mild anemia (hemoglobin levels usually >9 g/dL) are either normochromic, normocytic or hypochromic, normocytic. Although iron stores are adequate, impaired use of iron is evident by low serum iron concentrations and low iron-binding capacity. Ferritin levels are normal or elevated, and the reticulocyte count is inappropriately low. No specific cancer is associated with this anemia. Although unexplained, erythropoietin levels can be inappropriately low.

Treatment depends on controlling the underlying malignancy. Erythrocyte transfusions are given as needed. Administration of exogenous recombinant erythropoietin may ameliorate cancer-associated anemia, especially in patients with low erythropoietin levels. Effective regimens have used 150 U/kg of recombinant erythropoietin subcutaneously, 3 times weekly. An increased hematocrit count is expected within 2 to 4 weeks.

Pure erythrocyte aplasia: is a rare syndrome in which patients have a selective loss of erythrocyte precursors, with maintenance of other cell lines. Thymomas have been found in nearly 50% of all cases of erythrocyte cell aplasia; however, less than 10% of patients with thymoma have erythrocyte aplasia. In 25 to 30% of cases, thymectomy results in remission. The pathogenesis remains unknown.

Hemolytic anemia: of various origins has long been recognized as a complication of tumors. *Antibody-mediated* hemolytic anemia frequently is associated with B-cell neoplasms and occasionally with carcinomas, particularly ovarian. The failure of an autoimmune hemolytic anemia to respond to therapy should prompt a search for an underlying cause, such as malignancy. Successful treatment of the underlying tumor generally leads to resolution of the anemia. Corticosteroids generally are ineffective; occasionally, splenectomy is required in refractory cases.

Microangiopathic hemolysis: is an uncommon hematologic complication that occurs most frequently in patients with mucin-producing adenocarcinomas, especially gastric cancer. Evaluations reveal fragmented erythrocytes (schistocytes, helmet cells), a negative Coombs' test and, frequently, evidence of *disseminated intravascular coagulation* (DIC).

The mechanism of hemolysis is unclear but may be related to fibrin deposition caused by DIC or abnormal vascular endothelium caused by tumor emboli. Management includes erythrocyte transfusions (requirement may be substantial), management of DIC, and, most importantly, treatment of the underlying cancer. The use of heparin and antiplatelet agents remains controversial.

Erythrocytosis or polycythemia: secondary to inappropriate production of erythropoietin frequently is associated with an underlying malignancy.

Evaluations reveal increases in erythrocyte count and hematocrit count (men > 55% or women > 50% at sea level) and total erythrocyte mass. This syndrome is associated most frequently with renal tumors but also has been seen with *hepatomas, cerebellar hemangioblastomas, uterine tumors, adrenal cortical tumors, and, rarely, lung cancer*. The syndrome often is associated with increased erythropoietin levels, especially in patients with renal tumors.

Other possible causes include tumor-derived peptides, prostaglandins, or androgenic hormones that have erythropoietic effects.

This *erythrocytosis of malignancy* syndrome usually can be distinguished from *polycythemia vera* by bone marrow findings, the absence of leukocytosis, thrombocytosis, and splenomegaly. Serum erythropoietin levels often are increased, whereas in polycythemia vera they are typically decreased.

Further evaluations are focused on the kidneys (e.g., renal cell cancer or cysts) and the pelvic and neurologic examinations (especially cerebellar testing). The erythrocytosis usually resolves after successful treatment of the underlying malignancy. Additional treatment, such as phlebotomy, is rarely required.

The *leukemoid reaction (marked peripheral granulocytosis)* commonly accompanies cancer (especially breast, lung, or gastric cancer), particularly if liver metastases are present.

Elevations of granulocyte levels >20,000 mm^3 not associated with infection or inflammation are seen; occasionally, increases in monocyte and eosinophil levels are noted. The mechanism of increased granulocyte count is increased activity of tumor-derived colony-stimulating factors (granulocyte colony-stimulating factor, granulocyte-macrophage colony-stimulating factor, interleukin-3, and interleukin-1).

Unlike those with chronic myelocytic leukemia, patients with a leukemoid reaction have normal spleens, normal or elevated leukocyte alkaline phosphatase scores, absent (t9:22) translocation, and, generally, normal platelet counts. Granulocytosis is asymptomatic and specific therapy is not indicated.

HYPERCOAGULABLE STATE

The association between cancer and thrombosis has long been recognized. Patients with malignancy may present with a *recurrent migratory thrombophlebitis syndrome*.

Classically, pancreatic carcinoma is associated with migratory thrombophlebitis. The coagulation abnormalities associated with cancer include platelet disorders, alterations in coagulation and fibrinolytic proteins, DIC, and thrombosis, and can cause either bleeding or thrombosis. These hemostatic abnormalities are the second most common cause of death in patients with solid tumors. The malignancy-associated protein, cancer procoagulant (CP), is a cysteine protease that directly activates factor X to promote coagulation.

Although DIC is reportedly associated with almost every type of malignancy, mucin-secreting gastrointestinal adenocarcinomas and leukemia are the most frequent causes. Solid tumors are typically associated with *chronic DIC*, which clinically presents as mucocutaneous bleeding, easy bruising, or deep or superficial venous thrombosis. Classically, fibrin split products are elevated and platelets are decreased; less commonly, hypofibrinogenemia is present. This

DIC syndrome may be associated with a microangiopathic hemolytic anemia.

Acute DIC is seen in patients with acute or chronic leukemias. The most common leukemia associated with acute DIC is a subtype of acute myelogenous leukemia-acute promyelocytic leukemia (APL). In APL, the spontaneous or leukemia treatment-related release of procoagulant factors by progranulocyte granules induces the acute DIC. Signs and symptoms include petechiae, purpura, life-threatening hemorrhage, and oozing from venipuncture sites. Laboratory findings of acute DIC include reduced platelet counts and fibrinogen levels, prolonged prothrombin and partial thromboplastin times, and increased fibrin split products.

Heparin usually is reserved for patients with acute DIC, active thrombosis, or recurrent thromboembolic events. Long-term therapy with warfarin sodium usually is unsuccessful. Replacement therapy rarely is indicated in chronic DIC; however, it is indicated in acute DIC associated with active bleeding, markedly low fibrinogen level, or elevated prothrombin time.

Nonbacterial thrombotic endocarditis: is associated most commonly with gastric carcinoma and lung cancer, and is caused by deposition of fibrin and platelets on the valve leaflets of the left side of the heart.

Echocardiography is of little value because most vegetations are smaller than 2 mm and therefore difficult to detect. Transesophageal echocardiography is more sensitive, but still often non-diagnostic because of the size of the vegetations. Treatment of the underlying tumor is the mainstay of therapy. In some studies, heparin was more effective than warfarin sodium, likely due to the association with DIC. Quality of life was also improved with heparin anticoagulation.

Six

AIDS-related Malignancies

Malignancies have been detected in approximately 40% of all patients with acquired immunodeficiency syndrome (AIDS) sometime during the course of their illness. These cancers have been both a primary cause of death in some patients and also a source of considerable morbidity. In the current era of protease inhibitors and highly active antiretroviral therapy (HAART), patients infected with the human immunodeficiency virus (HIV) are surviving longer than ever. HAART appears to have substantially reduced the incidence of Kaposi's sarcoma (KS) and non-Hodgkin's lymphoma (NHL), and may enhance the efficacy of treatment for those patients who do develop these tumors. Unfortunately, HAART has not shown a similar effect on the development of other types of neoplasms, and the need to care for patients who develop malignancies as part of AIDS remains a challenge.

KAPOSI'S SARCOMA

KS has been the most common tumor associated with HIV infection, developing in approximately 10-13% of homosexual men with AIDS in the United States and 1-2% of other HIV-infected persons. The incidence of KS has declined substantially, from 4.8 per 100 person-years in 1990 to 1.5 per 100 person-years in 1997.

Epidemiology

Gender: Among AIDS patients in the United States, the incidence of KS is higher in males than in females. There is also a higher incidence of KS in men relative to women in Africa (male-female ratio, 3:1), despite the equal prevalence of HIV infection among men and women.

Age: The age distribution of AIDS-KS follows the distribution of HIV infection. As such, AIDS-KS can occur in all age groups. In US adult males, the most common age of onset of AIDS-KS is 30-40 years old. No peak age has been reported.

Race: No racial or ethnic differences in the incidence of AIDS-KS have been observed.

Geography: In the United States, KS is seen in approximately 10-13% of homosexual men with AIDS and 1-2% of other persons with HIV infection. The proportion of KS among AIDS-defining diagnoses is lower in parts of Europe, where there are proportionately fewer male homosexual AIDS cases (e.g., 6.8% of Italian AIDS patients), and higher in parts of Africa, where KS is endemic in the non–HIV-infected population. Among AIDS cases in the United States, the proportion of patients with KS has declined from the beginning of the AIDS epidemic, possibly as a result of changes in high-risk sexual behavior among gay men and the wider use of more effective antiretroviral combination regimens.

Etiology and Risk Factors

In the United States, the observation that KS occurs predominantly in homosexual men and the epidemiologic evidence that KS has declined among AIDS patients in parallel with the declining incidence of sexually transmitted diseases (STDs) among gay men are cited as support for the theory that a sexually transmitted agent may be involved in the development of AIDS-related KS.

Viruses: In 1994, unique viral DNA sequences were identified in tumor tissues from patients with AIDS-KS, which led to the identification of a new virus called KS-associated herpesvirus (KSHV) or *human herpesvirus type 8 (HHV-8)*. HHV-8 has been found in > 90% of AIDS-KS tumors, as well as in classic KS, endemic African KS, and post–organ transplant-related KS. It has also been identified in body cavity–based lymphoma/primary effusion lymphoma, multicentric Castleman's disease, and angio-immunoblastic lymphadenopathy with dysproteinemia (AILD) in the HIV-infected patient.

HHV-8 may be transmitted through sexual contact or through blood products. Seroprevalence of HHV-8 in AIDS-KS is nearly 100%.

HHV-8 is critical in the pathogenesis of AIDS-KS. The mechanism by which HHV-8 induces KS in susceptible individuals is the subject of intense current investigations.

Environmental and host factors: Various environmental and host factors, including HIV- and HHV-8–induced cytokines, AIDS-associated infections, the host's hormonal milieu, and antiretroviral therapy, may induce or suppress the development of KS and alter its growth. The high male-female ratio among AIDS patients with KS in the United States and the higher incidence of KS among men compared to women in Africa, where equal numbers of males and females are infected with HIV, suggest that female gender and, possibly, female sex hormones may confer some protection against this tumor or, conversely, that male gender or male sex hormones may induce its development.

Signs and Symptoms

The manifestations of KS in patients with AIDS are variable and range from small innocuous-looking cutaneous lesions to symptom-producing visceral or oral lesions, which may be quite troublesome and even life-threatening. Just about every internal organ can occasionally be involved with KS in some instances. KS is rarely seen in the bone marrow or CNS.

Skin lesions: KS tumors typically begin as flat or raised lesions that may progress to plaque-like or nodular tumors. Lesions vary in size and shape but are generally nonpruritic and painless. They range in color from light pink to red to deep purple. KS lesions may be cosmetically disfiguring and may result in social stigmatization that far exceeds any actual physical impairment.

Dermal and lymphatic infiltration: with tumor can result in edema of the extremities, periorbital areas, and genitals and may be complicated by skin breakdown and bacterial cellulitis. Edema can be marked and may prevent the patient from wearing shoes and/or walking.

Lesions on the feet: can cause pain and hamper walking.

Oral lesions: are often asymptomatic but can produce pain and swallowing difficulties.

GI tract involvement: with KS is seen in up to 50% of patients. Most lesions are asymptomatic; however, obstruction, bleeding, or enteropathy can occur occasionally.

Pulmonary KS: usually presents as dyspnea without fever and may become severely debilitating and rapidly fatal if untreated.

Screening and Diagnosis

Currently there are no screening tests for KS. Although most KS lesions are readily recognized, early lesions may be difficult to diagnose, and the lesions of other diseases (e.g., bacillary angiomatosis) may mimic those of KS. Once clinically suspected, the diagnosis of KS is made by biopsy and histologic examination of skin lesions, an excised lymph node, or other tissue, or by presumptive diagnosis based on the bronchoscopic or endoscopic appearance of a visceral lesion.

GI KS: has a typical red, raised appearance and is difficult to diagnose by biopsy because of the submucosal location of many lesions.

Pulmonary KS: In patients with pulmonary KS, chest radiographs typically demonstrate diffuse, reticular-nodular infiltrates, mediastinal enlargement, and, sometimes, pleural effusion. Bronchoscopy may reveal extensive endobronchial involvement with tumor. Definitive diagnosis requires transbronchial or open-lung biopsy. Transbronchial biopsies, however, often yield negative results. A presumptive diagnosis of pulmonary KS may be made, in the absence of fever, based on typical radiographic and endobronchial findings of KS-appearing lesions and after the exclusion of infections.

Thallium and technetium-99m scanning may help differentiate KS from other pulmonary diseases. Patients with KS have been found to have thallium- and technetium-avid scans, whereas pulmonary lymphomas and infections are more typically gallium-avid.

Pathology

Cutaneous KS: is a lesion of the dermis comprised of a proliferation of aberrant vascular structures lined by abnormal-appearing, spindle-shaped endothelial cells and with extravasated erythrocytes and leukocytes within the structures. These spindle cells are generally sparse in early stages but become more numerous and stack up between the vascular structures as the tumor advances. Infiltration of mononuclear leukocytes, including plasma cells, T-cells, and monocytes, is more prominent in earlier lesions. The histologic appearance of KS in AIDS is similar to that seen in the non–HIV-infected patient.

Cell of origin: The KS tumor cell is believed to be of mesenchymal, endothelial origin. Several endothelial cell markers are positive in KS, including stains for ulex europaeus and EN-4. In addition, the tumor stains with factor VIIIa, CD-34, and a-actin.

Staging and Prognosis

Prognostic factors: Although it is difficult to predict from the initial presentation which patients are most likely to have rapidly progressive tumors, several retrospective studies have shown a correlation of survival with the degree of T-cell immunodeficiency, as reflected in the absolute number of T-helper cells. Prior opportunistic infections or the presence of such symptoms as fevers, night sweats, and weight loss (B symptoms) also portend a poor prognosis. Patients who develop KS or whose tumor growth accelerates after an opportunistic infection often have a more aggressive clinical course. Patients with pulmonary involvement generally have a poor prognosis.

Staging system: A tumor classification system has been proposed for AIDS-related KS by the oncology committee of the AIDS Clinical Trials Group (ACTG). This system segregates patients into good or poor prognostic groups based on tumor characteristics, immune system function, and systemic illness. A retrospective analysis of 294 patients with AIDS-KS has shown that the TIS system is a valid predictor for survival.

Gauging response to therapy: Given the heterogeneity and unpredictable growth of this tumor, it is often difficult to gauge objective responses. The peculiarities of this multicentric tumor make some subjectivity almost inevitable in gauging treatment responses.

Treatment

The treatment of AIDS-related KS requires an individualized approach, based on the extent and location of the lesions, the wishes and treatment needs of the patient, the presence of tumor-associated symptoms (e.g., pain, bleeding, edema), the presence of other AIDS-associated illnesses, and the patient's tolerance of medications. Nevertheless, the following general statements can be made:

- Patients with widespread symptomatic disease or life-threatening visceral involvement require prompt, cytoreductive treatment with one or more chemotherapeutic drugs.
- Even in the absence of symptomatic visceral disease, the disfigurement and emotional distress of having these visible reminders of AIDS may mandate treatment for psychological reasons.
- For patients with asymptomatic indolent lesions, aggressive treatment is not mandatory, but these patients may derive substantial benefits from investigational therapies that are directed against HIV or HHV-8, or that may interrupt the pathogenesis of KS and/or restore immune competence.

Treatment Options

With the introduction of protease inhibitors and nonnucleoside reverse transcriptase inhibitors for HIV, cases of KS regression with combination antiretroviral therapy have been reported. Because KS seems to be influenced by the state of HIV infection, we believe that all patients with AIDS-KS should have their HIV infection under optimal control. There is no one best anti-HIV regimen, and oncologists should consult with infectious disease specialists familiar with the treatment of HIV. Eventually, even with good anti-HIV therapy, most patients with AIDS-KS will require some form of treatment for their tumor.

Local treatments, including cryotherapy, topical retinoic acid, intralesional chemotherapy and other sclerosing agents, and local radiation can all produce good local control of tumors. Interferon-alfa (IFN-a [Intron A, Roferon-A]) and cytotoxic chemotherapy are effective systemic treatments in patients with more extensive or symptomatic disease. Single-agent or combination chemotherapy is effective in controlling tumors, even in patients with very extensive disease and severe immune deficiencies. The use of hematopoietic growth factors has facilitated the administration of myelosuppressive treatments, such as IFN-a and chemotherapy.

IFN-α

The first treatment licensed for AIDS-related KS was recombinant IFN-a. Tumor responses have been seen in approximately 30% of patients treated with SC interferon given either daily or 3 times weekly. Current practice is to administer IFN-α 3 times weekly by SC injection. Unmaintained response durations in trials of IFN-α monotherapy have ranged from 12 to 24 months in complete responders and from 8 to 12 months in partial responders.

Duration of therapy: The optimal duration of IFN-α treatment is unknown; however, many patients relapse within a few months after discontinuation of therapy. Reinduction of second responses with IFN-α after relapse may be unreliable and often is of short duration. It is therefore generally recommended that treatment with IFN-α be continued for as long as drug tolerance and tumor responses continue.

Dose: The optimal dose of IFN-α also has not been clearly established. IFN-α is generally administered at either 3 or 5 million units SC 3 times weekly, together with antiretroviral therapy.

Major dose-limiting toxicities: of IFN-α include fever, chills, rigor, and other flu-like symptoms. These are dose related and often observed at the initiation of treatment but lessen somewhat with continued use. Neutropenia, transaminase elevation, and peripheral neuropathy may also occur, especially when IFN-α is used in combination with various antiretroviral medications.

Other side effects: include headaches, minor cognitive impairments, paresthesias, and mild thrombocytopenia. As the subjective side effects of IFN-α are also common in HIV-related or other conditions, care must be taken to avoid ascribing all of these symptoms to drug toxicity and overlooking treatable infections and other conditions.

Factors correlating with response: Factors that appear to correlate with a greater likelihood of tumor regression to IFN-α include a negative history for opportunistic infections and the absence of B symptoms.

Alitretinoin

Alitretinoin gel 0.1% (9-*cis*-retinoic acid [Panretin]) has received FDA approval for the topical treatment of localized cutaneous KS. This compound inhibits the growth of KS and induces apoptosis of KS cells by binding to retinoic acid receptors on the cell surface.

Phase II clinical trials comparing 3-4 times daily application of alitretinoin vs placebo gel demonstrated a 35% rate of complete and partial responses in the alitretinoin-treated patients, as compared with a rate of 18% in controls. Median time to response to alitretinoin was 29-34 days, with a median duration of response of 12-16 weeks. Responses were seen in both untreated and previously treated KS patients and were not dependent on the patient's CD4 count.

Local cutaneous adverse reactions to alitretinoin include erythema, skin irritation, skin cracking, flaking, peeling, and desquamation. The severity of these reactions can be mitigated with topical vitamin E.

Alitretinoin should be reserved for patients who do not require systemic treatment for visceral disease. However, it may be used in conjunction with other treatments for cutaneous disease.

Chemotherapy

For patients with more widely disseminated, rapidly progressive, or symptomatic disease, systemic chemotherapy is generally warranted.

Antiretroviral drugs: A total of 15 anti-HIV drugs have received FDA approval, and more are in various stages of clinical development. When evaluated by an oncologist, the majority of HIV-infected individuals will be taking some anti-HIV drugs. The interactions between cytotoxic chemotherapy and the various anti-HIV drugs have not been fully studied as yet. Thus, oncologists treating patients with AIDS-KS should continue to monitor them frequently for side effects.

Combination regimens: The two most frequently utilized combination chemotherapy regimens are Adriamycin (doxorubicin), bleomycin (Blenoxane), and vincristine (ABV) and bleomycin and vincristine (BV). These regimens were initially reported to yield tumor response rates in excess of 70-90%, with good palliation of symptoms, including decreased edema, decreased pain, and, in patients with pulmonary KS, respiratory improvement and alleviation of obstructive symptoms. A beneficial effect of these combinations on survival has not been clearly demonstrated, however.

Early reports of a high response rate with these combination regimens have not been reproduced by later multicenter trials. A conservative response rate of 50-60% has been reported in more contemporary phase III trials. The discrepancy in response rates most likely stems from differences in the response criteria used.

Liposomal anthracyclines: (e.g., liposomal doxorubicin and liposomal daunorubicin) are also very effective in inducing tumor regression in KS. Clinical trials have shown that liposomal anthracyclines as single agents can achieve a response rate equal to or better than the ABV combination regimen. As such, the liposomal anthracyclines have become the first-line chemotherapy for AIDS-KS.

The dose-limiting toxicity is neutropenia, and many patients will require the use of granulocyte colony-stimulating factor (G-CSF, filgrastim [Neupogen]) after several cycles of treatment. Other common side effects include nausea, fatigue, anemia, and thrombocytopenia. A palmar-plantar syndrome, characterized by acute painful erythematous swelling of the hands and feet, has been reported with the use of liposomal doxorubicin. Once the symptoms resolved, readministration of liposomal doxorubicin did not necessarily reproduce the syndrome. Neither of the liposomal anthracyclines has been reported to depress left-ventricular function.

Paclitaxel (Taxol): has been shown to produce responses in both chemotherapy-naive KS patients and patients with refractory tumors, including those refractory to liposomal anthracyclines. Dosage is typically 100-135 mg/m^2 IV given over 3 hours every 2-4 weeks.

The dose-limiting toxicity is neutropenia. Other reported toxicities include anemia, stomatitis, alopecia, and fatigue. Neuropathy has not been a major problem with this low-dose approach.

Investigational agents: Other drugs under investigation for the treatment of KS include thalidomide (Thalomid), antiviral drugs, several antiangiogenesis compounds, and the camptothecin analogs. Studies of compounds that may inhibit HHV-8 are also in development.

Radiation Therapy

Radiation therapy is used in KS primarily as palliation for symptomatic disease or for cosmetic improvement of disfiguring lesions. More than 90% of lesions will respond (complete responses [CRs] and partial responses [PRs]). Local radiation therapy commonly alleviates pain and bleeding, lessens edema, and shrinks obstructing lesions.

Treatment technique: For most superficial lesions, a single, shaped enface beam of relatively limited penetration (approximately 100 kV) works well. A relatively low-energy electron beam (e.g., 6 MeV) often can be used with shielding as an alternative to superficial x-rays.

Large lesions For very large lesions, electron beams are used more often, due to the limited penetration of kilovoltage X-ray beams and the limited width of the treatment cones attached to most superficial X-ray units. For patients with more widespread tumors of the leg with edema, parallel opposed megavoltage X-ray beams and overlying bolus material are often used to provide homogeneous irradiation to the entire area.

Dose fractionation regimens: Several dose fractionation regimens have proven effective in AIDS-related KS. As this tumor is very radiosensitive, almost any dose of radiation therapy can produce some response.

For most cutaneous lesions, a single treatment of 800 cGy will produce a short-term response. For lesions on sensitive structures (e.g., penis, hands, conjunctivae), some radiation oncologists attenuate treatment to a total dose of 2,000 cGy administered in 300 cGy increments (accepting a 50% decrease in CR rate), whereas 3,000 cGy delivered over 2 weeks is more typically used for lesions in general.

Prospectively acquired data clearly demonstrate a dose-response relationship for radiation therapy in AIDS-related KS. A dose of 4,000 cGy delivered in 20 fractions over 4 weeks was significantly more effective than 2,000 cGy in 10 fractions or 800 cGy in 1 fraction, as measured by higher response rate, longer duration of tumor control, and the absence of residual hyperpigmentation. However, the short- and medium-term effects of moderately intense but briefer regimens, such as 3,000 cGy in 10 fractions over 2 weeks, probably are equivalent to higher, more protracted regimens, and the moderately intense regimens require only half the time to deliver.

For patients with an anticipated survival of <3 months, in whom the response duration may be of less overall importance, a single fraction of 800 cGy is likely to provide the same benefit as the more intensive regimens. In contrast, small lesions in patients who are expected to survive for at least 1 year should be treated with fractionated radiation therapy, such as 3,000 cGy in 10 fractions over 2 weeks.

NON-HODGKIN'S LYMPHOMA

The incidence of NHL is 60 times higher in individuals with HIV infection than in the general population. The occurrence of lymphoma as a manifestation of AIDS has increased as treatment of HIV and opportunistic infections has prolonged survival. As many as 20% of all cases of NHL in the United States are HIV-related.

While NHL currently comprises approximately 5% of all initial AIDS-defining conditions, it accounts for as many as 12-16% of all AIDS-related deaths. The majority of patients present with advanced-stage, high- or intermediate-grade, B-cell lymphoma and have a high frequency of extranodal involvement. Primary CNS lymphoma occurs in approximately 0.5% of patients with AIDS.

The majority of patients with AIDS-related lymphoma have advanced HIV disease. Median CD4 counts in patients with systemic lymphoma range from 100 to 200 cells/mm^3, while CD4 counts < 50 cells/mm^3 are found in nearly all patients with primary CNS lymphoma.

Epidemiology

At-risk groups: NHL occurs with approximately equal frequency in all population groups infected by HIV, including IV drug users, homosexual-bisexual men, transfusion recipients, and patients with hemophilia. In a group of 1,295 HIV-infected men who had hemophilia, 5.5% developed NHL, with a mean latency period of 59 months between initial HIV infection and NHL.

Gender and race: AIDS-related NHL is seen more frequently in men than in women and occurs more often in whites than in blacks.

Age: The age distribution of AIDS-related NHL follows the distribution of HIV infection. Primary CNS lymphoma occurs with the same frequency in all age groups.

Geography: Current data do not indicate any geographic differences in the incidence of AIDS-related NHL.

Etiology and Risk Factors

AIDS-related NHL is believed to arise as a consequence of continued stimulation of B-cell proliferation as a result of HIV, Epstein-Barr virus (EBV), and other infections, all of which occur in the setting of profound T-cell immunodeficiency. HIV also induces the expression of a number of cytokines (e.g., interleukin-6 [IL-6] and interleukin-10 [IL-10]) that can further increase B-cell activation.

Small noncleaved lymphomas: Genetic errors are increased in the setting of chronic B-cell proliferation, and a variety of chromosomal translocations resulting in oncogene activation can lead to polyclonal and monoclonal B-cell expression. Other molecular biological abnormalities associated with small noncleaved lymphomas include expression of an abnormal p53 tumor-suppressor gene and the c-*myc* or *ras* oncogene.

Immunoblastic lymphoma: The pathogenesis of AIDS-related immunoblastic lymphoma appears to be distinct from that of small noncleaved lymphoma, and is more likely related to EBV infection without c-*myc* dysregulation. Clonal integration of EBV within tumor cells, with expression of various latent EBV proteins, has been demonstrated in essentially all cases of AIDS-related primary CNS lymphoma and in as many as two-thirds of systemic lymphomas.

Diffuse large cell lymphoma The specific molecular aberrations described in patients with AIDS-related diffuse large cell lymphoma appear distinct as well, with recent descriptions of abnormal bcl-6 expression in approximately 40% of cases.

Body cavity–based lymphoma/primary effusion lymphoma: appears to be highly associated with HHV-8 and EBV. The tumor cells stain positive for CD45. The disease appears to occur predominantly in males and may coexist with KS in patients with AIDS.

Signs and Symptoms

B symptoms: (i.e., fevers, weight loss, and night sweats) are seen in approximately 80% of patients with systemic AIDS-related NHL. In these patients, it is mandatory to exclude the presence of occult opportunistic infections before ascribing B symptoms to the lymphoma itself.

Extranodal involvement: Advanced-stage disease is expected in the majority of patients, with extranodal involvement reported in 60-90% of patients in most series. Common sites of extranodal involvement include the CNS (occurring in approximately 30% of patients), GI tract (25%), and bone marrow (25%). Essentially any other site in the body can also be involved, including the rectum, soft tissue, oral cavity, lung, and heart.

CNS *lymphoma* Patients with primary CNS lymphoma often present with focal neurologic deficits, seizures, and/or altered mental status. Any site in the brain may be involved, and one to four space-occupying lesions are usually seen on MRI or CT scan.

Other sites Changes in bowel habits, GI bleeding, weight loss, pain, and hepatomegaly are common presenting symptoms in patients with GI involvement. Pancytopenia may indicate bone marrow involvement.

Primary effusion lymphoma Patients usually present with pleural or pericardial effusion without an identifiable mass. Pain, shortness of breath, and B symptoms are the main initial complaints.

Screening and Diagnosis

Diagnosis of NHL in the patient with AIDS requires histologic confirmation by biopsy with immunophenotypic and/or molecular gene rearrangement studies.

A complete staging evaluation: should be done in all patients. This should include:

- CT or MRI of the head and chest/abdomen
- Bone marrow aspiration and biopsy
- Liver function studies
- spinal fluid analysis

Assessing spinal fluid for EBV: The presence of EBV DNA in CSF, as determined by polymerase chain reaction (PCR), appears to have a high specificity and sensitivity for the diagnosis of primary CNS lymphoma. The use of thallium single-photon emission computed tomography (SPECT) may further increase the diagnostic yield.

Pathology

Common tumor types: Over 95% of AIDS-related NHL cases are of B-lymphocyte origin. Most AIDS-NHL tumors are high-grade types, including the immunoblastic and small non-cleaved lymphomas. Diffuse large cell lymphoma constitutes up to 30% of AIDS-lymphomas.

Less common tumor types: Although not considered part of the AIDS epidemic, several cases of T-cell lymphoma occurring in HIV-infected patients have been described. In addition, cases of Ki-1–positive, large cell anaplastic lymphoma have been reported in HIV-infected patients. The clinical and pathologic characteristics of these forms of lymphoma are similar to those seen in non–HIV-infected individuals.

CNS lymphomas: are typically of the immunoblastic or large cell type.

GI and oral cavity lymphomas: Large cell or immunoblastic lymphomas are also more likely to involve the GI tract and oral cavity than are small noncleaved lymphomas.

Primary effusion lymphoma: The cells are large and pleomorphic with prominent nucleoli and immunoblastic morphology. Clonal immunoglobulin DNA rearrangement demonstrates clonality of the tumor cells but not surface immunoglobulin expression.

Staging and Prognosis

Staging system: Staging of AIDS-related NHL is the same as that for non–AIDS-related NHL. The Ann Arbor classification system for staging of NHL is utilized, and the staging work-up includes imaging studies, as well as bone marrow and CNS evaluation for lymphomas.

Prognostic factors: Four factors have been shown to correlate most closely with survival in patients with systemic AIDS-related NHL:

- a history of opportunistic infection prior to the lymphoma
- CD4 count < 100 cells/mm^3
- Karnofsky performance score < 70
- Stage IV disease, especially if due to bone marrow or meningeal involvement

In patients who lack these findings, median survival is typically 11-12 months, as compared with a median survival of approximately 4-5 months in those with one or more adverse prognostic features.

Three factors correlate with *better* survival in patients with primary CNS lymphoma:

- Karnofsky score > 70
- Age < 35 years
- Adequate dose of radiation therapy

Type of lymphoma: To date, no major differences have been seen in response or survival among the various pathologic types of systemic AIDS-related NHL. Patients with polyclonal lymphomas appear to have better tumor responses to chemotherapy and better survival. Patients with primary CNS lymphoma have an extremely poor prognosis, with a median survival of only 2-3 months despite therapy. Prognosis for patients with primary effusion lymphoma is also poor, with a median survival of only 5 months.

TREATMENT

Treatment of Systemic NHL

Chemotherapy

The mainstay of treatment for patients with systemic AIDS-related NHL is chemotherapy. As the likelihood of dissemination is great, AIDS patients who develop NHL must be assumed to have widespread disease at presentation and should be treated with systemic chemotherapy, even if dissemination is not confirmed on routine staging and evaluation.

CNS prophylaxis with either intrathecal cytarabine (Ara-C; 50 mg) or intrathecal methotrexate (10-12 mg) every week for 4 treatments has been shown to be effective in reducing the incidence of CNS relapse.

Dose intensity: A randomized trial (ACTG 142) showed no differences between standard-dose m-BACOD (methotrexate, bleomycin, Adriamycin, cyclophosphamide, Oncovin, and dexamethasone) and reduced-dose m-BACOD with respect to complete response rate, time to disease progression, or overall survival. Sub-analysis using a CD4 count of 100 cells/mm^3 as the cut-off point also showed no statistical differences in these end points in the two treatment groups. The standard-dose arm showed a statistically significant increase in toxicity, especially neutropenia. Therefore, the prudent approach for the treatment of patients with AIDS-NHL is to use low- or standard-dose regimens, such as CHOP or m-BACOD, with myeloid growth factor support.

Certain subsets of patients with high CD4 counts (> 100 cells/mm^3), no B symptoms, lower disease stage at presentation (stage I or II), and good performance status (0 or 1) may enjoy prolonged survival (> 2 years) when treated with either standard-dose or intensive, high-dose regimens. However, until more data are available to clearly identify these patient subsets, the intensive, high-dose approach is not recommended outside of clinical trial settings.

A small series of six HIV-infected patients treated with autologous bone marrow transplantation (BMT) is available from France. Four patients died of relapsed disease, and there was no survival benefit for the whole group. Autologous BMT for AIDS-lymphoma should only be attempted in a clinical trial setting. Studies are also in progress to evaluate high-dose chemotherapy with peripheral stem-cell support in high-risk and relapsed patients.

Growth factor support: The major dose-limiting toxic effect of multiagent chemotherapy regimens is myelosuppression. Studies of m-BACOD or CHOP (cyclophosphamide, doxorubicin HCl, Oncovin, and prednisone) chemotherapy demonstrated that coadministration of myeloid hematopoietic growth factors enhanced patient tolerance of these regimens.

Salvage chemotherapy: Patients in whom initial treatment fails or who relapse after initial remission rarely achieve a prolonged second remission. Recently, mitoguazone, given at a dose of 60 mg/m^2 on days 1 and 8 and then every 2 weeks, achieved a CR in 11.5% of patients with primary refractory or relapsed disease. The median survival for the whole group was 2.6 months, whereas a median survival of 21.5 months was noted in the complete responders.

Other agents under investigation for maintenance therapy include anti-CD20 antibody, interleukin-2 (IL-2 [Proleukin]), or interleukin-12 (IL-12). All patients who are at high risk for relapse or who have refractory or relapsed disease should be encouraged to participate in clinical trials.

Radiation Therapy

The role of radiotherapy in systemic lymphoma is limited to consolidation of the effects of chemotherapy. Treatment principles are similar to those used for aggressive NHL in the non-HIV setting and typically involve the use of involved or extended fields only.

Lymphomatous meningitis: For patients with lymphomatous meningitis and/or radiographically detectable cerebral deposits, "step-brain" irradiation (including the covering meninges) is administered, along with intrathecal chemotherapy to control microscopic spinal disease. Focal radiation therapy may be required for known tumor deposits in the spine. Unfortunately, many such patients develop multiple deposits anywhere along the spinal axis, either synchronously or metachronously.

Fractionated doses of 3,000-4,500 cGy may be used to control local lymphoma deposits in nodal areas. Patients who have lymphomatous meningitis typically have a poor prognosis and are best treated with regimens that do not unduly occupy their time (e.g., 3,000 cGy in 10 fractions over 2 weeks).

TREATMENT OF PRIMARY CNS LYMPHOMA

A very effective therapy for patients with AIDS-related CNS lymphoma has not yet been found.

Radiation Therapy

The conventional standard of treatment is step-brain irradiation, which can result in response rates of 50% and improve survival, as compared with untreated patients, even when adjusted for antiretroviral therapy, CD4 cell count, and time to diagnosis. Treatment is directed to the entire cranial contents, including the meninges down to C2.

Doses equivalent to 3,900 cGy (or more) delivered at 200 cGy/fraction appear to be associated with increased survival. Better Karnofsky performance scores and younger age at the time of treatment are also associated with longer survival. Mean survival ranges from 2 to 6 months, with death often due to complicating opportunistic infections.

Chemotherapy

As HAART has changed the biological behavior of AIDS, there has been more interest in using high-dose methotrexate, based on evidence of activity in non–AIDS-associated disease. Studies to evaluate short courses of combination chemotherapy or the use of less myelosuppressive single agents followed by whole-brain irradiation are currently in progress. Although these approaches appear to be efficacious in non–HIV-infected patients with primary CNS lymphoma, there are insufficient data to suggest that this approach is superior to CNS irradiation alone in AIDS patients.

CERVICAL CARCINOMA

Cervical carcinoma in the setting of HIV infection has been recognized as an AIDS-defining malignancy since 1993. Unfortunately, in some women, cervical carcinoma may be the first indication that they have HIV infection.

Cervical intraepithelial neoplasia (CIN) is also seen in association with HIV infection. These premalignant lesions, also known as squamous intraepithelial lesions (SILs), may foretell a higher incidence of cervical carcinoma among HIV-infected women. SILs have been associated with human papillomavirus (HPV), particularly those subtypes with greater oncogenic potential, such as serotypes 16, 18, 31, 33, and 35.

Epidemiology

Prevalence of HIV infection and cervical abnormalities: The risk of HIV infection in women with an abnormal Pap smear varies with the prevalence of HIV infection in the given population. Screening in clinics in high-prevalence areas has yielded HIV-positivity rates of between 6% and 7%. In such high-prevalence areas, among women under the age of 50 years with cervical carcinoma, up to 19% of women were found to be HIV positive. HIV-positive women have up to a 10-fold increased risk of abnormal cervical cytology. Several centers have reported abnormal cytology rates of 30-60% in HIV-positive women and Pap smears consistent with cervical dysplasia in 15-40%. The prevalence of cervical dysplasia increases with declining CD4 numbers in HIV-infected women.

Nationwide, invasive cervical carcinoma was found in 1.3% of women with AIDS. In New York, invasive cervical carcinoma constitutes 4% of AIDS-defining illnesses in women. Recent findings from linkage studies in the US and Italy clearly have shown increased rates of cervical cancer in women with HIV.

Race and geography: The prevalence of invasive cervical carcinoma among US Hispanic and black women is lower than in white women. However, this difference may stem from a difference in access to health care. The southern and northeastern sections of the United States have a higher reported number of cases of HIV-associated invasive cervical carcinoma.

Etiology and Risk Factors

The severe cellular immunodeficiency associated with advanced HIV infection may allow oncogenic viruses to flourish and may also compromise the body's immunologic defenses that control the development of these tumors.

HPV: There is abundant evidence that HPV infection is related to malignant and premalignant neoplasia in the lower genital tract. HPV serotypes 16, 18, 31, 33, and 35 are the most oncogenic and have been associated with invasive cervical carcinoma and progressive dysplasia. The prevalence of cervical SILs among HIV-infected women may be as high as 20-30%, with many having higher cytologic and histologic grade lesions.

Signs and Symptoms

The majority of cervical SILs are detected on routine cytologic evaluation of Pap smears in women with HIV infection.

Advanced invasive disease: Postcoital bleeding with serosanguineous and/or foul-smelling vaginal discharge is usually the first symptom of more advanced invasive disease. Lumbosacral pain or urinary obstructive symptoms may indicate advanced disease.

Screening and Diagnosis

Because the majority of patients with cervical dysplasia or early invasive cancer are asymptomatic, frequent cytologic screening of women at risk for HIV infection must be undertaken.

Screening of HIV-positive women: Current screening recommendations call for women with HIV infection to have pelvic examinations and cytologic screening every 6 months. Pap smears indicating cervical SIL must be taken very seriously, and abnormalities justify immediate colposcopic evaluation. Although abnormalities are sometimes missed by relying solely on cytologic screening, recommendations for the use of routine colposcopy have not yet been established.

Screening of women with a history of cervical SIL: For women who have a history of cervical SIL, more frequent reevaluation and cytologic screening should be undertaken. Since these women are at high risk for recurrence or development of lesions in other areas of the lower genital tract, post-therapy surveillance with repeat colposcopy also is warranted.

Work-up of women with invasive carcinoma: For women with invasive carcinoma, complete staging should be undertaken; this should include pelvic examination, CT of the pelvis and abdomen, chest X-ray, and screening laboratory tests for hepatic and bone disease. In addition, full evaluation and treatment for HIV and related complications should be initiated.

Pathology

Squamous cell carcinoma: Most cases of cervical carcinoma are of the squamous cell type.

Staging and Prognosis

The staging classification for cervical carcinoma, as adopted by the International Federation of Gynecology and Obstetrics (FIGO), also applies to the AIDS patient.

Cervical dysplasia in HIV-infected women is often of higher cytologic and histologic grade. These women are more likely to have CIN II-III lesions with extensive cervical involvement, multisite (vagina, vulva, and perianal) involvement, and endocervical lesions.

HIV-infected women with cervical carcinoma typically present with more advanced disease and appear to have a more aggressive clinical course. Tumors are typically high grade with a higher proportion of lymph node and visceral involvement at presentation. Mean time to recurrence after primary treatment is short, and many patients have persistent disease after primary therapy. Median time to death in one series was 10 months in HIV-infected women, as compared with 23 months in HIV-negative patients.

Treatment

Treatment of Preinvasive Disease

Cryotherapy, laser therapy, cone biopsy, and excision have all been used to treat preinvasive disease in HIV-infected patients. Short-term recurrence rates of 40-60% have been reported.

Determinants of recurrence: Immune status of the patient seems to be the most important determining factor for recurrence. Close surveillance after initial therapy is critical, and repetitive treatment may be necessary to prevent progression to more invasive disease.

Treatment of Cervical Carcinoma

The same principles that guide oncologic management of the immunocompetent patient with cervical carcinoma are utilized in AIDS patients with this cancer.

Surgery: can be undertaken for the usual indications, and surgical decisions should be based on oncologic appropriateness and not on HIV status.

Radiation therapy: As most AIDS patients with cervical cancer present with advanced disease, radiation therapy is indicated more often than surgery. If the patient's overall physical condition permits, treatment regimens are identical to those used for the same stage disease in uninfected individuals. It is important to note that the standard of care for advanced carcinoma of the cervix (stages III-IV, without hematogenous dissemination) has changed within the past year from radiation alone to a combination of radiation and concurrent cisplatin (Platinol)-based chemotherapy. At present, there is insufficient evidence to suggest any decrease in effectiveness of radiation therapy or other treatments in the AIDS patient compared with similarly non–HIV-infected individuals.

Chemotherapy: regimens, such as cisplatin (50 mg/m^2) or carboplatin (Paraplatin; 200 mg/m^2), bleomycin (20 U/m^2; maximum, 30 U), and vincristine (1 mg/m^2) have been used in patients with metastatic or recurrent disease. Vigorous management of side effects and complications of these treatments and of AIDS itself must be provided.

ANAL CARCINOMA

Although anal carcinoma is not currently an AIDS-defining illness, the incidence of this tumor is increasing in the population at risk for HIV infection. The incidence of anal carcinoma in homosexual men in a San Francisco study was estimated at between 25-87 cases per 100,000, compared with 0.7 case per 100,000 in the entire male population.

Etiology and Risk Factors

HPV: Precursor lesions of anal intraepithelial neoplasia (AIN), also known as anal SILs, have been found to be associated with HPV infection, typically with oncogenic serotypes, e.g., types

16 and 18. Abnormal cytology may predict the later development of invasive carcinoma.

Other STDs and sexual practices: Individuals with a history of perianal herpes simplex, anal condylomas, or practice of anal receptive behavior with multiple sexual partners are at greater risk of developing this tumor.

Signs and Symptoms

Rectal pain, bleeding, discharge, and symptoms of obstruction or a mass lesion are the most frequent presenting symptoms.

Screening and Diagnosis

Studies to evaluate the usefulness of anoscopy with frequent anal cytology have been undertaken to determine whether early detection of AIN may result in interventions that would prevent the development of invasive tumors.

Work-up of patients with anal carcinoma: For patients with anal carcinoma, determination of local disease extent, as well as full staging for dissemination, should be undertaken.

Squamous cell carcinoma: The majority of anal carcinomas are of the squamous cell type.

Histologic grading: The grading for AIN is similar to that for CIN, with AIN-1 denoting low-grade dysplasia and AIN-2 and AIN-3, higher-grade dysplastic lesions. The gross appearance of lesions on anoscopy does not predict histologic grade. Higher-grade dysplastic lesions are seen in patients with lower CD4 counts.

Staging and Prognosis

The staging of squamous cell carcinoma of the anus in HIV-infected individuals is the same as that in non–HIV-infected patients. Patients with severe immunosuppression, i.e., CD4 count < 50 cells/mm^3, may present with more advanced, more aggressive disease. The true natural history of this tumor in the AIDS population has yet to be defined, however.

Treatment

Treatment of Anal Intraepithelial Neoplasia and Carcinoma In Situ

Treatment of patients with local intraepithelial neoplasia is similar to that of women with CIN. Ablative therapy may be used.

Treatment of Invasive Anal Squamous Cell Carcinoma

For patients with squamous cell carcinoma of the anus, chemotherapy with mitomycin (Mutamycin; 10 mg/m^2 on day 1) and fluorouracil (1,000 mg/m^2 by continuous infusion on days 1-4) combined with radiation therapy can produce high rates of complete remission. Tolerance to treatment seen in patients who have relatively intact immune systems is similar to that seen in HIV-infected patients. However, the appropriate dose of radiation therapy for patients with anal carcinoma in the context of HIV infection remains somewhat unsettled. Patients who are unable to tolerate chemoradiation and those in whom treatment fails (defined as a positive biopsy after CR), should be considered for abdominoperineal resection.

OTHER NON–AIDS-DEFINING MALIGNANCIES

Case reports of other malignant tumors occurring in HIV-infected individuals include Hodgkin's disease, nonmelanomatous skin cancers, lung cancer, germ-cell tumors, myeloid or lymphoid leukemias, multiple myeloma, renal cell carcinoma, breast cancer, head and neck cancer, brain tumors, squamous tumor of the conjunctiva, and leiomyosarcoma in pediatric patients. Most of the case reports describe only a few affected individuals, and there are insufficient numbers of patients to confirm an increased risk of developing these malignancies among HIV-infected individuals, with the possible exceptions of Hodgkin's disease, nonmelanomatous skin cancers, and pediatric leiomyosarcoma.

As HIV-infected individuals are surviving longer with currently available combination anti-HIV drugs, clinicians should anticipate seeing the development of more tumors in these patients. Greater vigilance for these tumors is warranted.

Hodgkin's disease: Most of the studies showing a possible increased incidence of Hodgkin's disease in HIV-infected individuals are from European countries, especially Italy and Spain. The most common histology is mixed cellularity and lymphocyte-depleted. Male predominance, a higher prevalence of B symptoms, and more extranodal disease on presentation are the main characteristics of Hodgkin's disease in HIV patients.

Chemotherapy is recommended for this group of patients, due to the high proportion of stage III or IV disease. Standard treatments include ABVD (Adriamycin, bleomycin, vinblastine, and dacarbazine) or ABVD alternating with MOPP (mechlorethamine, Oncovin, procarbazine, and prednisone).

Nonmelanomatous skin cancers: As in the general population, basal cell carcinoma is more common than squamous cell carcinoma in the setting of HIV infection. The risk factors for the development of these tumors are the same as in the general population; namely, fair skin, history of sun exposure, and family history. A study from San Francisco demonstrated that these skin cancers can be treated successfully with standard local therapy, with a recurrence rate indistinguishable from that of the general population of approximately 6%.

Pediatric leiomyosarcoma: Cases of aggressive leiomyosarcoma developing in HIV-positive children have been reported. Leiomyosarcoma is a very rare tumor, occurring in < 2 cases per 10 million non–HIV-infected children. However, a much higher than expected frequency of leiomyosarcoma has been reported in HIV-infected children. Visceral sites are commonly involved, e.g., the lung, spleen, and GI tract.

Seven

Radiotherapy

Radiotherapy also called radiation therapy, is the treatment of cancer and other diseases with ionizing radiation. Ionizing radiation deposits energy that injures or destroys cells in the area being treated (the "target tissue") by damaging their genetic material, making it impossible for these cells to continue to grow. Although radiation damages both cancer cells and normal cells, the latter are able to repair themselves and function properly. Radiotherapy may be used to treat localized solid tumors, such as cancers of the skin, tongue, larynx, brain, breast, or uterine cervix. It can also be used to treat leukemia and lymphoma (cancers of the blood-forming cells and lymphatic system, respectively).

One type of radiation therapy commonly used involves photons, "packets" of energy. X-rays were the first form of photon radiation to be used to treat cancer. Depending on the amount of energy they possess, the rays can be used to destroy cancer cells on the surface of or deeper in the body. The higher the energy of the X-ray beam, the deeper the X-rays can go into the target tissue. Linear accelerators and betatrons are machines that produce X-rays of increasingly greater energy. The use of machines to focus radiation (such as X-rays) on a cancer site is called external beam radiotherapy.

Gamma rays are another form of photons used in radiotherapy. Gamma rays are produced spontaneously as certain elements (such as radium, uranium, and cobalt 60) release radiation as they decompose, or decay. Each element decays at a specific rate and gives off energy in the form of gamma rays and other particles. X-rays and gamma rays have the same effect on cancer cells.

Another technique for delivering radiation to cancer cells is to place radioactive implants directly in a tumor or body cavity. This is called internal radiotherapy. (Brachytherapy, interstitial irradiation, and intracavitary irradiation are types of internal radiotherapy). In this treatment, the radiation dose is concentrated in a small area, and the patient stays in the hospital for a few days. Internal radiotherapy is frequently used for cancers of the tongue, uterus, and cervix.

Several new approaches to radiation therapy are being evaluated to determine their effectiveness in treating cancer. One such technique is intraoperative irradiation, in which a large dose of external radiation is directed at the tumor and surrounding tissue during surgery.

Another investigational approach is particle beam radiation therapy. This type of therapy differs from photon radiotherapy in that it involves the use of fast-moving subatomic particles to treat localized cancers. A very sophisticated machine is needed to produce and accelerate the particles required for this procedure. Some particles (neutrons, pions, and heavy ions) deposit more energy along the path they take through tissue than do X-rays or gamma rays, thus causing more damage to the cells they hit. This type of radiation is often referred to as high linear energy transfer (high LET) radiation.

Scientists also are looking for ways to increase the effectiveness of radiation therapy. Two types of investigational drugs are being studied for their effect on cells undergoing radiation. Radiosensitizers make the tumor cells more likely to be damaged, and radioprotectors protect normal tissues from the effects of radiation. Hyperthermia, the use of heat, is also being studied for its effectiveness in sensitizing tissue to radiation.

Other recent radiotherapy research has focused on the use of radiolabeled antibodies to deliver doses of radiation directly to the cancer site (radioimmunotherapy). Some tumor cells contain specific antigens that trigger the production of tumor-specific antibodies. Large quantities of these antibodies can be made in the laboratory and attached to radioactive substances (a process known as radiolabeling). Once injected into the body, the antibodies actively seek out the cancer cells, which are destroyed by the cell-killing (cytotoxic) action of the radiation. This approach can minimize the risk of radiation damage to healthy cells. The success of this technique will depend upon both the identification of appropriate radioactive substances and determination of the safe and effective dose of radiation that can be delivered in this way.

EXTERNAL BEAM RADIOTHERAPY

External radiotherapy is normally given as a series of short daily treatments in the radiotherapy department, using equipment similar to a large X-ray machine.

The treatments are usually given from Monday to Friday, leaving patients to rest at the weekend. Each treatment is called a *fraction*. Giving the treatment in fractions ensures that less damage is done to normal cells than to cancer cells. The damage to normal cells is mainly temporary, but is the reason why radiotherapy has some side effects.

The number of treatments you have depends on several factors, including:

- Your general health
- The site and type of cancer being treated
- Whether or not you have had, or are going to have, surgery, chemotherapy or hormonal therapy as part of your treatment.

For these reasons, treatment is planned for each patient individually, and even people with the same type of cancer may have different treatments.

External radiotherapy does not make you radioactive, and it is perfectly safe for you to be with other people, including children, throughout your treatment.

A course of curative (radical) treatment may be given every weekday from two to six weeks. Instead of having one treatment a day or having a rest at the weekend, some people will have different treatment plans. They may have more than one treatment a day or treatment every day for two weeks. Giving radiotherapy in this way is known as continuous hyperfractionated radiotherapy (often called CHART).

Sometimes treatment may be given on only three days each week (for example, on Mondays, Wednesdays and Fridays).

Palliative treatment (for symptom control) may involve only one or two sessions of treatment, or up to five sessions.

The different types of radiotherapy machine work in slightly different ways. Some are better for treating cancers near the surface of the skin, while others work best on cancers deeper in the body.

The type of radiotherapy machine used will be carefully chosen by your specialist and physicist to give you the most appropriate treatment. Some machines are quicker than others and may give treatment in a very short time, such as a few seconds. Usually, radiotherapy treatment (including the time taken to position you) takes 10-15 minutes or less, on any machine.

The radiotherapy machine does not normally touch you and the treatment itself is painless, although it may gradually cause some uncomfortable side effects. If you have a specific type of radiotherapy known as electron treatment, a small applicator may be used, which touches a small area of skin.

GENERAL SIDE EFFECTS

While radiotherapy can destroy cancer cells, it can also have an effect on some of the surrounding normal cells. The side effects that may occur are described in the following pages. It is important to remember that no person will have more than a few of them, and for many people they may be very mild.

As radiotherapy affects people in different ways, it is difficult to predict exactly how you will react to your treatment. Before you start your treatment the staff will discuss with you any likely side effects of the particular treatment you are having, and can give tips on how to deal with them and how they can be treated. Being aware of side effects in advance can help you to cope with any problems that arise.

Most side effects of radiotherapy disappear gradually once the course of treatment is over. However, side effects may continue for a few weeks.

Tiredness

You may find that you feel very tired during your radiotherapy. This can often be made worse by having to travel to your treatment each day. Listen to your body, and if necessary, allow yourself extra time to rest, perhaps by taking a nap in the afternoons. It may help if you spread chores out over the week, sit down to do them, wherever possible, and accept any offers of help. Tiredness can be a problem for some months after your treatment has finished. See information on coping with fatigue.

Eating and Drinking

As always during treatment of any kind, it is important to maintain a healthy diet and drink plenty of fluids. At times you probably won't feel like eating, or you may find that your eating habits change. It may be easier to have small snacks throughout the day rather than large meals. It is not unusual to lose a little weight during radiotherapy, but if you are having any problems with eating it is important to tell the radiotherapy staff. They can arrange for you to talk to the dietitian.

Changes in the Blood

Radiotherapy to some parts of the body can sometimes affect bone marrow, which produces the different types of blood cells. If this is thought likely to happen in your case you will have regular blood tests during your treatment to check your blood counts (the number of cells in your blood). If your blood counts are low, you may feel tired and 'run down'. If your blood count becomes very low (which is unlikely), it may be necessary to have a short rest from treatment so that your blood cell level can return to normal. You may also need to have a blood transfusion.

It is very important to let your doctors know if you feel very unwell, or if your temperature goes above 38°C (100.4°F), or if you start feeling cold and shaky.

Skin Care

Some people develop a skin reaction, similar to sunburn, while having external radiotherapy. This normally happens after three to four weeks. People with pale skin may find that the skin in the treatment area becomes red and sore or itchy.

People with darker skin may find that their skin becomes darker and can have a blue or black tinge. The amount of the reaction depends on the area being treated and the individual person's skin. Some people have no skin problems at all. Your radiographers will be looking for these reactions but you should also let them know as soon as you feel any soreness.

Do not apply creams or dressings unless they have been prescribed or recommended by your specialist.

Occasionally, if the skin reaction is severe, your treatment may have to be delayed for a short time to allow the area to recover.

Staff at your radiotherapy department will be able to give you advice on how to look after the skin in the area that is being treated. The care of the skin varies according to the part of the body that is being treated and the dose of radiotherapy that the skin is receiving. You may be asked not to wash the treatment area at all while you are having treatment. Alternatively, you may be advised to use only tepid water to wash the area (and not to soak too long in the bath), and then to dry it by patting gently with a soft towel. Instead you could dry your skin with a hairdryer on the coolest setting. Do not rub the area as this may make it sore.

Soaps, talcs, deodorants and perfumes may also make your skin sore and should not be used. The staff at the hospital may suggest that you gently apply simple moisturisers, such as E45 cream or aqueous cream, to the area. After your treatment, simple soap and simple moisturisers are often recommended. Aloe vera cream or arnica cream can sometimes help the skin to heal. Always check with the radiotherapy staff before applying anything to your skin.

It is very important that any marks put on your skin to mark the treatment area are not removed. If the marks do fade or disappear, do not try to replace them yourself but let the radiotherapy staff know.

Men who are having radiotherapy to the head and neck should use an electric razor, rather than wet-shaving.

These restrictions apply only to the treatment area, and the rest of your skin can be treated normally. Your skin may peel after the redness has faded, but it should heal quickly. Skin reactions usually settle down two to four weeks after the treatment has finished, but the skin area may remain slightly darker than the surrounding skin.

Avoiding the Sun

Because the treated area is so sensitive it should not be exposed to the sun or cold winds. If you are having radiotherapy to the head or neck, try wearing a silk or cotton scarf when you go outside.

It is very important to cover the treated area if you go out in strong sunshine for at least the first year after your radiotherapy. Wear clothing made of cotton or natural fibres which have a closer weave and offer more protection against the sun. Even after this time the skin will be more delicate, so extra care should be taken. Use a sun-screen (of at least factor 15) and wear a hat and a long-sleeved shirt. It is important to remember that you can burn even through clothing if you are out in hot sun for a long time.

You can swim as soon as any skin reaction has settled down, usually within a month of finishing treatment. But if you are swimming out of doors, do not stay in the water too long, and do not forget to use a waterproof sunblock.

Clothing

Loose-fitting clothes, preferably in natural fibres rather than man-made materials, are more comfortable and less irritating to the skin. If you are having radiotherapy to your neck you should avoid tight collars and ties.

Shoulder straps and bra straps can also cause irritation if they are rubbing treated skin. If your breast area is being treated, you may be more comfortable not wearing a bra or wearing a cropped top or vest.

Smoking

Stopping smoking during and after radiotherapy is very worthwhile. Research has shown that it may make the radiotherapy more effective as well as reducing the side effects. It will also improve your general health and reduce your risk of developing other cancers. Stopping smoking or even cutting down at such a stressful time can be very difficult, but do your best. If you want help or advice talk to your specialist, GP or a specialist nurse, who will be able to suggest ways of stopping.

INTERNAL RADIOTHERAPY

Internal radiotherapy is used mainly to treat cancers in the head and neck area, the cervix, the womb, the prostate gland or the skin.

Treatment is given in one of two ways: either by putting solid radioactive material (the source) close to or inside the tumour for a limited period of time, or by using a radioactive liquid, which the patient takes either as a drink or as an injection into a vein.

If you have internal radiotherapy, you may have to stay in hospital for a few days and some special precautions will have to be taken while the radioactive material is in place in your body. Once the treatment is over there is no risk of exposing your family or friends to radiation.

The process of putting solid radioactive material close to or inside the tumour is called brachytherapy

Giving a radioactive liquid, either as a drink, a capsule, or as an injection into a vein is called radioisotope treatment

CAESIUM INSERTION

This type of internal radiotherapy treatment is used for treating cancer of the cervix, uterus or vagina. The radioactive source most commonly used is called caesium-137. The advantage of caesium insertion treatment is that it gives a high dose of radiotherapy directly to the tumour, but gives a low dose to normal tissues.

The caesium source has to be put inside an applicator (there may be more than one) to keep it in place. The applicator, is inserted into the vagina, while you are under a general anaesthetic or sedation in the operating room. At the same time, a flexible tube called a urinary catheter may be put into your bladder to drain off urine. This means you don't have to get on and off bedpans and risk moving the applicators. Once the applicators are in place an X-ray will be taken to check they are in the correct position. Sometimes the radioactive source is put into the applicator while you are in the operating room, but more commonly it will be put in place once you are back on the ward. You may hear this referred to as 'afterloading'.

The applicators are kept in place by a pack (cotton/gauze padding) inside your vagina. This can be uncomfortable and you may need to ask your nurse for regular painkillers.

Once the source is put into the applicators you have to stay in bed. This helps to keep them in the correct position. If you need anything, you can call a member of staff by using the call bell by your bed. If the source does get dislodged, you should call the staff on the ward immediately.

In some hospitals a machine, which may be called a Curitron or Selectron or similar name, is used to put the radioactive material into the applicators. The machine is attached by tubes to the applicators. When the machine is switched on it passes small radioactive sources into the applicators. If the machine is switched off, the source is pulled back inside the machine. The machine is kept switched on throughout your treatment, except when someone needs to go into your room. It can then be turned off, so reducing their exposure to the rays. However, safety measures and visiting restrictions are still necessary. The time you spend on the machine varies but it is usually between 12 and 48 hours. Sometimes a machine called a Microselectron can be used to give internal radiotherapy. This gives the radiotherapy more quickly, so the treatments last for only a few minutes .

CAESIUM OR IRIDIUM IMPLANTS

These can be used to treat a number of tumours including those in the mouth, lip and breast. Very fine needles, wires or tubes carry the radioactive source, and are inserted while you are in the operating room under a general anaesthetic.

An X-ray may be taken to ensure that they are in the correct position. You will be nursed in a separate room, and safety measures will be applied until the wires are removed, usually between three and eight days. Sometime this is done under general anaesthetic.

Implants in the mouth can be uncomfortable, and can make eating and talking difficult. A soft or liquid diet may be necessary while the needles are in place. Your nurse will show you how to keep your mouth clean, using regular mouth-washes. If eating is a problem you may be fed through a thin tube (nasogastric tube) which is passed via your nose and into your stomach.

The implant is removed once the correct dose of radiation has been received. This may be after two days, if the treatment is given as a booster after external treatment, or up to one week if given as the only form of treatment.

Once the implant has been removed the area will feel sore for up to two or three weeks afterwards. Your specialist will prescribe pain killers that you can take regularly until this improves.

Radioactive seed implants are occasionally used to treat small tumours of the prostate gland.

BRACHYTHERAPY

Intracavity Radiotherapy

This type of internal radiotherapy treatment is used for treating cancer of the cervix, uterus or vagina. The radioactive source most commonly used is called caesium-137. The advantage of caesium insertion treatment is that it gives a high dose of radiotherapy directly to the tumour, but a low dose to normal tissues.

Side Effects

It is not unusual to have slight bleeding or discharge once the radiotherapy treatment has ended. If it continues or becomes heavy it is important to let your doctor or nurse know.

Radiotherapy to the pelvic area can cause side effects such as tiredness, diarrhoea and a burning sensation when passing urine. These side effects can be mild or more troublesome depending on the strength of the radiotherapy dose and the length of your treatment. Your oncologist will be able to advise you what to expect.

Most of these side effects can be treated with medicines, which your oncologist will provide. Any side effects should gradually disappear once your treatment is over.

It is important that you drink plenty of fluids and maintain a healthy diet during your treatment. If your diarrhoea is not controlled with medicines you can ask to see a dietitian, who can advise you on what to eat to reduce diarrhoea. You may feel sick but this is not common. If you don't feel like eating, you can replace meals with nutritious high-calorie drinks, which are available from most chemists and can be prescribed by your GP.

Radiotherapy for cancer of the cervix affects the ovaries, unfortunately, and this brings on the menopause, usually about three months after the treatment starts. This means that your periods will stop and you will have menopausal side effects such as hot flushes, a dry skin and possibly loss of concentration. Some women become less interested in sex and notice that their vagina is dry. Sometimes radiotherapy causes a narrowing of the vagina, which can make sexual intercourse uncomfortable. See page 42 for advice on how to deal with the effects on your sex life and fertility.

The caesium source has to be put inside an applicator (perhaps more than one) to keep it in place. The applicator is inserted into the vagina while you are under a general anaesthetic or sedation in the operating room. At the same time, a flexible tube called a urinary catheter may be put into your bladder to drain off urine. This means you will not have to get on and off bedpans, which could dislodge the applicators.

Once the applicators are in place, an X-ray will be taken to check they are in the correct position. Sometimes the radioactive source is put into the applicator while you are in the operating room, but more commonly it will be put in place once you are back on the ward. You may hear this referred to as 'afterloading'.

The applicators are kept in place by a pack (cotton/gauze padding) inside your vagina. This can be uncomfortable and you may need to ask your nurse for regular painkillers.

Once the source is put into the applicators you have to stay in bed, which helps keep them in the correct position. If you need anything, you can call a member of staff by using the bell by your bed. If the source does get dislodged, you should call the staff on the ward immediately.

Possible Long Term Side Effects

Radiotherapy to the pelvic area has sometimes led to long-term side effects. However, improvements in the treatment-planning have made these much less likely.

In a small number of people, the bowel or bladder may be permanently affected by the radiotherapy. If this happens the increased bowel motions and diarrhoea may continue, or the patient may need to pass urine more often than before. The blood vessels in the bowel and bladder can become more fragile after radiotherapy treatment and this can cause blood to appear in the urine or bowel movements. This can take many months or even years to occur.

Caesium or Irridium Wires

These can be used to treat a number of tumours including those in the mouth, lip, cervix and breast. Very thin radioactive needles, wires or tubes are inserted while you are under general anaesthetic in the operating room.

An X-ray may be taken to ensure that the needles are in the correct position. You will be nursed in a separate room, and the safety measures described in the internal radiotherpy section will be used until the wires are removed—usually after three to eight days. Sometimes this is done under general anaesthetic.

Implants in the mouth can be uncomfortable, and can make eating and talking difficult. A soft or liquid diet will be necessary while the needles are in place.

Eight

Breast Diseases and Conditions

- Congenital abnormalities and disorders of development and involution
- Breast infection
- Breast trauma
- Neoplastic
- Gynaecomastia.

Breast Problems: Congenital, Developmental and Involutional

Congenital:
- Extra nipples and breasts
- Absence/hypoplasia of the breast.

Aberrations of breast development:
- Juvenile or virginal hypertrophy
- Fibroadenomas.

Aberrations of involution:
- Fibroadenosis
  - cystic disease
  - sclerosis
- Duct ectasia
- Galactocoele
- Epithelial hyperplasia.

Congenital Breast Abnormalities

The breasts are identical in boys and girls until puberty. Growth of the breast then begins in girls at about the age of 10. This growth may begin asymmetrically and may appear to be a breast lump. It should however not be biopsied as there is a risk of damaging the breast bud.

Accessory Nipples and Breasts

These may affect 1-5% of men and women, and they occur along the milk lines running from each axilla to the groin. Accessory nipples most commonly occur below the normal breast, whilst accessory breast tissue most commonly occurs in the lower axilla.

Treatment may be required for cosmetic reasons.

Nipple Disorders

Nipple disorders include:
- Inversion
- Eczema
- Discharge.

Nipple Inversion

Nipple inversion can be caused by:
- Congenital deformation
- Carcinoma
- Mammary duct ectasia with periductal fibrosis.

Nipple Eczema

Nipple eczema may be caused by:
- Paget's disease of the nipple
- Eczema.

Nipple Discharge

Nipple discharge can be of varied form:

- Clear—physiological
- Milky:
  - pregnancy—normal lactation
  - hyperprolactinaemia resulting in galactorrhoea.
- Brown or green:
  - perimenopausal
  - mammary duct ectasia
  - fibroadenosis.
- bloodstained:
  - carcinoma
  - intraductal papilloma.

Aberrations of Breast Development

Breasts develop throughout puberty and then continue to undergo cyclical changes with the menstrual cycle. In the event of pregnancy the breasts double their weight at term.

Many benign conditions in the developing and mature phases of the life cycle of the breast occur so often that they might be considered to be aberrations rather than disease.

Juvenile Breast Hypertrophy

This commonly presents in women under 25 whose breasts have grown normally throughout puberty but then continue to grow.

Their large breasts may cause them embarrassment, pain, discomfort and prevent them from performing everyday tasks.

No endocrine abnormality can be detected in these patients and treatment is with reduction mammoplasty, often resulting in a much improved quality of life.

Fibroadenoma of the Breast

While often considered a benign neoplasm, fibroadenomas may be thought of as aberrations of normal development. Unlike neoplasms breast fibroadenomas develop from a whole lobule rather than a single cell, and like normal breast tissue they remain responsive to hormonal control. Fibroadenomas are composed of both fibrous and glandular tissue.

Fibroadenomas are common and account for 13% of all symptomatic breast lumps. They are most common in women in their second or third decade, accounting for 60% of breast lumps in this younger population.

The tumour is well demarcated from the surrounding breast tissue by a condensed connective tissue capsule.

The tumour develops from a whole lobule and not from a single cell. Microscopically, the tumour comprises proliferation of the connective tissue stroma and atypical multiplication of ducts and acini.

Two histological patterns are noted:

- Pericanicular—connective tissue stroma surrounds small islands of glandular tissue, in a whorled pattern.
- Intracanicular—connective tissue stroma predominates and compresses the gland spaces; the epithelial elements appear as narrow strands or cords of epithelium lying within the fibrous tissue.

Clinical Features and Diagnosis

Presentation is usually as a discrete, firm, nontender and highly mobile nodule within the breast. Small lesions may slip away from the examining hand during palpation giving rise to their description as "breast mice." A few patients may present with multiple fibroadenomas.

Diagnosis may be made with a combination of clinical assessment, ultrasonography and fine needle aspiration cytology. Fibroadenomas in older patients may calcify and give characteristic mammographic appearances.

Management

Less than 5% of fibroadenomas increase in size and about 25% either get smaller or completely disappear.

The difficulty in management however is to ensure that breast cancer is not missed, and some would advocate that all such lumps should be excised, thus providing both diagnosis and treatment.

Others however would argue that for women under 40 years old, with a fibroadenoma diagnosed clinically, with ultrasound and with fine needle aspiration cytology, excision is not required unless the lump is over 4 cms in diameter. For women over 40 years old, all lumps should be excised.

Fibrocystic Disease of Breast

Fibroadenosis or fibrocystic disease is the most common cause of breast lumps in women of reproductive age. The peak incidence is between 35 and 50 years of age. It is rare before 25 years.

The term embraces a spectrum of histologic changes, and may encompass many patients who have cystic lesions detected clinically or sclerotic breast lesions detected on mammography as discussed elsewhere.

Histologically it is characterized by overgrowth of both fibrous stroma, and of epithelial elements i.e. ducts and lobules, in differing proportions. These changes may be considered as abberations of normal breast involution and not part of a disease process. The condition may be due to a disordered or imbalanced response to endogenous sex hormones.

Only in those cases showing marked epithelial hyperplasia—epitheliosis—is the risk of breast carcinoma thought to be increased.

Pathology

A variety of changes may be noted including:

- Cysts:
  - microcysts—less than 1 cm in diameter
  - macrocysts—up to 5 cm in diameter; includes the blue domed cysts of Bloodgood which unopened, appear brown to blue due to the contained fluid.
- Apocrine metaplasia—the normal ductular epithelium that lines the cyst proliferates to resemble that of apocrine sweat glands.
- Fibrosis—proliferation of fibrous tissue without epithelial change.
- Adenosis:
  - simple adenosis—hyperplastic proliferation of lobular acini/ductules.
  - sclerosing adenosis—proliferation of fibrous tissue accompanies that of the acini, splitting them apart.

Clinical Features

Typically, patients present with one or more lumps in the breast which may be painful, and frequently, bilateral. The size and pain usually vary with the menstrual cycle. One or more of these elements may be absent.

Cysts are more common in perimenopausal women. They are usually single. The presence of multiple, diffuse cysts may be referred to as Schimmelbusch's disease. The discharge varies from clear to green but should not be blood-stained.

On palpation, a cyst may be recognised by its smooth texture and characteristic tense fluctuation.

Management

Carcinoma must be excluded:

A discrete lump thought clinically to be a cyst should be aspirated. The lesion is benign if:

- The fluid is not bloodstained
- The lump completely disappears
- The cyst does not refill
- Cytology is negative.

If the lump is solid, or one of the above conditions is not upheld, mammography or preferably, excision biopsy is indicated.

Pain that is localised, is normally relieved by excision. Pain that is diffuse, cannot be relieved by excision. In these cases, bromocriptine, or danazol, may be helpful.

Aberrations of Involution

After pregnancy or in nulliparous women after the age of 30, the breast begins to involute.

During this process the breast stroma—the fibrous connective tissue which supports the glandular tissue of the breast—is gradually replaced by fat. This results in the breasts becoming less radiodense, softer and allowing them to droop. The glandular elements of the breast also change with areas of fibrosis, the formation of small cysts and an increase in the number of glandular elements or adenosis.

Duct Ectasia (Mammary)

Mammary duct ectasia refers to dilatation of the large and intermediate breast ducts. It results from the shortening and dilation of subareola ducts as they involute. In a small proportion of individuals excessively dilated ducts may present with a breast lump or nipple discharge.

Clinical Features

Patients are most commonly in the decade around the menopause or older. It has been estimated that by the age of 70, 40% of women have a substantial degree of duct ectasia.

Presentation is usually with a hard or doughy tender lump beneath or close to the areola, and nipple discharge which is often cheesy but may be green or blood stained. There may be slit-like nipple retraction.

The condition may be complicated by secondary infection.

Dilated ducts may be seen on mammography.

Differentiation from carcinoma may be difficult clinically.

Management

Surgery may be required to exclude malignancy, if the discharge is troublesome or to evert the nipple. Sub-areolar excision of all the major ducts may be necessary if the ectasia is extensive.

Galactocoele

A galactocoele is a cystic lesion of the breast which occurs after the cessation of lactation. It is due to obstruction of a lactiferous duct which becomes distended with milk and epithelial cells.

Patients usually present with a subareolar mass and milky nipple discharge. Secondary infection may produce foci of acute mastitis or abscess formation.

Treatment is by excision.

Epithelial Hyperplasia (Breast)

This condition is identified histologically by an increase in the number of cells lining the terminal duct lobular unit. Hyperplasia may be graded as mild, moderate or florid and there may be atypia.

The presence of atypia is associated with a significantly increased risk of subsequent breast carcinoma.

BREAST INFECTION

1. *Lactating Breast Infection*

Breast feeding may cause abrasion of the skin around the breast and, on occasion, cracking of the nipple. This permits the entry of infective organisms, most commonly Staphylococcus aureus but also Staphylococcus epidermidis and streptococci. This may result in a circumareolar breast abscess, or deep infection of the lactiferous ducts.

Uncommonly, infections arise in the sebaceous glands (of Montgomery) of the areola.

Clinical Features

The initial presentation is that of a diffuse cellulitis which localises into an abscess after several days.

The patient may be generally unwell with a spiking fever. The affected area of the breast is painful and tender, red and warm. There may be a purulent discharge if the lesion is extensive.

Management

Breast milk should be obtained for culture and sensitivity.

Blind therapy is with flucloxacillin, assuming infection with staphylococcus. Other antibiotics which may adversely effect the baby should of course be avoided. Use erythromycin if penicillin-allergic.

Continuing breast feeding should be encouraged as this helps to drain the affected segment of the breast. It is important to empty the affected breast and if it is too tender for feeding to continue, the baby should be fed from the non-infected breast and milk expressed from the infected one.

If the infection persists after an initial course of flucloxacillin (and results of culture and sensitivity are not available), then co-amoxiclav, which has a wider spectrum of action, may be tried.

Any abscess which develops should be recurrently aspirated or incised and drained.

If inflammation or an associated mass persists, the possibility of underlying breast carcinoma should be considered and investigated with further imaging or needle biopsy.

Non-lactating Breast Infection

Breast infection in non-lactating women most commonly occurs in the periareolar region of the breast. Less commonly however, in patients with certain pre-existing conditions such as diabetes, infection may also be seen in peripheral breast tissue.

A. Periareolar Non-lactating Breast Infection

This is a condition where non-dilated subareolar breasts ducts become infected. It most commonly affects young women, with a mean age of 32 years.

The condition may present with periareolar inflammation, and. the breast may be tender. There may be a history of nipple discharge and on examination the nipple may be retracted and there may be an associated inflammatory mass or abscess.

As with other breast infections treatment is with appropriate antibiotics, and abscesses should be aspirated or incised and drained.Any residual inflammation or masses following treatment should be further investigated to exclude a neoplasm.Recurrent breast infection or abscesses require surgery to remove the diseased duct.A common complication of draining a periareolar abscess is the formation of a mammary duct fistula.

B. Peripheral Non-lactating Breast Infection

Infections affecting peripheral portions of the breast are uncommon, but when they occur they are often associated with a pre-existing condition such as diabetes, rheumatoid arthritis, steroid treatment and trauma. Infections may also occur as part of a condition known as granulomatous lobular mastitis.

Pilonidal abscesses may also affect the breasts, particularly in sheep shearers and hairdressers.

Infective organisms may be aerobic or anaerobic and include Staphylococcus aureus, Enterococci, Anaerobic streptococci and Bacteroides species.

As with other breast infections antibiotics should be prescribed, and if there are abscesses these should be recurrently aspirated or incised and drained.

3. Skin Associated Breast Infection

The skin of the breast may become affected by cellulitis or abscess formation following direct infection often by Staphylococcus aureus or rarely certain fungi.

Such infections occur in women whose skin has been damaged by previous surgery or radiotherapy, but also occur in women predisposed to infection due to being overweight, having large breasts or due to poor personal hygiene.Treatment is with appropriate antibiotics and the aspiration or incision and drainage of abscesses.

Advice may be given if necessary about weight loss, keeping the breasts as clean and dry as possible i.e. avoiding talc, skin creams and the wearing of a cotton bra or cotton T shirt under a bra.

In cases of hidradenitis suppurativa, excision of affected skin prevents further infection in a proportion of patients.

BREAST NEOPLASMS

Classification:

- Benign
- Pre-malignant
- Malignant:
  - primary:
    - § carcinoma in situ
    - § invasive breast carcinoma
  - secondary.

Benign Breast Tumours

Classification:

- Epithelial:
  - intraduct papilloma
  - adenoma i.e. an excess of ductules.
- Mesenchymal:
  - lipoma
  - fibroma.
- Mixed:
  - fibroadenomas
  - Phyllodes tumours.

Note fibroadenomas though included here are not true neoplasms. They originate from a whole group of cells and are so common that they are best considered as abberations of normal development rather than neoplastic in origin.

Intraductal Papilloma

Intraductal papillomas are localised areas of epithelial proliferation within large mammary or lactiferous ducts. The lesions may occur singly or as part of the multiple intraductal papillomatosis syndrome which has an increased risk of malignancy.

Patient's are generally premenopausal and present with nipple discharge and bleeding. A small, painful subareolar nodule is present in 30% of cases.

The condition must be distinguished from Paget's disease, adenoma of the nipple, and carcinoma. A mammogram is indicated. The injection of contrast—ductography—may identify the papilloma as a filling defect.

Treatment is by surgical excision of the affected segment of breast tissue—microdochectomy.

Phyllodes Tumours

Phyllodes tumours consist of mixed epithelial and connective tissue elements but have greater stromal cellularity than fibroadenomas.

Benign and malignant tumours are recognised. Distinction is made on cytological grounds such as cellular irregularity and mitotic activity. Most of the tumours previously termed cytosarcoma phyllodes fall into the benign group.

Phyllodes tumours usually develop in women over the age of 35 years but may occur in young girls around the menarche.

Presentation is usually with a bulky, lobulated mass which greatly enlarges and distorts the breast. The overlying skin is red and warm, reflecting the increased vascularity.

In large tumours, pressure skin necrosis may develop. In these, the capsule of the tumour may rupture, and the growth fungate through the skin as an irregular mass.

Management depends on the age of the patient. In those less than 20 years of age, malignant transformation is rare so that the condition may be regarded as benign. Simple enucleation through a submammary incision is sufficient.

Phyllodes tumours in older patients show a marked tendency to local recurrence. Treatment is by local excision with a good clearance. Mastectomy may be indicated for extensive lesions, older patients, or in patients with small breasts. Local treatment is identical for benign and malignant tumours.

The prognosis for benign phyllodes tumour after surgery is excellent. That for malignant phyllodes tumour depends on the size of the lesion and the histological findings. It is poor for tumours greater than 10 cm diameter and with more than ten mitoses per ten high power fields.

Breast Carcinoma in Situ

In situ carcinoma of the breast is characterised by the proliferation of malignant epithelial cells within the ducts or lobules without invasion of the surrounding stroma. It represents the earliest stage of breast cancer, and probably, the best opportunity for cure.

Two patterns are defined:

- Ductal carcinoma *in situ*
- Lobular carcinoma *in situ.*

Ductal Carcinoma in Situ of Breast

In ductal carcinoma in situ, the malignant cells are epithelial, confined to the ducts and do not invade the basement membrane. It is associated with an increased risk of invasive breast carcinoma. The risk of invasive carcinoma is increased in proportion to the extent of in situ disease.

In the general population, the incidence of ductal carcinoma *in situ* is about 5%. However, in populations screened mammographically, this increases to 15-20% due to the tendency to produce conspicuous microcalcification. Most cases are detected by mammography whilst asymptomatic. Previously, diagnosis was made at a late stage when the lesion was palpable e.g. a firm mass or 'ropy' cords, or had caused other symptoms, as in Paget's disease. Usually, only one breast is affected.

The introduction of breast screening has seen a 3-4 fold increase in the diagnosis of DCIS.

Two broad types of ductal carcinoma in situ are recognised:

- Comedo-type tumours are characterised by:
  - pleomorphic cells ductal epithelial cells obliterate the lumina of the ducts and grow along them.
  - eventually solid cords of anaplastic cells
  - central necrosis
  - microcalcification
  - associated with multicentric disease
  - high expression of C-erb2 oncogene.
- Non-comedo type tumours are characterised by:
  - variable histology:
    - § cribriform
    - § micropapillary
    - § clinging
    - § solid.
  - less frequent:
  - mitoses
    - § necrosis
    - § calcification.

Often, comedo and non-comedo types occur simultaneously.

Management

Untreated, DCIS is associated with a substantially increased risk of developing invasive carcinoma:

- Comedo type—50% become invasive within 3 years.
- Non-comedo type—30% become invasive within 10-15 years.

The optimal therapy remains controversial but should involve local resection with pathologically clear margins. This may be combined with various combinations of radiotherapy and/or tamoxifen. Regular follow-up with clinical examination and mammography is advised.

For women with widespread or multifocal microcalcifications, with Paget's disease, or who are elderly, a simple mastectomy may be preferred.

Lobular Carcinoma in Situ of Breast

LCIS commonly occurs in premenopausal women. The incidence is unknown as there are no distinctive clinical or radiologic features. The condition is usually discovered as an incidental finding when a biopsy is made for otherwise benign disease. There are no clear mammographic features. Clinically, it is not palpable and does not tend to metastasize.

LCIS is frequently bilateral and multicentric. It is associated with an eleven-fold increased risk of subsequent invasive carcinoma. There is no relation between the breast in which LCIS is detected and that in which invasive carcinoma occurs. LCIS is regarded as a marker of increased risk anywhere in the breast. Thirty percent of patients develop invasive carcinoma within 15-20 years. This is a lower relative risk than ductal carcinoma *in situ*.

Management consists of lifelong surveillance by annual mammography and clinical examination. As the majority of patients are premenopausal, the use of Tamoxifen may alter the hormonal milieu and diminish the risk of invasive carcinoma.

BREAST CANCER

Breast cancer is the commonest malignancy in women, accounting for 20% of all cancer deaths in females.

One in eleven women will suffer from breast cancer. The annual age adjusted death rate is approximately 27 per 100,000.

These statistics and the accessibility of the breast to screening procedures have provided the impetus for national breast cancer screening programmes.

Risk Factors

The clearest risks for invasive breast cancer are:
- Female sex
- The presence of preinvasive cancer:
  - lobular carcinoma *in situ*
  - ductal carcinoma *in situ.*
- Previous breast cancer

Other risk factors (classified as increased risk above normal) include:
- family history of breast cancer—the risk of breast cancer in a woman has been quantified with respect to the number of affected first degree relatives and by the age of affected first degree relative (1).

Table 8.1: Relative risk for breast cancer by number of affected first degree female relatives

Number of women first degree relatives	*Relative risk for women < 50 years (99% CI)*	*Relative risk for >= 50 years (CI)*
1	2.14 (1.92 to 2.38)	1.65 (1.53 to 1.78)
2	3.84 (2.37 to 6.22)	2.61 (2.03 to 3.34)
3	12.05 (1.70 to 85.16)	2.65 (1.29 to 5.46)

Table 8.2: Relative risk for breast cancer by age of affected first degree relative

Age at time of diagnosis in first years degree relatives	*Relative risk for women < 50 years (99% CI)*	*Relative risk for women >= 50 (CI)*
< 40 years	13.5 (3.4 to 53.9)	3.9 (1.8 to 8.6)
>= 40 years	7.8 (2.4 to 25.0)	2.6 (1.8 to 3.7)

- Age—peak incidence 45-75 years but any age postmenarche >> 4x.
- Country of residence—high in West > 4x e.g. UK, low in East e.g. Japan

- Previous breast cancer > 4x.
- Irradiation of chest—shows a linear dose-response relationship 2-4x.
- Social class (I vs. V) 2-4x.
- Race—more common in Caucasians < 2x.
- Previous ovarian or endometrial cancer < 2x.
- Early menarche or late menopause < 2x.
- Nulliparity or older than 30 years before first child < 2x.
- Hormonal supplementation < 2x.
- Obesity—oestrogen synthesis in adipose tissue.
- Alcohol consumption.

In the male, Klinefelter's syndrome is a risk factor for breast cancer.

Histological Classification

- Carcinoma of no special type ("ductal") 60-70%
- Carcinoma of special type:
  - Tubular 1-5%
  - medullary < 5%
  - mucinous < 5%
  - papillary 1%.
- Infiltrating lobular carcinoma 10-20% (may be bilateral).
- Mixed—ductal, lobular, rare types 10%.

Grading of a tumour is based on—degree of glandular formation, mitotic rate, nuclear pleomorphism; each scored from 1-3. Score.

- Well differentiated—grade I (3-5).
- Moderately differentiated—grade II (6-7).
- Poorly differentiated—grade III (8-9).

Clinical Presentation

Breast cancer may be asymptomatic, occurring as an impalpable lesion on screening mammogram. (Upto 70% of important mammographic lesions are impalpable).

In other cases, patients may present with:

- Palpable breast lump:
  - 40-50% in the upper outer quadrant
  - 70-80% scirrhous i.e. hard and encapsulated
  - may be tethered to superficial or deep structures
  - does not fluctuate or transilluminate
  - 15-40% multicentric
  - bilateral in up to 30% of cases of lobular carcinoma
  - frequently, patient detected.
- Skin changes:
  - dimpling
  - peau d'orange
  - nipple "eczema" in Paget's
  - visible lump
  - surface ulceration; neglected carcinoma in elderly.
- Recent nipple inversion.
- Bloodstained nipple discharge—uncommon.
- Non-cyclic breast pain—usually, a late sign.
- Disseminated disease:
  - Bone pain, pathological fracture
  - Dyspnoea, pleural effusion
  - Hepatomegaly, jaundice.

Diagnosis

The diagnosis of breast cancer must be made with certainty before surgery can be undertaken. The diagnosis cannot be made on history and examination alone.

Investigative measures to confirm the diagnosis include:

- Imaging:
  - mammography
  - ultrasound
  - ductography.
- Biopsy:
  - fine needle aspiration biopsy
  - core needle biopsy
  - localisation biopsy
  - open biopsy.
- Detection of metastatic disease:
  - liver function tests
  - serum calcium
  - chest radiograph
  - isotope bone scan

– liver ultrasound scan
– CT brain.

The yield from an extensive search for metastatic disease is poor except in cases where suspicion is great clinically. Hence, symptoms of metastasis or patients with stage III disease should have a bone scan, chest X-ray and liver ultrasound. A CT scan of the brain should only be carried out when the history or examination is suggestive of metastasis e.g. fits.

TNM Staging of Breast Cancer

- T0—no evidence of primary tumour.
- T1—the tumour is 2 cm or less in diameter, with no skin involvement—except in the case of Paget's disease where confined to the nipple—and no nipple retraction or fixation.
- T2—tumour greater than 2 cm but less than 5 cm.
- T3—tumour greater than 5 cm in greatest diameter, less than 10 cm.
- T4—greater than 10 cm or skin or chest wall involvement or peau d'orange.
- N0—no palpable ipsilateral axillary nodes.
- N1—palpable, ipsilateral axillary nodes.
- N2—ipsilateral axillary nodal metastases fixed to one another or to other structures.
- N3—metastases to ipsilateral internal mammary nodes.
- M0—no evidence of metastases.
- M1—distant metastases (includes ipsilateral supraclavicular nodes).

Management of Breast Cancer

The management of breast cancer is determined by the stage of the disease and in part, the patient's wishes. Patient involvement has been shown to reduce the incidence of anxiety and depression after treatment.

Breast cancer management in recent years has moved away from radical to conservative surgery. This has occured due to a change in theory of how breast cancer disseminates—see submenu.

Management requires a multidisciplinary approach entailing input from:

- Surgeon
- Breast care nurse
- Pathologist e.g. FNAC at time of clinic
- Radiologist e.g. mammography
- Oncologist e.g. in advanced disease
- Psychiatrist e.g. in event of depressive illness
- Plastic surgeon e.g. for breast reconstruction.

Management may be considered to consist of a combination of:

- Local treatments to control local disease
- Systemic treatments to treat micrometastatic disease.

The aims of local management are to:

- Remove the local tumour reducing local growth
- Eliminate the risk of this deposit seeding distant sites.
- Provide an aesthetic result.

There has been a tendency to move away from radical operations to breast conservation. This has resulted from a realisation that prognosis is not altered greatly by more extensive excisions yet morbidity is increased.

Equally, for conservative surgery there has been a realisation that adjuvant radiotherapy to the breast is a necessity. Local recurrence rates of up to a third at 8 years occur in simple excision without radiotherapy. The rates with radiotherapy are between 10 and 20%.

Management of disease in the breast must be combined with a consideration of management of:

- Axillary disease
- Distant metastases.

Breast Conservation Surgery

Breast conservation surgery may involve either wide local excision or a quadrantectomy:

- Wide local excision involves removal of the tumour with at least a 1 cm margin of normal breast tissue.

- Quadrantectomy is more extensive and involves removal of a whole quadrant of the breast.

Breast conservation is often combined with axillary node dissection and/or local radiotherapy. The wider the excision the lower the recurrence rate, but the poorer the cosmetic result. However, cosmetic results are better generally than mastectomy and breast reconstruction is not usually required.

Alternative terms for operations involving breast conservation include lumpectomy, tumourectomy and tylectomy. They all imply removal of the tumour with a peripheral rim of normal tissue.

Breast tumours suitable for breast conservation include:

- Tumours where there is a single clinical and mammographic lesion.
- Tumour size:
  - less than 3-4 cm in diameter
  - dependent on the size of the breast:
    - § in small breasts, tumours greater than 2cm diameter may be impossible to remove without a cosmetic result that is similar to that of mastectomy.
    - § in large breasts, tumours slightly greater than 4cm diameter may be treated conservatively as the cosmetic results are generally favourable and prognosis is not thought to be greatly different from mastectomy.
- No sign of local advancement e.g. fixation to overlying skin or deeper muscle.

Mastectomy

A third of localised breast tumours are unsuitable for treatment by breast conservation. A number of procedures may be performed:

- Simple mastectomy:
  - removal of breast, nipple, areola and skin. Nodes may be removed separately. Chest wall muscles left intact
  - enables later reconstruction
- Modified radical mastectomy (Patey's operation):
  - removal of breast, nipple, areola, skin and level I and II axillary nodes plus pectoralis minor; pectoralis major muscle is preserved

Mutilating operations now rarely performed:

- Halsted radical mastectomy—removal of breast, nipple, areola, major and minor pectoralis muscles, axillary nodes
- Urban extended radical mastectomy—as above plus removal of internal mammary nodes, medial costal cartilages and part of sternum

The last two procedures are used only in advanced disease where their associated morbidity is less than that from radiotherapy

The tumours best treated with mastectomy include:

- Patient preference:
  - small tumours may be amenable to conservative treatment, but the patient may have a strong feeling that mastectomy will provide more peace of mind
  - patient may prefer to avoid radiotherapy with its attendant complications
- Size of tumour:
  - tumours greater than 2-3 cm in small breasts; generally, removal of masses greater than this size results in a cosmetic defect that is unacceptable
  - in larger breasts, masses up to 4 cm have been treated with breast conservation with little aesthetic deficit and what is believed to be little influence on prognosis
- Those with clinical or radiographic evidence of more than one tumour:
  - more prevalent with lobular carcinoma
  - multifocal disease:
    - § presence of synchronous tumour within the the same quadrant
    - § increases with increasing primary tumour size

§ widespread multifocal disease is probably best treated with mastectomy.
– multicentric disease: presence of synchronous tumour outside of the same quadrant
• Poor tumour differentiation
þ centrally-located tumours:
– often difficult to excise by conservative measures without poor cosmesis due to loss of nipple
– many women prefer mastectomy to simple conservation if the nipple will be lost by both techniques.

Radiotherapy Treatment in Breast Cancer

Radiotherapy is commonly used in the management of breast cancer.

A meta-analysis has been shown that radiotherapy reduces the local recurrence rate by about two-thirds and significantly reduces breast cancer-related deaths (1).

However this study reveals that radiotherapy does increase other causes of death especially vascular disease—probably because the heart, coronaries and carotids are included in the irradiated field. Of note is that historical methods of radiation included overlapping fields, high daily doses, and larger irradiated volumes, all of which may increase mortality from causes other than breast cancer. This meta-analysis suggests that mortality from such causes may be lower when daily doses of < 2.2 Gy were employed.

This evidence suggests that many patients, especially those who are younger and node positive, should consider nodal irradiation, even when systemic treatment is given.

Systemic Treatments

Two types of systemic treatment are available:
• Hormonal therapy
• Cytotoxic chemotherapy

Hormonal therapy is best suited in the presence of slow growing disease, where the tumour is known to be oestrogen sensitive and since it is well tolerated it is ideal for elderly and unfit patients.

Cytotoxic chemotherapy is better suited where the tumour is rapidly progressive and when the tumour is oestrogen receptor negative.

Hormonal Therapy

Many breast cancer cells, particularly those which are oestrogen receptor positive require oestrogens to proliferate. Hormonal therapy aims to remove the proliferative oestrogen stimulus.

Hormonal therapy is used in two main circumstances:
• In advanced disease where surgery is not attempted or is not potentially curative
• In patients who have potentially curative surgery but who are at high risk of recurrence

Currently there are two approaches to reducing the oestrogen stimulus:
• Antioestrogens
• Aromatase inhibitors

Antioestrogens are used in the hormonal treatment of breast cancer. The gold standard is tamoxifen which is primarily an oestrogen receptor antagonist with some agonist acitivity.

Tamoxifen taken for 5 years following surgical treatment is a standard part of the treatment regime for postmenopausal women with hormone-receptor-positive breast cancer. If used in this context then tamoxifen:
• Increases the proportion of women who survive for at least 10 years from about 50 to 60% among those with lymph-node involvement
• Increases the proportion of women who survive for at least 10 years without lymph-node involvement from about 73 to 79%.
• Almost halves the risk of development of cancer in the contralateral breast.

Inhibition of aromatase prevents the synthesis of oestrogens.

Aminoglutethimide has been used in the past to produce a medical adrenalectomy, preventing the synthesis of adrenal oestrogens in patients post-oophorectomy. The clinically relevant activity of aminoglutethimide was aromatase inhibition. Recently specific inhibitors of aromatase have been developed which obviate the need for glucocorticoid replacement.

There are two classes of aromatase inhibitors:

- Non-steroidal:
  - anastozole
  - letrozole
  - are potent aromatase inhibitors which may be used in advanced breast cancer.
- Steroidal:
  - formestane
  - exemestane
  - may be used in advanced breast cancer.

Chemotherapy

Chemotherapy is indicated in two situations for the treatment of breast cancer:

- Adjuvant chemotherapy in patients at risk of micrometastasis.
- Treatment of known metastatic disease

First line treatment is with an anthracycline or mitozantrone. Resistant tumours may respond to a taxol compound.

Guidance from the National Institute of Clinical Excellence (NICE) states that both docetaxel (Taxotere) and paclitaxel (Taxol) should be available for the treatment of advanced breast cancer where initial cytotoxic chemotherapy (including anthracycline) has failed oris inappropriate.

Long Term Follow-up

The aim of follow up is three fold:

- To detect local recurrence
- To detect disease in the other breast
- To ensure that a close eye is kept on first degree relatives particularly if the patient is pre-menopausal.

Regular clinical examination and mammography are recommended. Follow up should be arranged according to the type of surgery performed.

After breast conservation surgery, recurrence occurs at a fixed rate each year and the patient should be reviewed every 6 months. For mastectomy however, recurrence decreases with time and thus after 2 years of 6 monthly follow up, the patient may be reviewed annually.

Prognosis

Overall 5 year survival is 80%.
Influencing factors include:

- Clinical staging (manchester system):
  - stage 1—80% 5 year survival
  - stage 2—68% "
  - stage 3—40% "
  - stage 4—10% "
- Size—small i.e. less than 2 cm—95% 5 year survival;—large i.e. more than 2 cm—80% 5 year survival.
- Tumour type—tubular and mucinous have best prognosis.
- Grade—high grade tumours carry poorer prognosis.
- Receptor status—oestrogen receptor positive tumours are are more likely to respond to hormone therapy.
- Age at diagnosis.

Breast Cancer in the Male

Male breast cancer accounts 1% of all breast cancer. Among men with Klinefelter's syndrome, the incidence is comparable to that of women.

Presentation is usually in the 6th decade with a lump beneath the areola.

Management is similar to that in female breast carcinoma. Early disease is treated by surgery and radiotherapy; late disease, by hormonal therapy. Orchidectomy is often effective.

Breast cancer in men generally has a poorer prognosis than that in women. The smaller amount of breast tissue allows for a more rapid dissemination of metastases into regional lymphatics.

PAGET'S DISEASE OF THE NIPPLE

Paget's disease of the nipple is a presentation of breast cancer that invariably, is associated with ductal carcinoma in situ (DCIS) or invasive carcinoma in the underlying breast. Typically, it presents as a unilateral red, bleeding, eczematous lesion of the nipple which is eventually eroded.

This condition occurs in approximately 1 in 50 breast cancers, and is most frequent among middle-aged and elderly women.

About 40% of cases present with a palpable lump, a relatively late stage.

Rarely Paget's disease may affect other apocrine gland-bearing areas such as the vulva.

Histologic examination of the nipple reveals multiple Paget cells:

- Clear
- Sited among the basal epidermal cells
- Typical ballooned appearance
- Pale cytoplasm
- Prominent nuclei
- Nucleus surrounded by halo—accumulation of intracellular mucopolysaccharide.

At the skin, the epidermis is invaded. The underlying dermis contains an inflammatory infiltrate.

In the vast majority of cases, careful study of the breast reveals an associated DCIS or invasive carcinoma.

A popular theory is that Paget's disease results from invasion of the nipple by malignant cells spreading down the ducts from the associated breast tumour.

Other theories propose that the Paget cells arise in the nipple from local epidermal cells, and that the concurrence of DCIS and nipple malignant cells are due to common carcinogenic influences.

Clinical Features

Classically, the condition is unilateral. The earliest symptoms are those of itching, tingling and discomfort.

Later, a small patch of redness or roughening is evident on the nipple that progresses to frank erosion with red granulation tissue and bleeding. The areola is often affected. There may be a palpable lump.

Changes occur slowly. It may take 4-5 years for the nipple to be fully eroded.

Less commonly, Paget's disease is characterised by a dry, red, scaly rash that spreads widely to involve much of the breast.

Management is concentrated on detecting and treating any associated malignancy.

Total mastectomy with axillary dissection may be preferable in older patients as it is rapid and reliable. In those who wish to avoid mastectomy, radiotherapy alone or after cone excision of the nipple, areola and underlying ducts may be offered.

Wide local excision without radiotherapy is unsatisfactory; it is associated with a 50% recurrence rate. Adjuvant therapy is indicated only for established invasive carcinoma.

Paget's disease with associated intraduct carcinoma only and no palpable lump, has an excellent prognosis, with a cure rate approaching 100%.

Nine

Endocrine Tumors

PARATHYROID DISEASES

HYPOPARATHYROIDISM

Hypoparathyroidism may arise whenever there is inadequate secretion of PTH or the hormone is biologically ineffective. Under these circumstances the diminished physiologic action of PTH on the kidney leads to hypocalcaemia and hyperphosphataemia. Reduced end-organ sensitivity to PTH may also induce hypoparathyroidism. A constellation of clinical changes is associated with hypoparathyroidism.

Aetiology

Parathyroid gland deficiency:

- *Primary deficiency:*
  - idiopathic/congenital pseudohypoparathyroidism
  - DiGeorge syndrome
- *Secondary deficiency:*
  - destruction during thyroid, parathyroid or laryngeal surgery; by far the most common cause
  - infiltration by iron in haemochromatosis or by metastases

Reduced secretory activity:

- Hypomagnesaemia-Mg necessary for PTH secretion
- Vitamin D excess

End organ resistance:

- Pseudohypoparathyroidism
- Hypomagnesaemia

Clinical Features

With milder expressions of the syndrome, the clinical manifestations are subtle. At the other extreme more overt expressions of acute hypocalcaemia may be present:

- Increased neuromuscular excitability:
  - may cause Chvostek's sign, tetany, carpopedal spasms, laryngeal stridor and convulsions
- Mental changes—ranging from irritability to depression and frank psychosis
- Neurological signs suggesting an intracranial tumour with elevated CSF pressure e.g. papilloedema
- Intracranial calcification visualised by skull radiology—particularly, in the basal ganglia

- Calcification of lens, leading to formation of cataracts
- Abnormalities of cardiac conduction—mainly prolonged Q-T intervals and T-wave changes
- Abnormalities of dentition with defective enamel, dental hypoplasia, and delayed eruption of teeth
- Alopecia with premature greying
- Chronic mucocutaneous candidiasis is common in autoimmune

Investigations

Diagnosis is based on:

- Low serum calcium
- Increased plasma phosphate—low in hypocalcaemia due to intestinal malabsorption or vitamin D deficiency
- Normal alkaline phosphatase—raised in hypocalcaemia due to chronic renal failure
- Skull radiology may reveal basal ganglia calcification
- PTH: low plasma levels
- Urinary cAMP excretion rises following administration of PTH

Treatment

Acute symptomatic hypocalcaemia requires urgent correction with intravenous calcium; oral calcium is rarely adequate to sustain normocalcaemia.

Permanent hypoparathyroidism and pseudohypoparathyroidism are treated with supraphysiological doses of vitamin D or one of its active metabolites; the metabolites are preferred since they have a relatively short half life and permit easier modification of the treatment regime.

Doses of 1.25-2.5 mg per day of vitamin D are required.

Maintenance doses of the metabolites are:

- 0.5 to 1.0 mcg per day 1,25 (OH)2 D
- 1.0 to 2.0 mcg per day 1 OH D

Supplementary calcium is only required if the diet provides less than 600 mg per day.

HYPERPARATHYROIDISM

Hyperparathyroidism is a condition in which there is excessive secretion of parathyroid hormone. The principal target organs are the kidney and bone, with a secondary effect on the gut through 1,25 dihydroxy vitamin D.

Hyperparathyroidism can be primary, secondary or tertiary according to the extent of excessive parathyroid hormone produced, and the degree of autonomy of the parathyroid glands.

Clinically, there may be effects of both hypercalcaemia and of hypocalcaemia.

Investigations should include serum calcium and phosphate, and parathyroid hormone.

PRIMARY HYPERPARATHYROIDISM

This may be defined as a circulating level of PTH which is inappropriately high for the prevailing level of calcium. Most patients are hypercalcaemic but the condition may equally occur in normocalcaemic patients with co-existent vitamin D deficiency. It implies hyperfunction of one or more parathyroid glands with a change in the set point for the control of calcium.

It has an incidence of 0.5 per 1000 and is most common between 40 and 60 years of age when it is twice as common in women than men. In other age groups, the sex incidence is roughly equal. In young people of either sex, it is important to investigate possible multiple endocrine neoplasia.

Aetiology

Over 80% of primary hyperparathyroidism cases are caused by a single parathyroid adenoma of the chief or clear cells of the parathyroid gland.

Other causes include:

- Multiple adenomas—5%
- Diffuse hyperplasia:
  - of chief cells—8%
  - of clear cells—4%
- Carcinoma—2%
- Ectopic PTH-secreting tumour

Co-existence of hypercalcaemia with hypertension and neurofibroma is suggestive of multiple endocrine neoplasia—MEN I or MEN IIa. Primary hyperthyroidism is rarely familial.

Pathology

In hyperparathyroidism, the principally affected sites are where the bone turnover is most active, for example the trabecular bone of the vertebrae, the phalanges, the ends of long bones and parts of the skull.

Macroscopically there is demineralisation of bone. Increased bone reabsorption leads to subperiosteal resorption of the phalanges, thinning of the cortex, and the formation of bone cysts or brown tumours. Deformities can lead to fracture or bending.

Microscopically there is an increased number of osteoclasts which increase the amount of bone resorption. The marrow spaces are filled with fibrous tissue producing osteitis fibrosa.

The increased osteoblast activity causes an increased woven-non-lamellar–bone trabeculae.

Clinical Features

"Bones, moans and stones" is the classical description of hyperparathyroidism but such clear cases are uncommon.

Clinical features due to excess PTH may include:

- Bone resorption leading to bone pain, pathological fracture, and rarely, osteitis fibrosa cystica; characteristic changes visible on radiography
- Renal calculi occur in 10-15% of patients with primary hyperparathyroidism
- Other features of metastatic calcification may be present such as nephrocalcinosis, and corneal calcification; occasionally, chondrocalcinosis may be evident on radiology
- Rarely, primary hyperparathyroidism may present as acute pancreatitis
- Polyuria, thirst, weakness, vomiting

Features attributable to hypercalcaemia may be evident in primary and tertiary hyperparathyroidism.

- In secondary hyperparathyroidism, the clinical picture may be complicated by hypocalcaemia. In chronic renal failure, co-existent osteomalacia results in renal osteodystrophy.

Investigations

The investigations in primary hyperparathyroidism include:

- Raised serum Ca with high or normal—but inappropriately high for the level of Ca—serum PTH
- Serum alkaline phosphatase—often normal but may be markedly increased in bone disease
- Serum phosphate:
  - decreased in about half of cases
  - a raised serum phosphate suggests nonparathyroid hypercalcaemia
  - a normal serum phosphate is not diagnostically useful
- Urine Ca—increased in most patients
- Metabolic acidosis is reflected by reduced plasma bicarbonate and high plasma chloride
- Bone radiographs abnormal—pathognomonic subperiosteal bone resorption of the phalanges; there may be loss of the lamina dura of the teeth; in severe cases osteitis fibrosa cystica is present
- Ultrasound of the neck may reveal a thyroid parathyroid adenoma; also may be shown by a radioactive thallium technetium scan
- Two-site radioimmunoassays for PTH can differentiate primary hyperparathyroidism—high PTH—from malignancy related hypercalcaemia (low PTH)
- Venous PTH sampling—may be employed to localise the the source of the PTH on occasions where it has not been identified during initial surgery

Radiology

The radiological changes in hyperparathyroidism are:

- Classically, subperiosteal bone resorption—most often on the radial aspect of the middle phalanges of the fingers; the extent correlates well with the increased serum alkaline phosphatase
- Loss of lamina dura—the thin layer of compact bone forming the sheath for the tooth socket—a late sign
- Extensive bone resorption in the skull gives a stippled 'pepper pot' appearance
- Cystic lesions—brown tumours—may occur elsewhere in the skeleton—appear as rounded radiolucent lesions which are trabeculated—but are less common and a late sign
- Resorption of metaphyseal bone in children gives rise to crippling skeletal deformities
- There may be diffuse osteopenia

Treatment

For primary hyperparathyroidism, surgery is indicated in all patients under the age of 60 years and in other patients with a serum calcium concentration above 3.00 mmol per litre.

Treated patients may show a mild transient state of hypoparathyroidism for several days or weeks afterwards until the remaining previously suppressed glands recover. Mild circumoral and digital paraesthesiae may occur and are easily controlled using iv or oral calcium.

Severe and prolonged low serum levels of calcium, magnesium, and phosphate may occur post-operatively and require an active vitamin D metabolite such as 1 HCC.

SECONDARY HYPERPARATHYROIDISM

Secondary hyperparathyroidism refers to hyperplasia of all four parathyroid glands secondary to prolonged hypocalcaemia or hyperphosphataemia. It is a normal homeostatic response and is the most common form of hyperparathyroidism. Serum calcium levels are replenished from skeletal stores, and by increasing both renal tubular reabsorption and gut absorption of calcium

Aetiology

Secondary hyperparathyroidism is due to chronic hypocalcaemia associated with:

- Chronic renal failure—defective absorption of calcium in the gut due to reduced levels of 1, 25 dihydroxy cholcalciferol
- Malabsorption and vitamin D deficiency

Clinical Features

Same as those in Primary Hyperparathyroidism.

Investigations

Investigations in secondary hyperparathyroidism show:

- Low or normal serum calcium
- PO4 is raised or normal in chronic renal failure; and lowered in malabsorption
- Serum alkaline phosphatase is elevated

Treatment

The aim in secondary hyperparathyroidism is to treat the underlying cause.

Skeletal calcium may be conserved by administering active metabolites of vitamin D such as:

- 1 hydroxy cholecalciferol—1 HCC—0.5-2.0 mcg per day
- 1,25 dihydroxy cholecalciferol—1,25 HCC—0.25-1.0 mcg per day

Both agents increase the intestinal absorption of calcium and directly inhibit the activity of parathyroid cells. Care is necessary to avoid precipitating hypercalcaemia.

TERTIARY HYPERPARATHYROIDISM

Tertiary hyperparathyroidism describes a condition in which autonomous parathyroid activity and hypercalcaemia occur following prolonged secondary hyperparathyroidism.

The set point at which serum calcium shuts off PTH production is raised. It is most commonly seen in patients undergoing maintenance renal dialysis. Tertiary hyperparathyroidism may also occur in patients with long standing malabsorption or chronic renal failure.

Associated Conditions

Tertiary hyperparathyroidism is associated with the following conditions:
- Renal dialysis
- Chronic renal failure
- Chronic malabsorption

Investigations

Investigations in tertiary hyperparathyroidism show:
- Raised Ca in the serum
- Albumin is normal or low
- PO4:
  - Decreased or normal in chronic renal failure
  - Decreased in malabsorption
- Serum alkaline phosphatase is raised
- Plasma PTH raised

Treatment

The intermittent administration of i.v. 1,25 (OH)2 D may postpone the evolution of secondary hyperparathyroidism to tertiary hyperparathyroidism.

The treatment of choice is subtotal parathyroidectomy leaving about 100 mg of parathyroid tissue. The tissue may be implanted into the arm or another accessible site to facilitate future surgery if required. Invasive tumour like overgrowth of the implants may occu

PSEUDOHYPOPARATHYROIDISM

Pseudohypoparathyroidism is a rare disorder characterised by failure of target cells to respond to parathyroid hormone. It is inherited in an autosomal dominant fashion.

Features are similar to hypoparathyroidism.

There is peripheral resistance to the action of PTH.

Classification

There are two main types of pseudohypoparathyroidism:
- *Type I:*
  - adenylate cyclase is not activated by PTH
  - urinary cAMP levels do not rise when PTH is administered
- *Type II:*
  - cells fail to respond to the intracellular cAMP signal
  - urinary cAMP levels rise when PTH is administered

Clinical Features

There are the usual clinical features of hypocalcaemia:
- Carpopedal spasm
- Paraesthesiae
- Abdominal cramps
- Papilloedema
- Epilepsy

Associated endocrine disorders include:
- Hypothyroidism
- Diabetes mellitus

Phenotypically pseudohypoparathyroidism is associated with:
- Short stature
- Mental retardation
- Obesity
- Strabismus
- Subcutaneous calcification—rare in acquired hypoparathyroidism
- Shortened metacarpals and metatarsals:
  - Brachydactyly
  - Especially 3rd, 4th and 5th rays
- Bowing of the legs

- Rounded moon face
- Cerebral calcification

Metacarpal shortening may easily be demonstrated by asking the patient to make a fist and observing that the relevant knuckles are absent.

Investigations

The laboratory results show:

- Low serum calcium
- increased plasma phosphate—low in Hypocalcaemia due to intestinal malabsorption or vitamin D deficiency
- Normal alkaline phosphatase—raised in hypocalcaemia due to chronic renal failure
- skull radiology may reveal basal ganglia calcification
- high PTH concentrations
- In type I pseudohypoparathyroidism, urinary cAMP fails to rise following administration of PTH
- In type II pseudohypoparathyroidism, urinary cAMP rises normally following PTH administration.

PSEUDOPSEUDOHYPOPARATHYROIDISM

This is used to describe patients whom present with the somatic abnormalities of pseudohypothyroidism but lack the biochemical ones.

The occurrence of pseudopseudohypoparathyroidism in the same families as pseudohypoparathyroidism has been reported. This may represent incomplete genetic expression of the same genetic abnormality.

THYROID DISEASES AND CONDITIONS

HYPERTHYROIDISM

Thyrotoxicosis is a disease caused by excessive concentrations of free thyroid hormones (most often T4).

Many of the clinical features of thyrotoxicosis are characterised by signs of sympathetic overactivity such as tremor, tachycardia, and sweating producing weight loss, fatigue and heat intolerance.

The level of catecholamines is normal but the excess thyroid hormones seem to potentiate the action of the catecholamines.

Hyperthyroidism is extremely common, affecting perhaps 2 to 5% of all females at some time in their lives. The vast majority of cases are caused by intrinsic thyroid disease; a pituitary cause is extremely rare.

Aetiology

- Primary:
  - due to pathology within the thyroid gland
  - most common.
- Pecondary:
  - a pathological process causes excessive stimulation of a normal thyroid gland.

Hyperthyroidism (Primary)

This is hyperthyroidism secondary to pathology within the thyroid gland. Ninety perent of cases are due to:

- Grave's disease
- Toxic nodular goitre:
  - —multinodular
  - single toxic nodule—usually an adenoma.

Other common causes:

- Thyroiditis
  - de Quervain's
  - silent/post-partum
  - Hashimoto's—hashitoxicosis may develop mid-course.

Uncommon:

- Intentional/factitious
- Overenthusiastic therapy
- Drug-induced
- Jod—Basedow.

Hyperthyroidism (Secondary)

Hyperthyroidism as a result of pathology in another organ which causes excess stimulation of the thyroid gland.

Excess TSH:

- Uncommon:
  - TSH secreting pituitary adenoma
  - pituitary stimulation due to excessive hypothalamic release of TRH.
- Rare:
  - hydatidiform moles
  - choriocarcinoma
  - embryonal testicular carcinoma.

Extraneous thyroid hormone—all rare:

- Struma ovarii—ovarian teratoma with thyroid tissue.
- Metastatic, well differentiated thyroid carcinoma.

Clinical Features of Hyperthyroidism

Typical presentations of thyrotoxicosis:

- Increased heat production—warm, moist skin, heat intolerance.
- Telangiectasia, palmar erythema, pretibial myxoedema, onycholysis.
- Weight loss, increased appetite, increased frequency of bowel movement but frank diarrhoea is uncommon; steatorrhoea may occur; dyspepsia; like juvenile-onset diabetes mellitus, may cause a decrease in weight despite an increased appetite.
- Oligomenorrhoea.
- Tachycardia, exertional dyspnoea, hyperdynamic circulation; systolic hypertension is common and diastolic hypertension can occur in up to 30% of patients.
- Tiredness, irritability, nervousness.
- Fine tremor, hyperkinesia.
- There are eye signs in Graves' disease.

Others:

- Occasionally, bone pain due to osteoporosis.
- In elderly patients, there may be atrial fibrillation or cardiac failure.
- Alopecia, pruritus, pretibial myxoedema, acropachy.

Atypical Presentations of Thyrotoxicosis

These may include:

- Atrial arrhythmias in middle aged patients.
- Severe proximal myopathy with normal CK values
- Deterioration or unmasking of myasthenia gravis
- Hypokalaemic periodic paralysis—especially in orientals.
- Chronic diarrhoea.
- Hypercalcaemia.
- Osteoporosis.
- Gynaecomastia (Fig. 9.1).

Differential Diagnosis

The differential diagnosis of hyperthyroidism includes:

- Anxiety states:
  - differentiation may be difficult clinically
  - positive findings for thyrotoxicosis are eye signs, proximal myopathy, wasting, hyperdynamic circulation with warm peripheries
  - anxiety tends to cause clammy hands.

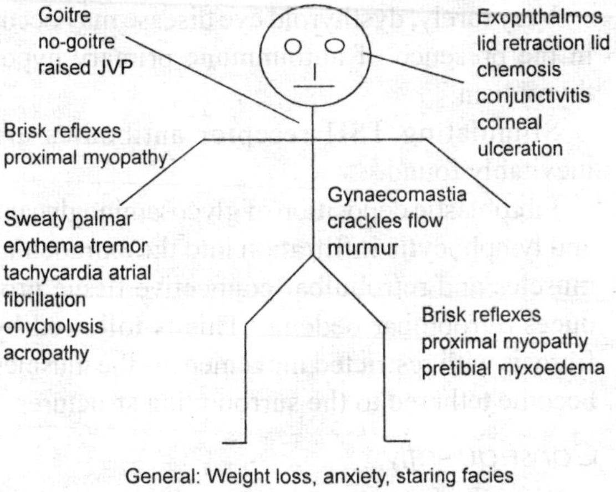

Fig. 9.1: Diagram of the clinical features of hyperthyroidism

- Phaeochromocytoma:
  – especially if the patient is hypertensive.

Investigations in Hyperthyroidism

Thyroid function tests consists of:
- T3 and T4 determination.
- TSH determination—normal serum TSH concentration nearly always excludes the diagnosis of thyrotoxicosis; the rare exceptions to this are a TSH-producing pituitary tumour or thyroid hormone resistance syndrome.
- TRH stimulation test (rarely performed)
- Radioisotope iodine scanning
- Serology.

Other investigations:

- FBC:
  – normochromic normocytic anaemia may be seen in Grave's disease.
- ESR:
  – raised in Grave's disease
  – high in subacute thyroiditis.
- Calcium—often raised
- LFTs—may be abnormal in Grave's disease.

Treatment Modalities

There are three treatment options available:
- Drug treatment
- Surgery
- Radioiodine.

1. *Drug Treatment*

- Beta blockers for acute symptomatic treatment.
- Antithyroid drugs for long term treatment
  – antithyroid drugs are prescribed either for the short-term control of thyrotoxicosis prior to definitive treatment, or in the hope of achieving remission in patients with Graves' disease, especially in those presenting under the age of 40. Generally a course of 18 months is recommended but the probability of achieving long-term remission is less than 50%.
  – rates of remission are lower in males, in older patients, and in those patients with severe hyperthyroidism.
  – antithyroid drugs are ineffective in thyroiditis (viral, postpartum or amiodarone induced)—this is because the action of the antithyroid drugs is to block production of thyroid hormones whereas the hyperthyroidism associated with thyroiditis is caused by release of stored thyroid hormone from damaged thyroid cells.

2. *Surgical or Radio-iodine Treatment in Thyrotoxicosis*

Indications for radioiodine treatment include:
- Radio-iodine treatment.
  – increasingly becoming the first-line treatment for adults with Graves' thyrotoxicosis.
  – treatment of choice for most patients with relapsed Graves' disease.
  – treatment of choice in patients with toxic nodular hyperthyroidism.
  – women of child-bearing age are advised to avoid pregnancy for four months after receiving radio-iodine treatment.

- the presence of Graves' ophthalmopathy is a relative contra-indication to radio-iodine therapy because it may deteriorate after radio-iodine treatment.

Specific indications for surgical intervention include:

- Patient choice
- Large goitre that is unlikely to resolve with antithyroid drugs.

Pregnancy and Thyrotoxicosis

Pregnant women with hyperthyroidism require management by a hospital specialist.

Antithyroid drugs are the treatment of choice in pregnancy but the "block and replace" regime is contraindicated.

In North America propylthiouracil is preferred as it is excreted less in breast milk and carbimazole may be associated with aplasia cutis. 'The suggested association of carbimazole with neonatal aplasia cutis has led some clinicians to prefer propylthiouracil for use during pregnancy (2).'

The smallest dose of antithyroid medication possible should be used because of the risk of fetal hypothyroidism—carbimazole 5-10 mg/day; propylthiouracil 50-100 mg/day. Generally treatment is withdrawn 4 weeks prior to delivery after which normal doses may be resumed.

Often hyperthyroidism due to Graves' disease improves spontaneously across pregnancy, so a smaller dose of antithyroid drug may be required.

Radio-iodine is contraindicated and pregnancy should be avoided for at least 4 months following receipt of I-131.

THYROID EYE DISEASE

Ophthalmologic involvement is common in Graves' disease, and it accounts for the majority of dysthyroid eye disease. Typically, it develops within 12 months of the onset of hyperthyroidism but may precede it or develop concurrently with it.

Very rarely, dysthyroid eye disease may occur in the presence of autoimmune primary hypothyroidism.

Stimulating TSH receptor antibodies are inevitably found.

Fibroblastic deposition of glycosaminoglycans and lymphocytic infiltration into the extraocular muscles and retrobulbar connective tissue produces retrobulbar oedema. This is followed by fibrosis with restricted movement as the muscles become tethered to the surrounding structures.

Consequently:

- The eye is pushed forwards and there is axial proptosis The cornea may become exposed with drying, irritation and later ulceration.
- Extraocular muscle movement is impaired.
- Increasing pressure is exerted on the optic nerve with loss of acuity and eventually, atrophy.
- Venous drainage from the orbit is impaired resulting in conjunctival and periorbital oedema, and conjunctival injection.

Clinical Features

- 5-10% cases are unilateral.

Presentation may include:

- Orbital pain
- Lacrimation
- Photophobia
- Blurred or double vision.

Features found on examination may include:

- Proptosis—usually bilateral, often asymmetric; less commonly, symmetrical.
- Lid retraction and lid lag.
- Periorbital puffiness.
- Impaired extraocular muscle function.
- Chemosis–conjunctival oedema–and injection
- Exposure keratitis; possibly, corneal ulceration.
- Ophthalmoplegia—generally superior rectus producing diplopia maximal on upward and outward gaze.

- Reduced visual acuity.
- Papilloedema; optic atrophy.
- Pretibial dermopathy (the least common manifestation of Grave's disease) occurs in patients with severe ophthalmology—generally occurs as a nodular or diffuse thickening of the skin of the anterior lower leg, but it can occur elsewhere.

The management of dysthyroid eye disease can be divided into immediate and longterm management.

The *immediate priorities* are to treat the endocrine disorder and render the patient euthyroid, prevent any visual loss and protect the cornea:

- Treatment of thyroid disease (although thyroid eye disease may occur before other signs of Graves' disease and does not always respond to treatment of thyroid disease); also thyroid eye disease may occur for the first time after hyperthyroidism treatment.
- Artificial tears are often required for lubrication
- eyelids can be taped closed or a lateral tarsorraphy can be undertaken (stitching the eyelids together at their outer corner).
- High dose steroids may facilitate medical decompression of the optic nerve (visual loss may occur due to compression of the optic nerve, particularly when there is minimal exopthalmos. Optic nerve function should be assessed in terms of colour vision and the presence of any central scotomas).
- Guanethidine eye-drops may reduce lid retraction (often patient does not tolerate longterm treatment)
- Surgical decompression may be employed—this surgery utilises space in ethmoidal, sphenoidal and maxillary sinuses.
- Orbital radiotherapy—this treatment modality is increasingly utilised at an early stage in management of thyroid eye disease.
- A Fresnel prism stuck to one lens of a spectable may be used in the management of diplopia—this lens is changed with respect to changes in exophthalmus.

Longterm management aims to restore external ocular muscle function and restore appearance.

There is evidence that thyroid eye disease may occasionally be made worse by treatment with radioiodine (1).

Treatment with bromocriptine, somatostatin analogues, plasmapharesis and acupuncture have been suggested for the management of this condition but a role for these agents requires confirmation (1).

Note that thyroid-eye disease generally goes into spontaneous remission with time (1).

Neonatal Hyperthyroidism

This uncommon condition results from transplacental passage of stimulating IgG TSH-receptor antibodies to the infant from a mother with a past or current history of Graves' disease.

The maternal concentration of stimulating TSH-receptor antibodies must be high for the neonate to be affected and maternal pre-tibial myxoedema serves a useful marker of the maternal state.

Clinical Features

Presentation is with:

- Goitre
- Exophthalmus
- Failure to thrive
- Fever
- Often marked tachycardia and cardiac failure if treatment is delayed.

Treatment

The condition is often self-limiting since the maternal immunoglobulins have a half-life of about three weeks in the infant.

Short term treatment with carbimazole and propranolol may be life saving.

Thyroid function tests should be regularly monitored in affected babies.

THYROID CANCER

Thyroid carcinoma is rare, having an annual incidence of about 3-5 per 100,000.

Thyroid cancer accounts for about 0.4% of all cancer deaths. Women are affected more commonly than men in a ratio of 2-3:1.

Types

- Papillary adenocarcinoma : 60—80%
- Follicular adenocarcinoma : 20—25%
- Medullary adenocarcinoma : 5%
- Anaplastic carcinoma : 5%
- Thyroid lymphoma : <1%.

Aetiology

Little is known about the aetiology of thyroid cancer. Low dose radiation may be an important factor as many cases have been reported 10-30 years after X-ray exposure.

There is evidence that individuals treated with radioiodine have a small but significant increase in the incidence of thyroid cancer (1).

Clinical Features

A rapidly growing hard thyroid mass with lymphadenopathy and indicators of extrathyroidal invasion e.g. hoarseness, dysphagia is suggestive of maligancy. Other important factors to elicit are a history of exposure to ionizing radiation and a family history of thyroid cancer.

The exact presentation varies with the type of tumour for example:

- Papillary—very slow growth; often spreads to lymph nodes in the neck. The most common thyroid cancer.
- follicular—usually middle aged women. Often spread to bones and lungs.
- medullary—20% of cases associated with MEN-II; raised calcitonin, cervical nodes often affected; may present with intractable diarrhoea and flushing anaplastic—usually in older patient; may present with a firm rapidly growing.

Investigations

- Fine needle biopsy—the most effective method of distinguishing benign from malignant nodules. Results usually expressed as positive, suspicious, non-diagnostic or negative.
- Tumour products—basal and pentagastrin-stimulated serum calcitonin distinguishes medullary carcinoma. Serum thyroglobulin is non-diagnostic and may be found in benign and malignant lesions
- Ultrasound—not useful as a primary test but may help to distinguish cystic lesions—nearly always benign—from solid lesions.
- Thyroid scanning with radioiodine—thyroid cancer is characteristically a 'cold nodule' on radioisotope scanning of the thyroid; hot nodules rarely malignant. Not a primary test (Fig. 9.2).

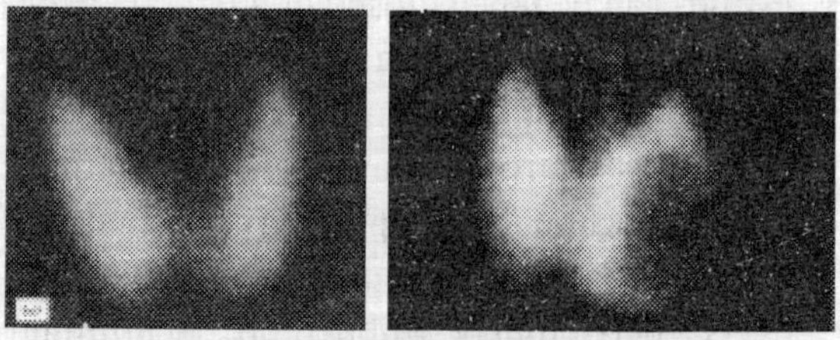

Fig. 9.2

Scintiscans of thyroid. The scan on the left is normal. A typical scan of a "cold" thyroid nodule failing to accumulate iodide isotope is shown on the right.

- Chest X-ray—lung secondaries
- Tthyroid mass, stridor, vocal

Management

Most thyroid tumours are treated surgically with follow up radioiodine ablation if the tumour will concentrate I^{131}.

Papillary and follicular tumours are usually treated by near total or total thyroidectomy. An ipsilateral total lobectomy and isthmusectomy is indicated if only one lobe is affected. Following surgery, most centres will then ablate all residual functioning thyroid tissue with radioactive iodine over a period of 6-12 months. Others would propose administering suppressive doses of thyroxine and monitoring the patient for possible recurrence but this has become less fashionable recently.

Medullary and anaplastic tumours do not generally take up I^{131} and are both treated by total thyroidectomy. Cervical lymph node dissection and external irradiation may also be performed.

Prognosis

Better differentiated tumours carry a better prognosis:

- Papillary—20 year survival is greater than 90% if the carcinoma is small and intra-thyroidal. The prognosis is is slightly worse in the elderly where there is a greater tendency to more aggressive disease and lung metastasis in the form of lymphangitis carcinomatosa.
- Follicular—20 year survival is 60-70%. Angioinvasion is associated with greater mortality
- Medullary—20 year survival is 70-80%. Less differentiated variants have a poorer survival.
- Anaplastic—20 year survival is less than 5%. Most die within 1 year.

Urgent Referral for Suspected Thyroid Cancer

Urgent referral:

- Hoarseness that persists for more than 6 weeks
- Ulceration of oral mucosa that persists for more than 3 weeks.
- Oral swellings that persist for more than 3 weeks
- If there are red or red and white patches seen on examination of the oral mucosa.
- Dysphagia that persists for 3 weeks.
- Unilateral nasal obstruction especially when associated with purulent discharge.
- If there is unexplained tooth mobility that is not associated with periodontal disease.
- Unresolving neck masses for more than 3 weeks
- The presence of cranial neuropathies.
- An orbital mass or orbital masses.

The level of suspicion is further increased if the patient is a heavy alcohol drinker or heavy smoker and is aged over 45 years and male. The chewing of tobacco (called Gutkha in India) or the chewing of Paan Masala or Betel should also increase the level of suspicion.

1. Papillary Adenocarcinoma of the Thyroid

This is the most commonly recognised thyroid cancer and the most easily diagnosed by fine needle biopsy. It accounts for over 60% of thyroid carcinoma. Women are affected more often than men. Papillary carcinomas occur rather evenly from the third to seventh decade and account for 80% of all thyroid cancer in individuals under 40 years of age.

Histologically, it shows papillae around a fibrovascular stalk and usually contains elements of follicular differentiation. It is slow growing and may be asymptomatic for many years. It is often multifocal. Local spread to regional nodes in the neck and mediastinum is common and 50% of patients show nodal metastases at the time of death.

It is not uncommon for a local lymph node metastasis to be detected before the primary tumour. Early metastases of this type have been termed "lateral aberrant thyroid".

Distant metastasis to the lungs or bone is rare.

2. Follicular Adenocarcinoma of the Thyroid

This accounts for 20-25% of thyroid cancer with females affected three times as frequently as males and with a peak incidence at 55 years of age. It is usually unifocal and rarely spreads to lymph nodes. It is angioinvasive to lungs and bone in over 50% of cases and this may be the first sign of malignancy.

It is a well differentiated tumour and shows reasonable response to TSH. It may take up iodine and may form thyroid hormones. Very rarely, it produces hyperthyroidism.

3. *Medullary Adenocarcinoma of the Thyroid*

This is a malignancy of the parafollicular cells of the thyroid.

This is a relatively uncommon thyroid carcinoma accounting for about 5% of thyroid malignancy. Both sexes are equally affected and the age of onset is variable. Aggressiveness is intermediate between that of well-differentiated and anaplastic lesions. About 80-90% of cases are sporadic; these usually affect adults and are unilateral. The other cases are familial, with an autosomal dominant inheritance; these tumours are typically bilateral and multifocal.

The medullary carcinoma arises from the parafollicular or C-cells of the thyroid which are of neural crest origin and form part of the APUD system. Calcitonin levels tend to be elevated and diagnostic. Levels of serum serotonin, ACTH and other peptides may also be raised. Spread to both regional lymph nodes and distant metastases to bone, liver and lung are common.

Diarrhoea and facial flushing are associated with medullary carcinomas of the thyroid.

Twenty percent of cases occur as part of the MEN-II syndrome.

4. *Anaplastic Carcinoma of the Thyroid*

This is seen most frequently in individuals over 60 years of age with an equal incidence in both sexes. It is an aggressive tumour which may arise from dedifferentiation of a papillary or follicular thyroid cancer. It accounts for about 5% of thyroid carcinomas.

Local invasion occurs to the trachea and to the oesophagous and the patient may present with dyspnoea or dysphagia respectively. Almost 80% of patients have a history of long-standing goitre.

Thyroid require total thyroidectomy and aggressive lymph node dissection.

Surgical Options

Partial Thyroid Lobectomy

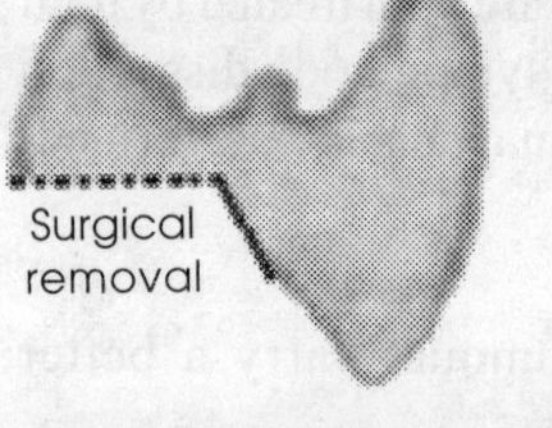

This operation is not performed very often because there are not many conditions which will allow this limited approach. Additionally, a benign lesion must be ideally located in the upper or lower portion of one lobe for this operation to be a choice.

Thyroid Lobectomy

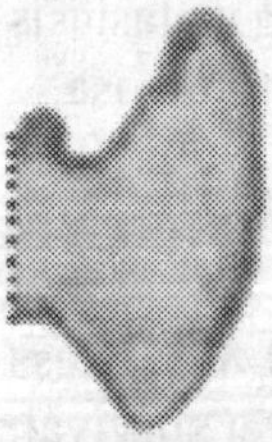

This is typically the "smallest" operation performed on the thyroid gland. It is performed for solitary dominant nodules which are worrisome for cancer or those which are indeterminate following fine needle biopsy. Also appropriate for follicular adenomas, solitary hot or cold nodules, or goiters which are isolated to one lobe (not common).

Thyroid Lobectomy with Isthmusectomy

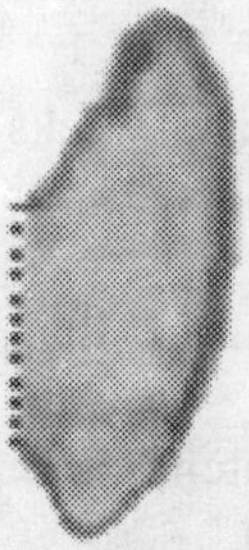

This simply means removal of a thyroid lobe and the isthmus (the part that connects the two lobes). This removes more thyroid tissue than a simple lobectomy, and is used when a larger margin of tissue is needed to assure that the "problem" has been removed.

Appropriate for those indications listed under thyroid lobectomy as well as for Hurthle cell tumors, and some very small and non-aggressive thyroid cancers.

Subtotal Thyroidectomy

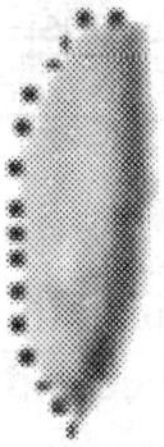

Just as the name implies, this operation removes all the "problem" side of the gland as well as the isthmus and the majority of the opposite lobe. This operation is typical for small, non-aggressive thyroid cancers. Also a common operation for goiters which are causing problems in the neck or even those which extend into the chest

Total Thyroidectomy

This operation is designed to remove all of the thyroid gland. It is the operation of choice for all thyroid cancers which are not small and non-aggressive in young patients. Many surgeons prefer this complete removal of thyroid tissue for *all* thyroid cancers regardless of the type.

GOITRE

A goitre is a non-specific term that is used to describe any enlargement of the thyroid (Fig. 9.3).

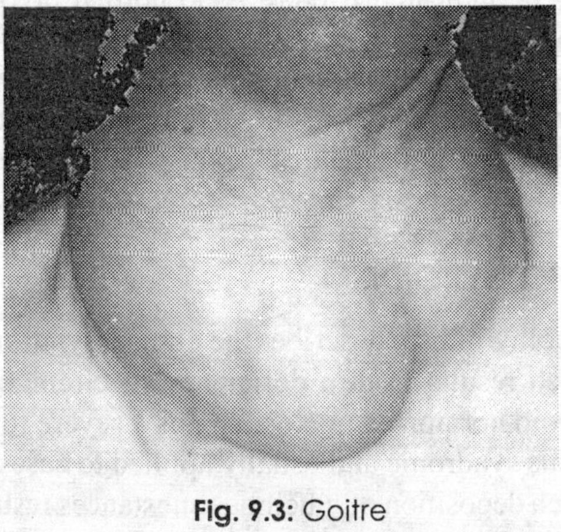

Fig. 9.3: Goitre

It is seen as a midline neck swelling which moves up on swallowing.

Goitres are more common in women than men.

Patterns of Thyroid Enlargement

Three patterns of thyroid enlargement are recognised:

- Diffuse:
  - painless:
  - iodine deficiency
  - simple goitre
  - goitrogens
  - dyshormogenesis
  - Grave's disease in remission
  - thyroiditis
  - infiltration, e.g. sarcoidosis
- Painful:
  - de Quervain's thyroiditis
  - Hashimoto's thyroiditis—rarely
- Multinodular
- Single nodule:
  - adenoma
  - carcinoma

Aetiology

Causes of goitre include:

- Physiological:
  - puberty—increased metabolic demand
  - pregnancy—increased demand; increased TBG
  - physiologic stress of any kind
- Autoimmune:
  - Graves' disease
  - Hashimoto's thyroiditis
- Thyroiditis:
  - subacute granulomatous/de Quervain's
  - subacute lymphocytic/silent
  - Riedel's thyroiditis—uncommon; gland usually shrinks
  - acute infective—transient
  - infiltrative e.g. sarcoidosis, tuberculosis
- Iodine deficiency—simple, endemic goitre

- Idiopathic—simple, sporadic goitre
- Multinodular goitre—develops from simple goitre
- Dyshormogenesis—including Pendred's syndrome:
  - Inability to use trapped iodine
  - Deficiency of peroxidase and dehalogenase
  - Abnormal protein binding in the plasma
    - § goitrogens
    - § thyroid cysts—rare
    - § thyroid tumour

History and Presentation

Many patients are asymptomatic. Features however, may include:

- Pain—in association with:
  - haemorrhage into a nodule
  - de Quervain's or rarely, Hashimoto's thyroiditis
  - rapidly growing neoplasm
- Choking attacks—which may occur even with quite small goitres

Large, retrosternal tumours may cause:

- Obstruction of the great veins
- Dysphagia
- Stridor—if more than 75% of the diameter of the trachea is compressed
- Recurrent laryngeal palsy—rare

Examination may reveal a bruit, especially in a toxic goitre

Investigations

Assessment of thyroid physiology:

- Thyroid function tests—TSH, T4 or T3; mandatory in all patients with goitre

Assessment of thyroid morphology:

- Chest X-ray—detection of tracheal compression
- Chest CT—if suspect malignant change in a retrosternal thyroid
- Ultrasound scan—differentiates solid, partly cystic and cystic changes

Assessment of thyroid pathology:

- Isotope scan—now technetium rather than radio-iodine.
- Fine needle aspiration biopsy: ultrasonographically-guided biopsy is both highly sensitive and specific for pathology when compared with definitive diagnosis at post-operative pathological examination

Management

Diffuse, non-toxic goitre—small goitres usually require little treatment apart from reassurance and possibly iodine supplements. Large goitres may be treated by subtotal thyroidectomy since thyroxine causes shrinkage in less than 30% of cases.

The treatment of choice for thyrotoxicosis caused by thyroid nodular disease is radioiodine (2).

Multinodular goitre—thyroxine is often successful in preventing progression and occasionally, in causing regression. *Surgery is indicated* if:

- There is retrosternal extension
- There is dysphagia attributed to the goitre
- There is marked tracheal deviation or stenosis
- There is a recurrent laryngeal palsy
- The goitre is cosmetically unacceptable
- The patient is hyperthyroid

A total thyroidectomy with lifelong thyroxine may be indicated if there is no normal thyroid tissue.

Solitary "cold" nodules"may be removed for cosmetic reasons or if shown to be malignant.

Solitary "hot" nodules—excised if associated with hyperthyroidism.

HYPOTHYROIDISM

Hypothyroidism describes the clinical syndrome which results from a deficiency of circulating thyroid hormones; myxoedema is a severe form of this syndrome and usually applied to cases in which deposition of mucinous substances results in thickening of the skin and subcutaneous tissues.

The prevalence is approximately 15 per 1000 in females and 1 per 1000 in males with a peak in the fifth or sixth decades. However, any age group may be affected.

Onset is extremely insidious and symptoms may be unnoticed for several years. Lethargy, fatigue and physical and mental slowness are common presenting features in adults; in children, cretinism may result.

Types

1. Congenital
2. Neonatal
3. Subclinical

Congenital Hypothyroidism

Congenital hypothyroidism occurs in about 1 in 4000 live births in the UK, twice as often in females than in males.

The development of the central nervous system is intrinsically reliant on thyroxine from early foetal life, and some infants may have developed irreversible brain damage before birth. However, neonatal screening with the commencement of thyroxine therapy within 2 weeks of birth has enabled many infants to attain normal intellectual development.

Infants with primary hypothyroidism have raised TSH and lowered thyroxine.

Presenting features include:

- Coarse facies, with macroglossia
- Dry skin
- Hoarse cry
- Hypotonia
- Hypothermia
- Umbilical hernia
- *Prolonged jaundice*
- Constipation
- Presence of a goitre suggests a goitrogen aetiology
- The *posterior fontanelle remains open*, and closure of the anterior fontanelle is delayed
- The infant may be *anaemic*
- If untreated mental retardation may develop.

Treatment

This is by replacement with thyroxine, at first 25 micrograms per kilogram per day. The risk of overtreatment is advancement of bone age and subsequent reduced adult height; monitoring is therefore with growth measurement, bone age assessment and levels of free T4 and TSH.

With a stable clinical scenario children might require monitoring every few months in the first couple of years of life, falling to yearly monitoring after the 3rd birthday.

With such an apparently well child it is sometimes difficult for parents to remember to give thyroxine daily, but their memory may improve near to a clinic visit, relected by a normal T4 but a high TSH; the latter reflects a longer time period since it takes a longer time to correct.

Screening for congenital hypothyroidism : involves looking for high concentrations of neonatal blood TSH—this test discriminates better than low blood thyroxine, although it accepts a failure to recognise congenital pituitary hypothyroidism.

The screening works in parallel to the PKU screening program, so allowing it to be implemented at minimal extra cost and organisation.

The prevalence of this condition appears to have increased since the introduction of the program, and it is hard to decide if this is a true increase in prevalence or a reflection of overdiagnosis or previous underdiagnosis.

The test is repeated in those being treated with a withdrawal of the treatment at one year.

Neonatal Hypothyroidism

Hypothyroidism late in foetal life—for example, from maternal iodine deficiency late in pregnancy—or during infancy affects somatic rather than neurological development. The hallmark of so called myxoedematous cretinism is marked growth retardation; intellectual development may not be impaired as thyroxine levels in the early critical phases of brain development are normal.

Diagnosis of neonatal hypothyroidism is readily confirmed by thyroid function tests and the condition responds well to thyroxine or iodine supplementation.

Subclinical Hypothyroidism

This is defined as an elevated serum TSH but a normal serum thyroxine concentration in an asymptomatic patient. The most common cause is chronic autoimmune thyroiditis (occurs in 3% of adults and 10% of postmenopausal women). Some patients with subclinical hypothyroidism will have common and nonspecific symptoms such as tiredness or weight gain.

The rate of progression from subclinical to overt hypothyroidism has been stated as less than 3% per annum (1). However, in those patients with positive thyroid antibodies, it can be that up to 80% of patients will develop overt hypothyroidism over a four year period (2).

Management

- Some authorities suggest it is better to treat subclinical hypothyroidism before overt hypothyroidism develops, especially in patients with positive thyroid antibodies as the rate of progression to overt hypothyroidism is much higher in these patients.
- In patients with only slightly raised TSH (less than 10 mU/L), without antithyroid antibodies (thyroid peroxidase autoantibodies), treatment may be deferred as the conversion rate to overt hypothyroidism is less than 3% per year (1).
- Increased TSH may be transient and may reflect a non-thyroidal illness or transient thyroiditis from which the patient is recovering.
  - do not start treatment on the basis of a single raised TSH level in people who are antibody negative (1,3)—it is prudent to repeat the measurement after about 3 months (2,3).
- Prodigy guidance suggests treatment should usually be commenced if diagnosis is confirmed on repeat testing 3 months later (3).
  - however if the TSH level is only slightly raised (less than 10 mU/l), and antithyroid antibodies are not present, then treatment may be deferred (providing follow-up is assured) (3).
- The aims of treatment is to restore serum TSH concentration to within the reference range; levels below this range may be associated with an increased risk of developing atrial fibrillation. However overall, the risks of thyroxine therapy are probably minimal provided the TSH is kept within the normal range, and a trial of treatment in symptomatic patients with subclinical hypothyroidism may be acceptable (2).
  - if thyroxine therapy is initiated then a usual starting dose would be 50-100 mcg per day (although 25 mcg per day may be sufficient).
  - start with 25 mcg daily and increase cautiously if coexistent heart disease or the elderly (3).

Aetiology

Hypothyroidism may be classified into:

- Primary hypothyroidism where the pathology affect the thyroid gland itself.
- Secondary hypothyroidism where the thyroid gland is normal but the production of stimulatory factors is disordered.

Investigations in hypothyroidism

- Primary hypothyroidism is indicated by a reduction in free and total T4, and elevated serum TSH.
- Elevated serum TSH with normal serum T4 indicates subclinical hypothyroidism.

- Free or total serum T3 is generally unhelpful since it may be only slightly reduced in severe hypothyroidism, or may be elevated by illness unrelated to thyroid function, or as a consequence of incorrect drug therapy.
- Secondary hypothyroidism is suggested by reduced free or total T4 and TSH below or within normal range; other tests for hypothalamic/ pituitary function are necessary.
- Other tests of thyroid function—e.g. thyroidal uptake tests, serum cholesterol have limited value in the diagnosis.
- Primary myxoedema may demonstrate a normal or exaggerated response of TSH to TRH; a negative TSH response excludes primary hypothyroidism but not a secondary cause.
- Antithyroid antibodies are suggestive of aetiology only.

Other possible features:

- Normochromic macrocytic anaemia.
- CK, AST and LDH may be elevated (due to abnormal muscle membranes).

Treatment of Hypothyroidism

Symptomatic patients are treated with thyroxine. Initially a relatively small dose of thyroxine (25–50 microgrammes per day) is given for the first four weeks and then this is altered depending on response. Normally, a single oral dose of 50-150 microgrammes per day is effective long term treatment.

Special consideration should be given to patients with ischaemic heart disease because the resultant increase in heart rate may precipitate worsening angina, myocardial infarction or even death. Thyroxine should be given in low dose—25 microgrammes daily or on alternate days—and in conjunction with beta blockers e.g. propranolol.

Dosage is increased gradually until euthyroidism is reached. Note that the half-life of thyroxine is approximately 7 days and therefore any change in dosage will take approximately 4 weeks to be assessed accurately by TSH test (TSH had a half-life on approximately 1 hour).

THYROIDITIS

The most common and well characterised forms of thyroiditis are:

- Hashimoto's or autoimmune thyroiditis
- De Quervains or subacute granulomatous thyroiditis
- subacute lymphocytic or painless thyroiditis
- Riedel's thyroiditis

Less common and less characterised forms are:

- Acute or infective thyroiditis
- Infiltrative thyroiditis e.g. sarcoidosis, tuberculosis.

Hashimoto's Thyroiditis

This is an autoimmune disorder characterised by extensive infiltration of the thyroid parenchyma by lymphocytes and plasma cells, with the formation of germinal centres. It is the most common cause of sporadic goitrous hypothyroidism in non-iodine deficient areas. Peak incidence is between 30 and 50 years of age with a female predominance of 15:1.

Pathogenesis

The basic defect in Hashimoto's disease appears to be a deficiency of antigen-specific suppressor T cells. This permits uncontrolled attack on the follicular cells by cytotoxic T cells with simultaneous unregulated T helper cell participation in the formation of autoantibodies by B-cells.

The autoantibodies most consistently found in Hashimoto's disease are to the TSH receptor and to thyroid microsomes. Those to the TSH receptor are thyroid growth stimulating immunoglobulins. Less commonly, there are autoantibodies to thyroglobulin and to follicular cell membranes.

Thyroid enlargement probably reflects:

- Thyroid growth without increased hormone synthesis.
- Lymphocytic infiltration.
- Occasionally, increased TSH levels.

The thyroglobulin and thyroid microsomal antibodies are probably secondary to follicular cell damage initiated by cytotoxic T cells.

The association with the HLA-DR5 genotype may indicate a genetic predisposition to this pattern of autoantibody production.

It is associated with the HLA-DR5 genotype.

Morphology

Classically, the gland is symmetrically enlarged with the capsule intact and rarely adherent to the surrounding structures. Microscopically, there is extensive replacement of the gland by lymphocytes, plasma cells and macrophages with the formation of lymphoid germinal centres. Fibrosis is rare and confined to the interlobula septa.

The less common fibrosing variant shows less thyroid enlargement, less lymphoid infiltration and more fibrosis. Unlike Riedel's thyroiditis, however, the fibrosis does not extend beyond the capsule.

Clinical Features

Classically, presentation is with a goitre or hypothyroidism or both.

The thyroid may be barely palpable or greatly enlarged. Characteristically, it is firm, and well defined with an enlarged pyramidal lobe and palpable neighbouring lymph nodes. Enlargement is usually slow and painless.but rarely, may be more rapid and painful.

At presentation, 75% of patients are euthyroid, 20% are hypothyroid, and 5% are hyperthyroid—a disease known as hashitoxicosis. About 50% eventually become hypothyroid because of destruction of the thyroid gland.

There appears to be an increased incidence of lymphoma but not of thyroid carcinoma.

Associated Conditions

Other autoimmune disorders associated with the disease include:

- Systemic lupus erythematous
- Rheumatoid arthritis
- Pernicious anaemia
- Vitiligo
- Type II diabetes mellitus
- Grave's disease
- Turner's syndrome—females with Turner's syndrome have a much higher incidence of autoimmune thyroiditis than the general population.

Diagnosis

The condition may be suspected clinically on the basis of the goitre with or without hypothyroidism.

Serum TSH is usually raised.

Measurement of antithyroid antibodies reveal:

- Antithyroid peroxidase antibodies (previously known as thyroid microsomal antibodies)—high titre.
- Thyroglobulin antibodies—low titre.

The gland may feel lumpy or irregular and biopsy may be necessary to distinguish it from a carcinoma of the thyroid. Surgical incision has been likened to cutting through an unripe pear.

If the patient is hypothyroid then oral thyroxine may keep the patient euthyroid and lead to resolution of the goitre.

de Quervain's Thyroiditis

This is a distinctive form of self-limited thyroiditis noted for painful enlargement of the thyroid gland in association with fever and hyperthyroidism. It most commonly affects people in the second to fifth decade, with a female predominance of 3:1. The condition is widely believed to be triggered by a virus infection—

mumps, influenza, Coxsackie, adenovirus or ECHO.

Characteristically, levels of T3 and T4 are increased but the uptake of radioactive iodine is low or absent.

Pathophysiology

The early stages are characterised by glandular enlargement, follicular disruption and neutrophilic invasion. Later, macrophages and multinucleate giant cells are seen enveloping fragments of colloid. These resemble granulomas.

Viral antibodies are detectable in about half of cases.

The initial transient hyperthyroidism is produced by the leakage of preformed thyroid hormones from the damaged follicular cells. Follicular disruption also explains the low or absent uptake of radioactive iodine.

The ensuing transient hypothyroidism is due to gland destruction. Regeneration of the follicles, usually from the edges of the most severely affected areas, results in restoration of thyroid function.

Clinical Features

Presentation is with:

- Sudden, painful enlargement of the thyroid mimicking a "sore throat" or "ear ache"
- Flu-like symptoms
- General features of hyperthyroidism

Typically, both lobes are enlarged but rarely, one lobe is affected. Painful dysphagia is common.

Blood tests reveal high ESR, raised T4 and T3, and suppressed TSH. Uptake of radioactive iodine is low.

Characteristically, the condition progresses through a phase of transient hyperthyroidism, followed 4-6 weeks later by a similar period of transient hypothyroidism. The patient is usually euthyroid 4-6 months after the onset of the illness.

Management

- Beta blockers may be required to control toxic symptoms in the hyperthyroid phase.
- Pain in the thyroid usually responds to aspirin but in more severe cases, may require a short course of prednisolone.

Relapses occur in up to 47% of patients, usually in the first year.

Subacute Lymphocytic Thyroiditis

- Subacute lymphocytic thyroiditis may present with painless goitrous enlargement or hyperthyroidism, or both. Generally, the levels of T3 and T4 are raised, while thyroid uptake of radioactive iodine is low.
- The condition is relatively common in the USA where it may account for 15% of all cases of hyperthyroidism. It is less common in the UK. Silent thyroiditis may occur at any age but is most frequently reported in the 12 months following childbirth—so called postpartum thyroiditis.
- Aetiology is obscure. There is no clear association with viral infection, de Quervains thyroiditis, Hashimoto's disease or primary hypothyroidism. This condition is mediated by antithyroid peroxidase antibodies (formerly known as antimicrosomal antibodies) and thyroid stimulating immunoglobulin (as seen in Graves' disease) are not present (1).
- Morphologically, it is characterised by foci of lymphocytic infiltration, sometimes with increased interstitial fibrous tissue. There are no lymphoid germinal centres and few, if any, plasma cells
- The condition is self-limiting. Hyperthyroidism is commonly followed by a phase of hypothyroidism may become permanent in 25% of patients (1).
- Patients with this condition are referred for pecialist management.
- Antithyroid drugs and radioiodine are unhelpful—this is because hyperthyroidism is

secondary to thyroid distruction causing increased thyroxine release. Beta blockers may provide symptomatic relief.

Riedel's Thyroiditis

This is an extremely rare sclerosing disease of unknown aetiology. It is characterised by replacement of the thyroid parenchyma with dense fibrous tissue which extends beyond the thyroid capsule into surrounding structures in the neck. Peak incidence is in the fourth to seventh decade with a female predominance of 3:1.

Usually, the main complaint is of a painless lump in the neck. Rarely, there may be dysphagia, dyspnoea, stridor, or suffocation. Hypothyroidism occurs in 25-50% of cases. The thyroid is woody or iron-hard. It is usually markedly contracted and difficult to palpate. Rarely, it may be of normal size or slightly enlarged. Occasionally there may be features of compression.

The condition may resemble an infiltrating carcinoma and may be associated with other idiopathic fibrosing conditions such as sclerosing cholangitis and fibrous mediastinitis.

Surgery may be needed to relieve pressure on the trachea. It is uncommon for thyroidectomy to be required.

Thyroiditis (Acute)

Infection of the thyroid is rare. It usually occurs in young children or debilitated patients. Most often, it occurs secondary to infection elsewhere.

Bacterial infection is most common. Agents include staphylococcal aureus—in one third of cases—streptococci, Salmonella, Enterobacter and mycobacteria. Fungal infection is rare.

Presentation is usually with painful enlargement of the thyroid gland.

The condition is usually transient. It may be treated with surgical drainage and antibiotics.

Long term thyroid dysfunction is rare.

ADRENAL GLAND DISEASES

PHAEOCHROMOCYTOMA

Phaeochromocytomas are functional tumours that arise from chromaffin cells in the adrenal medulla. They account for 0.1-0.2% of cases of systemic hypertension.

Phaeochromocytomas usually secrete a combination of noradrenaline and adrenaline, but some tumours may also secrete dopamine and rarely ACTH causing Cushing's syndrome.

Neoplasms of chromaffin cells may also arise in other parts of the body. By convention those arising outside the adrenal gland are referred to as extra-adrenal paragangliomas. Of these, chromaffin tumours arising from aortico-sympathetic paraganglia have histologic, biochemical and clinical similarities to phaeochromocytomas and are sometimes referred to as extra-adrenal phaeochromocytomas.

TEN PERCENT RULE

Phaeochromocytomas may be referred to as the 10% tumour:

- 10% are extra-adrenal, most commonly, in the organ of Zuckerkandl, located in the aortic bifurcation. Less than 1% are extra-abdominal.
- 10% are bilateral, increasing to 70% in familial cases.
- 10% are malignant, but the risk of malignancy in women is three fold that in men.

- 10% are multiple.
- 10% occur in children, but 25-30% of children have extra-adrenal and/or bilateral tumors.

Aetiology

The aetiology is not known but a significant genetic component is recognised. Ten percent are familial. These are invariably adrenal in origin, and are bilateral in 70%.

Phaechromocytomas may be associated with:

- Multiple endocrine neoplasia—MEN IIa, MEN IIb
- Other neuroectodermal disease:
  - neurofibromatosis—in 5% of cases of phaeochromocytoma.
  - von Hippel Lindau syndrome—rarely.
  - tuberous sclerosis.

Tumours that arise in association with MEN-II or von Hippel Lindau syndrome, in general, affect younger age groups.

Pathology

Phaeochromocytomas may arise as one or more discrete neoplasms within the adrenal medulla and particularly in MEN syndromes there may be surrounding diffuse or nodular hyperplasia.

The tumour mass varies widely but on average is approximately 100 gms. Large tumours may be encapsulated by connective tissue, and may contain areas of haemorrhage, necrosis or cyst formation. The cut surface may be grey or brown in colour, and the tumour due to its stored catecholamines reacts histochemically to dichromate producing a brown-black colouring.

Tumour cells resemble those of the normal adrenal medulla by being arranged in nests. There may be mitotic figures or nuclear pleomorphism, and tumour cells may be found in capillaries or sinusoids. None of these features however indicate that the tumour is one of the ten percent of phaeochromocytomas that are malignant. Malignancy may only be proved by the finding of distal metastases.

Clinical Features

All ages and races can be affected. The peak incidence is in the third and fourth decades of life. Men and women are equally affected.

Hypertension is the usual presenting feature. This may be sustained or paroxysmal with intervening periods of normotension.

Other symptoms related to catecholamine excess may present acutely as a hypertensive crisis, with features such as:

- Headache
- Palpitations
- Tachycardia
- Sweating
- Anxiety
- Panic attacks
- Tremor
- Nausea and vomiting
- Fever.

Virtually any stress can precipitate an attack, for example, exercise, emotion, postural changes, diagnostic procedures, or surgery. Occasionally, attacks occur spontaneously. Rarely, they are fatal.

Patients may show typical cardiovascular, cerebrovascular, and renal effects of prolonged hypertension, such as congestive heart failure with pulmonary oedema.

The diagnosis of phaeochromocytoma should be suspected:

- In any hypertensive with orthostatic hypotension and tachycardia.
- In any hypertensive whose symptoms respond poorly to anti-hypertensive treatment.
- In any patient whose blood pressure fluctuates widely.
- In any hypertensive with cafe au lait spots.

Diagnosis

A diagnosis of phaeochromocytoma can be confirmed from:

- 24 hour urinary free catecholamines, VMA's
- High performance liquid chromatography assay of plasma adrenaline and noradrenaline. Samples must be taken from an indwelling catheter to avoid the consequences of stress at the time of venepuncture. However, this is said to be the most reliable method of diagnosis.
- Clonidine suppression test
- pentolinium suppression test.

The tumour may be localised by:

- Abdominal CT
- MIBG scanning
- Adrenal angiography.

Differential Diagnosis

Phaeochromocytoma is a great mimic. Its differential diagnosis includes:

- Essential hypertension
- Migraine
- Thyrotoxicosis
- Alcohol withdrawal
- Carcinoid syndrome
- Hypoglycaemia
- Angina pectoris
- Pre-eclampsia, eclampsia or simple hypertension of pregnancy.

Management

Initial pharmacological treatment permits optimal surgical interventions. Alpha adrenoreceptor blockade with phenoxybenzamine is commenced a few days before beta blockade with propranolol. The intravascular hypovolaemia is corrected over 7-10 days prior to surgery.

The tumour is localised using the following imaging methods:

- CT scan—which can detect tumours greater than 1 cm in diameter.
- 131 I-meta-iodobenzylguanidine (MIBG) scintigraphy:
  - more sensitive than CT
  - MIBG is specifically concentrated in adrenergic cells and is useful for assessing metastases.

Surgery is curative in 75% of cases.

Excessive handling of the tumour peroperatively should be avoided as this may release large amounts of catecholamine into the circulation resulting in severe, acute hypertension.

Vasodilators such as sodium nitroprusside, and intra-venous alpha- and beta-blockers should be available during surgery in the event of a hypertensive crisis.

Operative mortality is at least 3%.

When surgery is not possible, consider treatment with:

- Phenoxybenzamine and propranolol
- Alpha-methyl-p-tyrosine—inhibits the hydroxylation of tyrosine to dopa and so, reduces synthesis of adrenaline and noradrenaline.

Prognosis

Prognosis is dependent on the presence or absence of complications of hypertension e.g. cerebrovascular accident, renal impairment.

- Mortality from elective surgery—less than 2%; approximately 80% of patients become normotensive following surgery.
- Ninety six percent 5-year survival with benign disease.
- Forty five percent 5-year survival with malignant disease.
- Recurrence rate—less than 10%.

ADRENOCORTICAL TUMOURS

Adrenocortical tumours account for about 25% of the cases of hypercortisolism. About 50% of adrenocortical tumours are malignant.

Clinical Features

Adrenocortical tumours may cause:

- Hypercortisolism

- Virilising or feminising syndromes, including pseudoprecocious puberty
- They can also be a cause of hyperaldosteronism.

Treatment of Adrenocortical Tumours

Treatment is by surgical excision.

Treatment of recurrent tumours can be achieved by drug therapy, for example metyrapone for Cushing's syndrome due to adrenal adenoma, op'-DDD used for treatment of Cushing's syndrome due to adrenal carcinoma. Patients with Conn's syndrome which is the result of an inoperable tumour may be treated with spironolactone—an aldosterone antagonist.

Ten

Brain Tumors

It is possible for any type of cell within the brain or spinal cord to undergo neoplastic change. The bony confines of the skull means that mere growth and displacement of existing tissue causes disturbance-hence the phrase space occupying lesion; mass effects and focal signs result. Some are invasive and replace normal tissue.

The most common primary brain tumour is the glioma. Primary tumours of the neurones are rare. Secondary metastases are common, spreading through the bloodstream or by direct invasion.

Children and adults tend to be affected by different tumours. Medulloblastomas, pilocytic cerebellar astrocytomas, teratomas, pinealomas and craniopharyngiomas are confined to children and adolescents. Gliomas of the hemispheres, meningiomas, neurinomas, pituitary adenomas are seen in adult life into old age.

INCIDENCE

Brain tumours may be histologically malignant but rarely metastasise outside the brain. About 20% are secondary metastases-most commonly, lung then breast and kidney. Of the primaries, the majority are gliomas (43%), followed by meningiomas (10%), and pituitary adenomas (10%). Others are comparatively rare.

Their incidence shows two age peaks-in children between 5-9 years of age, and in late middle age. In children, medulloblastomas of the posterior fossa are the dominant cerebral tumour whilst in adults, gliomas, meningiomas and metastases are the most common.

Pathology

- Neuroepithelial
- Nerve sheath
- Meninges
- Blood vessel-haemangioblastoma
- Germ cell-germinoma, teratoma
- Tumours of maldevelopment
- Anterior pituitary-adenoma, adenocarcinoma
- Local extension to nervous system
- Primary malignant lymphoma
- Metastases distribution
- Cerebral hemispheres:
  - extrinsic-meningioma, cysts (dermoid, epidermoid, arachnoid)
  - intrinsic-astrocytoma, glioblastoma, oligodendroglioma, primary lymphoma, metastasis
- Hypothalamus:
  - astrocytoma
- Sellar/suprasellar region:
  - pituitary adenoma, craniopharyngioma, meningioma, optic nerve glioma, cysts (dermoid, epidermoid)
- Skull base and sinuses:
  - carcinomatous meningitis, chordoma, glomus, osteoma

- Ventricular system:
  - colloid cyst, choroid plexus papilloma, ependymoma, germinoma, teratoma, meningioma
- Pineal region:
  - ependymoma, germinoma, teratoma, meningioma, pineal cytoma/blastoma, astrocytoma
- Posterior fossa:
  - extrinsic-trigeminal and acoustic neuroma, meningioma, cysts (dermoid, epidermoid, arachnoid), metastasis
  - intrinsic-metastases, haemangioblastoma, medulloblastoma, astrocytoma

Clinical Features

The clinical features of intracranial tumours vary according to the site of the lesion and its type. Symptoms usually occur insidiously over weeks or years with often only minor intellectual and emotional impairment; more rarely, they may present acutely due to haemorrhage or the development of hydrocephalus.

Mass effects of intracranial tumours:

- Raised intracranial pressure and brain shift due to space occupying lesion or to obstructive hydrocephalus, leading to:
  - supratentorial-tentorial herniation
  - infratentorial-tonsillar herniation

Focal Damage

- Seizures-present in over one third of patients with intrinsic tumours of the cerebral hemispheres. Late onset-in the third decade or later-and of no obvious cause should raise the suspicion of a brain tumour. Epileptiform convulsions are more frequent with slow growing than rapidly growing tumours. Epilepsy is infrequent with tumours of the posterior fossa or brainstem.
- Disturbed function:
  - supratentorial-cerebral-cranial nerves I-VI damage
  - infratentorial-cerebellar-cranial nerves III-XII damage

Differential Diagnosis

The differential diagnosis will vary in detail according to the particular tumour being considered, but in general should include all other causes of intracranial mass lesions:

- Vascular origin:
  - haematoma
  - giant aneurysm
  - arteriovenous malformation
  - infarction with oedema
  - venous thrombosis
  - (migraine-vascular aetiology still uncertain)
- Trauma:
  - haematoma
  - contusion
- Infection:
  - abscess
  - tuberculoma
  - sarcoidosis
  - encephalitis
- Cysts

There are several broad symptomatological clues that restrict the choice of differentials:

- Vascular lesions, e.g. infarction/haemorrhage, are rapid in onset, produce a substantial deficit initially, and generally improve with time.
- Migraine rarely presents for the first time in adult life and may give a history of intermittent headache of duration longer than one year.
- Abscesses usually have a short history from the onset of symptoms, may be secondary to an obvious penetrating focus, and can present with no systemic signs of infection.
- *Cysts:* arachnoid cysts are not usually progressive; parasitic cysts usually have a history of geographical exposure to the infective agent.

Investigations

The aim of investigating intracranial tumours is to confirm their presence, the site of growth, and pathology.

- Chest X-ray, ESR } helps establish whether a primary tumor or metastasis
- Skull X-ray-look for signs of raised intracranial pressure, e.g. suture separation; calcification,

e.g. hyperostosis of adjacent bone in meningioma; erosion of posterior clinoids, e.g. craniopharyngioma; osteolytic lesions, e.g. dermoid, epidermoid, meningiomas
- CT scan-the investigation of choice for many tumours; note site, e.g. frontal/occipital, extrinsic/intrinsic; mass effects, e.g. midline shift; multiplicity of lesions; effect of contrast enhancement
- MRI-particularly valuable for tumours around the skull base and in the posterior fossa
- Angiography-helps differentiate certain tumours, e.g. meningiomas, secondary tumours and gliomas; also used to exclude arteriovenous malformations/aneurysms
- Biopsy-burr hole, stereotactic, open with decompression
- CSF examination-lumbar puncture is often contraindicated because of raised ICP, but CSF may be obtained from other sources, e.g. ventricular drainage on shunt insertion
- Tumour markers-alpha-fetoprotein and human chorionic gonadotrophin are reliable markers for germinomas

Management

There are no definitive guidelines for the management of intracranial tumours. Each lesion requires due consideration of:
- Grade-benign or malignant
- Site-how approachable
- Type-is this known with certainty and if so, does it lend itself to conservative treatment.

In general, conservative therapy is the treatment of choice wherever specific measures exist, e.g. pituitary adenomas.

Benign tumours are best treated by excision except where they are inaccessible or are attached to adjacent structures.

The management of malignant tumours and non-excisable benign lesions is more complex. Any existing oedema may be reduced using steroids such as dexamethasone with diuretics such as mannitol to lower ICP. The difficulty is then of deciding when and how to operate. Monitoring with repeat CT scans may be appropriate for small, asymptomatic tumours; the initial CT provides a baseline against which to assess the progress of the tumour.

Burr hole or stereotactic biopsy may be performed to further identify the histology of the lesion. Depending upon the nature and site of the tumour, this may then be followed by partial or complete removal.

Radiotherapy is often used either alone or following surgery. Many but not all intracranial tumours are radiosensitive.

Chemotherapy has to date been disappointing. The main difficulty is in finding a drug which will cross the blood brain barrier. BCNU, CCNU, vincristine and methotrexate may be used depending upon the tumour type.

Urgent Referral

- Progressive subacute neurological deficit developing over days to weeks (e.g. weakness, sensory loss, ataxia, dysphasia)
- New onset seizures characterised by one or more of the following:
  - characteristic focal seizures
  - prolonged focal post-ictal deficit (longer than one hour)
  - status epilepticus
  - the presence of an inter-ictal focal neurological deficit
- Patients with vomiting, headache AND papilloedema
- Cranial nerve palsy (e.g. visual failure including optician defined visual field loss, diplopia, unilateral sensorineural deafness)

Consider Urgent Referral

Patients with non-migranous headaches of recent onset, that have been present for at least one month, when accompanied by features suggestive of raised intra cranial pressure (e.g. patient woken by headache; drowsiness; vomiting).

Eleven

Hematologic Malignancies

MULTIPLE MYELOMA AND OTHER PLASMA CELL DYSCRASIAS

Multiple Myeloma

Multiple myeloma is a disseminated malignancy of monoclonal plasma cells that accounts for 8% of all hematologic cancers. In the year 2001, an estimated 14,400 new cases will be diagnosed in the United States and another 11,200 Americans will die of this disease. In the early 90s the incidence rates for myeloma decreased (13.1% in males and 8.7% in females), however, the mortality rate has increased (5.6% in men and 3.8% in women).

Epidemiology

Gender: Males are affected more frequently than females (1.4:1 ratio).

Age: The median age at presentation is 65 years, according to most tumor registries, although the median age reported in studies is approximately 60 years.

Race: The annual incidence per 100,000 population is 4.9 among white men and 3.4 among white women. Among black men and women, the frequency doubles to 9.8 and 8.0, respectively, per 100,000. This racial difference is not explained by socioeconomic factors and is presumably due to unknown genetic factors.

Geography: There is no clear geographic distribution of multiple myeloma. In Europe, the highest rates are noted in the Nordic countries, the United Kingdom, Switzerland, and Israel. France, Germany, Austria, and Slovenia have a lower incidence, and developing countries have the lowest incidence. This higher relative incidence in more developed countries probably results from the combination of a longer life expectancy and more frequent medical surveillance.

Survival: The 5-year survival rate for all patients treated with conventional therapy is approximately 25-30%. The 5-year survival rate is lower among patients ? 65 years old (20-25%) than in those < 65 years of age (30-35%).

Etiology and Risk Factors

No predisposing factors for the development of multiple myeloma have been confirmed.

Environment: Some causative factors that have been suggested include radiation exposure (radiologists and radium dial workers), occupational exposure (agricultural, chemical, metallurgical, rubber plant, pulp, and paper workers and leather tanners), and chemical exposure to benzene, formaldehyde, epichlorohydrin, hair dyes, paint sprays, and asbestos. None of these associations has proven to be statistically significant, and all have been contradicted by negative correlations. The initial report that survivors of the atomic bombings in Japan had an increased risk of developing myeloma has been refuted by longer follow-up.

Viruses: A preliminary report in a limited number of patients noted the presence of herpesvirus 8 in the dendritic cells of the bone marrow in patients with multiple myeloma. Further investigation is necessary to determine the significance of this infection, since interleukin-6 levels are high in patients with the virus and this cytokine is the major cell growth stimulus for myeloma.

Genetic factors: Although multiple myeloma is not an inherited disease, there have been numerous case reports of multiple incidence in the same family. However, a case-control study revealed no significant increase in incidence among relatives of patients who had multiple myeloma, other hematologic malignancies, or other cancers.

Monoclonal gammopathy of unknown significance (MGUS): Patients with MGUS develop myeloma, macroglobulinemic lymphoma, or amyloidosis at a rate of 1.5% per year.

Signs and Symptoms

The clinical features of multiple myeloma are quite variable. Findings that suggest the diagnosis include lytic bone lesions, anemia, azotemia, hypercalcemia, and recurrent infections. Approximately 20% of patients are free of symptoms and are diagnosed by chance.

Bone disease: Bone pain, especially from compression fractures of the vertebrae or ribs, is the most common symptom. At diagnosis, 70% of patients have lytic lesions, which are due to accelerated osteoclast formation resulting from cytokines that increase bone resorption in areas infiltrated with plasma cells.

Anemia: A normocytic, normochromic anemia is present in 60% of patients at diagnosis. This is due primarily to the decreased production of RBCs by marrow infiltrated with plasma cells. Patients with or without renal failure may also have decreased levels of erythropoietin, which may worsen the degree of anemia.

Hypercalcemia: Among newly diagnosed patients, 20% have hypercalcemia (corrected serum calcium level, > 11.5 mg/dL) secondary to progressive bone destruction, which may be exacerbated by prolonged immobility. Hypercalcemia should be suspected in patients with myeloma who have nausea, fatigue, confusion, polyuria, or constipation.

Renal failure: Approximately 20% of patients present with renal insufficiency and another 20% develop this complication in later phases of the disease. Casts of Bence Jones protein in the distal tubule are the most common cause of renal failure, but hypercalcemia, dehydration, and hyperuricemia are contributing factors. Uncommonly, amyloidosis or light-chain deposition disease may contribute to renal failure.

Infections: Many patients with myeloma develop bacterial infections that may be serious. In the past, gram-positive organisms (e.g., *Streptococcus pneumoniae, Staphylococcus aureus*) and *Hemophilus influenzae* were the most common pathogens. More recently, however, gram-negative organisms have become more frequent. The increased susceptibility of myeloma patients to bacterial infections has been attributed to impairments of host-defense mechanisms, such as hypogammaglobulinemia, granulocytopenia, and low cell-mediated immunity.

Screening and Diagnosis

No screening measures for multiple myeloma have been proven to provide any benefit.

The diagnosis usually requires the presence of bone marrow plasmacytosis and a monoclonal protein in the urine and/or serum (Table 11.1). One immunoglobulin class is produced in excess while the other immunoglobulin classes are usually depressed.

Table 11.1: Common laboratory features of plasma cell dyscrasias

Multiple myeloma
Marrow plasmacytosis > 15%
Monoclonal immunoglobulin peak (usually > 30 g/dL)
Decreased levels of uninvolved immunoglobulins
Presence of Bence Jones protein
Lytic bone lesions or diffuse osteopenia
Smouldering myeloma
Same as multiple myeloma but without symptoms
Hemoglobin > 10.5 g/dL
Monoclonal immunoglobulin peak (< 4.5 g/dL)
Normal serum calcium and creatinine levels
No lytic bone lesions
Solitary plasmacytoma of bone (SPB)
Solitary bone lesion due to plasma cell tumor
Normal bone marrow plasmacytosis
No anemia, hypercalcemia, or renal disease
Preserved levels of uninvolved immunoglobulins
Monoclonal gammopathy of unknown significance (MGUS)
Monoclonal immunoglobulin level < 3.0 g/dL
Bone marrow plasma cells < 10%
No none lesions
No symptoms due to plasma cell dyscrasia
Usually proserved levels of uninvolved immunoglobulins
Amyloidosis without myeloma
Same as MGUS plus evidence of amyloidosis on biopsy

Initial work-up The initial work-up for patients suspected of having a plasma cell dyscrasia should include:

- CBC with differential and platelets
- Routine serum chemistry panel (e.g., calcium, BUN, creatinine)
- Bone marrow aspirate to assess plasmacytosis
- Serum protein electrophoresis and immunofixation to define protein type
- 24-hour urine protein and electrophoresis
- Quantitative immunoglobulin levels
- Skeletal survey (bone scans contribute little since isotope uptake is often low in purely lytic bone disease)
- Cytogenetics

MRI is an excellent tool for evaluation of spinal cord compression/impingement. In addition, MRI identifies generalized signal abnormalities and focal lesions that can be monitored after therapy. MRI is especially useful in staging nonsecretory disease presenting as macrofocal lesions.

In addition, prognostic factors, such as β_2-microglobulin (β2M), C-reactive protein, lactate dehydrogenase (LDH), plasma cell labeling index, and ploidy, may provide useful data.

Laboratory and Pathologic Features

Peripheral blood: The peripheral blood smear may reveal a normocytic, normochromic anemia with rouleaux formation.

Bone marrow: Bone marrow examination usually reveals an increased number of plasma cells (> 15%). These cells are strongly positive for CD138, and cytoplasmic immunoglobulin (cIg) and are negative for CD5, CD20, and surface immunoglobulin (sIg) expression. Whereas normal plasma cells express CD19, malignant plasma cells lose this expression, and this may be related to loss of *Pax-5* gene expression. CD10 expression is generally negative but has sometimes been noted in advanced disease. Monoclonality may be demonstrated by immunoperoxidase staining with k and l antibodies.

The pattern of bone marrow involvement in plasma cell myeloma may be macrofocal. As a result, plasma cell count may be normal when an aspirate misses the focal aggregates of plasma cells that are better visualized radiographically or on direct needle biopsy.

Monoclonal proteins: The types of monoclonal protein produced are IgG (60%), IgA

(20%), IgD (2%), IgE (< 0.1%), or only light-chain k or l (18%). Biclonal elevations of myeloma proteins occur in < 1% of patients, and < 5% of patients are considered to have nonsecretory disease because their plasma cells do not secrete detectable levels of monoclonal immunoglobulin.

Staging and Prognosis

Different criteria have been used to stage myeloma at different institutions, primarily due to the lack of standard definitions and consistency among investigators. However, the Durie-Salmon staging system is employed most frequently. The variability in interpretation of staging criteria has resulted, in part, from imprecise quantification of the extent of bone lesions and from factors other than myeloma that contribute to hypercalcemia (e.g., immobility) or anemia (e.g., renal failure).

Prognosis

Cytogenetic abnormalities: Chromosomal abnormalities, especially loss of whole chromosome 13 (monosomy) or deletions of parts of chromosome 13 (13q), have been associated with inferior survival after both standard chemotherapy and high-dose therapy. Multivariate analysis has shown these chromosomal changes to be most the important predictors of survival.

β2M level: Serum β2M level is an important and convenient prognostic indicator. When cytogenetic changes are not studied, β2M is consistently the most important prognostic indicator on multivariate analysis. Because β2M is excreted by the kidneys, high levels are present in patients with renal failure; this complicates the interpretation of an elevated value.

LDH level: High LDH levels also have been associated with lymphoma-like extraosseous disease, plasma cell leukemia, plasma cell hypodiploidy, drug resistance, and shortened survival.

Other indicators: of shortened survival include elevated C-reactive protein, DNA hypodiploidy, low plasma cell RNA levels, high plasma cell labeling indices, plasmablastic histology, and expression of the common acute lymphoblastic leukemia antigen (cALLA). Patients with decreased plasma cell RNA or DNA hypodiploidy also are less likely to respond to chemotherapy.

Treatment Response Criteria

Since the criteria for treatment response among patients with multiple myeloma have varied among institutions, response rates have been difficult to compare. Bence Jones protein is reduced more rapidly in responders than is serum myeloma protein because of the rapid renal catabolism of light chains.

The University of Arkansas criteria for partial response (PR) are:

- > 75% reduction in serum myeloma protein
- > 95% reduction in Bence Jones protein to < 50 mg/24 h
- < 5% bone marrow plasma cells
- Criteria for complete response include:
- Disappearance of serum myeloma protein and Bence Jones protein by immunofixation
- No monoclonal plasma cells in bone marrow

Treatment

Exciting advances in tumor biology and micro-environment?and their potential interaction? Should identify unique targets for rational intervention therapeutics. The rational design of therapy hopefully will improve its outcome, which has not improved with conventional chemotherapy over the last 3 decades. Only 5-10% of myeloma patients live longer than 10 years and there is no hint of a cured subgroup.

PREVIOUSLY UNTREATED PATIENTS

Chemotherapy

MP: The combination of melphalan (Alkeran) and prednisone (MP) remains the standard regimen. The combination of multiple alkylating agents is not convincingly superior to MP. A meta-analysis of 18 published randomized trials comparing MP to other combination regimens arrived at the same conclusion. Combination chemotherapy is probably not superior to MP even in poor-risk patients. Approximately 40% of patients have responded to the MP regimen, with a median remission of 2 years and an overall median survival of 3 years.

Melphalan and other alkylating agents should be used sparingly or completely avoided in patients who are candidates for high-dose therapy, as prior therapy affects stem-cell procurement. Extensive use of alkylating agents may also predispose patients to the subsequent development of myelodysplastic syndrome (MDS) or acute myeloid leukemia (AML).

To standardize dosage for differences in melphalan absorption, evidence of adequate myelosuppression should be confirmed after 2-3 weeks. If the myeloma has failed to respond, the dose should be increased by 20% increments every 4-5 weeks until adequate myelosuppression occurs.

VAD-based regimens: are stem cell-sparing and do not impair stem-cell collection; these regimens are preferably employed for induction prior to high-dose therapy. Such regimens produced a response rate of 55% in untreated patients without an improvement in overall survival. Responses occurred more rapidly than with MP; these rapid responses provide an advantage in patients with hypercalcemia, renal failure, or severe bone pain. No dosage adjustment is necessary for renal failure.

Pulse dexamethasone: alone has also been useful in patients who need vertebral radiotherapy for spinal cord compression or for painful vertebral compressions that require immediate irradiation, as this approach avoids severe myelosuppression.

High-dose Therapy Following Induction

Employed after remission induction in newly diagnosed patients, high-dose therapy achieves a high complete response rate (30-50%). Significantly prolonged event-free and overall survival rates were observed in a randomized study, which enrolled patients < 65 years old. Older individuals tolerate high-dose therapy with peripheral stem-cell support well, without excess mortality. Moreover, outcome, in terms of event-free and overall survival, is comparable to that in matched cohorts < 65 years old. Hence, older individuals (? 65 years old) are also candidates for high-dose therapy. More recently, older patients receiving intermediate-dose melphalan (100 mg/m^2) with stem-cell support have been shown to have a better outcome, compared with matched controls receiving conventional therapy.

High-dose akylating agents combined with peripheral blood stem-cell support is now considered to be standard treatment of symptomatic myeloma patients without excessive comorbidity.

Radiotherapy

Higher doses of radiotherapy (40 Gy-50 Gy) are employed in local control and cure of solitary plasmacytoma of bone and extramedullary plasmacytoma. Lower doses (10 Gy-20 Gy) may be employed for palliation of local bone pain from tumor infiltration, pathologic fractures, and spinal cord compression. It should be emphasized that excellent pain relief may be obtained by prompt institution of high-dose corticosteroid therapy, especially in newly diagnosed patients.

Radiotherapy should be employed sparingly, as irradiation of multiple sites may impair stem-cell mobilization in patients who are candidates for high-dose therapy. Employment of high doses of radiation may preclude the subsequent use of total-body irradiation (TBI) as a conditioning regimen for high-dose therapy. TBI has been administered along with high-dose chemotherapy and stem-cell support. TBI contributes to a slight increase in mortality and morbidity. Registry studies suggest that addition of TBI may result in inferior survival , and there is no convincing evidence of its benefit. A randomized trial in progress should clarify this issue.

REMISSION MAINTENANCE

Alkylating agents

Maintenance therapy with alkylating agents has not prolonged remission and survival times, compared with no maintenance therapy followed by the resumption of MP upon disease relapse. Continued alkylating agent treatment also exposes approximately 2% of patients to the risk of myelodysplasia or acute leukemia. However, patients at high risk of early relapse may benefit from maintenance therapy.

REFRACTORY OR RELAPSING DISEASE

Approximately 50% of patients with newly diagnosed multiple myeloma have disease that is unresponsive to chemotherapy. Moreover, in virtually all patients who respond initially (with the exception of those few who die of unrelated diseases), the myeloma will relapse. Of patients who relapse after an unmaintained remission, approximately 60% achieve a second, shorter remission or maintain a stable tumor load with resumption of the original therapy.

VAD

VAD is the treatment of choice for disease relapsing after MP therapy. VAD produced responses in 40% of patients with relapsing disease, compared with 25% of patients with primary unresponsive disease.

Pulse dexamethasone (Decadron) alone induced results similar to VAD in patients with primary resistant disease (response rate, 25% vs 25-30%), but was inferior to VAD in relapsing patients (response rate, 25% vs 40%).

VAD-RESISTANT DISEASE

Combination Chemotherapy

High doses of alkylating agents, alone or in combination, have been effective in approximately one-third of patients with VAD-refractory disease. Intravenous melphalan (100 mg/m^2) or the combination of high-dose cyclophosphamide (Cytoxan, Neosar) and etoposide are two examples of such regimens.

Thalidomide

The striking activity of thalidomide (Thalomid) as a single agent in refractory disease has been confirmed in 180 patients treated on a dose-escalating schedule from 200 mg-800 mg in 200-mg increments. At least a 25% reduction in paraprotein occurred in 64 patients (36%) and 54 (33%) had > 50% reduction in paraprotein. More than 75% of patients achieved the second dose level and 50% received the highest dose level. The majority of patients had received previous high-dose therapy. The median duration of remission in responding patients was > 12 months. The main toxicities included constipation, sedation, and symptoms of peripheral neuropathy.

Other New Agents

Liposomal daunorubicin (DaunoXome, DNX) administered at a dose of 100 mg/m^2 every 3 weeks elicited a partial response in 33% of 18 patients. Toxicities were mainly hematologic and included grade 3 and 4 neutropenia and thrombocytopenia; one patient died of neutropenic sepsis, one patient each developed congestive heart failure, pericarditis and renal failure.

Vinorelbine (Navelbine) 25 mg/m^2 employed with dexamethasone 40 mg on days 1-4 and 9-12 every 3 weeks elicited a parital response in

18 of 39 patients (43%), however, dexamethasone is an active drug and the contribution of vinorelbine to this response is being assessed in a phase III trial. Topotecan (Hycamtin) as a single agent elicited a response rate of 16% in refractory and relapsed myeloma; futher evaluation of this agent in combination is necessary.

CD20 is expressed on tumor cells in a minority of patients and these are candidates for a trial with rituximab (Rituxan). Administration of interferon with rituximab to upregulate CD20 expression may increase the response.

Primary resistant disease: For patients with primary resistant disease, myeloablative therapy with autologous bone marrow or peripheral blood stem-cell support has improved both remission duration and longevity when compared with standard therapy (median survival, 83 vs 37 months).

Resistant relapse: Myeloablative therapy with autologous stem-cell support does not appear to be of clear benefit in patients with disease in resistant relapse. Treatment with two sequential transplants is currently being investigated in these settings.

In view of the high mortality with myeloablative therapy supported by allogeneic transplantation (30-50% during the first year), this procedure appears to be contraindicated in patients with disease in an early phase when given in the standard manner. For patients with disease in resistant relapse or with poor prognosis (i.e., deletion of chromosome 13), new nonmyeloablative procedures that reduce mortality and exploit a graft-vs-tumor effect are now being studied.

Supportive Therapies

Various supportive therapies may be beneficial in patients with multiple myeloma.

Chronic anemia: Patients with chronic symptomatic anemia and inappropriately low erythropoietin levels (often with renal failure) may benefit from a trial of erythropoietin (epoetin alfa [Epogen, Procrit]), 40,000 units given by SC injection once weekly.

Infection: Infectious complications secondary to prolonged neutropenia after intensive chemotherapy may be reduced with granulocyte colony-stimulating factor (G-CSF, [Neupogen]). Recurrent bacterial infections associated with a marked reduction in normal IgG (sometimes estimated from the depression of IgM or IgA) may be reduced with monthly gamma globulin.

Results of one study suggest that trimethoprim-sulfamethoxazole (TMP-SMX) prophylaxis during induction therapy may decrease bacterial infections. This study also noted a higher incidence of nausea and skin rash in patients taking TMP-SMX compared to controls. Further study of antibiotic prophylaxis is necessary to determine its role in patients with myeloma.

Bone pain or imminent fracture: Therapy with bisphosphonates, such as pamidronate (Aredia) or alendronate (Fosamax), may prevent or delay bone pain or recurrent or imminent pathologic fractures in stage III patients with at least one bone lesion. Pamidronate administered over the long term (21 monthly treatments) to stage III multiple myeloma patients with at least one lytic lesion has been shown to reduce skeletal events and decrease the need for radiation. Moreover, patients without lytic lesions also show a decrease in bone mineral density, and this decrease persists despite therapy. These patients may also benefit from therapy with pamidronate.

Several clinical and preclinical studies suggest that pamidronate may have an antimyeloma effect. Patients who were receiving salvage therapy and were given pamidronate to decrease bone morbidity demonstrated an improvement in survival, as compared with patients receiving placebo. These facts support the use of pamidronate as an adjuvant to chemotherapy in patients with multiple myeloma.

Percutaneous verebroplasty provides pain relief that is not only rapid, but sustained, and it also strenghtens the vertebral bodies. This procedure consists of injection of polymethyl methacrylate, the principal component of bone cement, in the vertebral body. It is performed under general or local anesthesia. Transient worsening of pain and fever may occur and are responsive to nonsteroidal anti-inflammatory agents.

Absolute contraindications for percutaneous verebroplasty include coagulation disorders and lack of emergency decompressive surgery. Decompressive surgery is essential, as the most significant complication of the procedure is epidural or foraminal leakages that cause spinal cord and root compressions.

A relative contraindication is vertebral compressions, which result in loss of more than 30% of original vertebral height. This makes the procedure technically complicated; however, experienced invasive radiologists perform this procedure more readily in the last few years.

Smouldering Myeloma

In 20% of patients with multiple myeloma, the disease is asymptomatic and is diagnosed by the chance finding of an elevated serum protein concentration during a screening examination.

Laboratory features: Features of low tumor mass are usually present, without renal disease, hypercalcemia, or lytic bone lesions (Table 11.1).

Treatment: Chemotherapy should be withheld until there is a risk of a complication, except in those few patients with more advanced disease (stage II or III), who should receive chemotherapy promptly.

Prognostic factors: Recent studies have helped define prognostic criteria for groups at high risk of early disease progression (e.g., cytogenetic changes [especially chromosome 13], labeling index of plasma cells [> 0.4%], β2M levels [4 mgL], and diffuse disease activity or multiple focal lesions on MRI evaluation). Such criteria, along with the presence of lytic lesions, serum myeloma protein > 5 g/dL, and Bence Jones protein > 500 mg/24 h, identify patients at high risk of progression, in whom the early commencement of chemotherapy may be beneficial.

OTHER PLASMA CELL DYSCRASIAS

Other plasma cell dyscrasias include monoclonal gammopathy of unknown significance (MGUS), solitary plasmacytoma of bone (SPB), asymptomatic myeloma, Walden_s_trms macroglobulinemia, amyloidosis, the POEMS (polyneuropathy, organomegaly, endocrinopathy, monoclonal gammopathy, and skin changes) syndrome, and heavy-chain disease. Monoclonal gammopathy of unknown significance. MGUS occurs in 1% of normal individuals > 40 years old and rises progressively in frequency with age.

Laboratory features: Common laboratory features of MGUS are:

Treatment: Approximately 25% of patients with this disorder develop multiple myeloma, macroglobulinemia, or non-Hodgkin?s lymphoma over a time span of 20 years. The long period of stability supports the value of annual monitoring with serum electrophoreses and blood counts, and suggests that chemotherapy may be withheld until there is evidence of a serious disorder.

Solitary Plasmacytoma of Bone

Approximately 3% of patients with myeloma have an SPB.

Laboratory features: All patients have either no myeloma protein or a very low level in serum or urine. MRI may reveal abnormalities not detected by bone survey and may upstage patients to multiple myeloma.

Treatment: for SPB consists of radiation therapy (at least 45 Gy). Multiple myeloma becomes evident in most patients over time, so that only 20% remain free of disease for more than 10 years. The median time for disease progression is 2 years.

Solitary Extramedullary Plasmacytoma

In contrast to SPB, solitary extramedullary plasmacytomas are often truly localized and can be cured in most patients with localized radiation therapy (45-50 Gy).

Waldenström's Macroglobulinemia

This uncommon disease is characterized by lymphoplasmacytic bone marrow and tissue infiltrate in addition to elevated IgM production. The mutation pattern analysis suggests that final transformation occurs in postgerminal center IgM memory B cell. Corresponding with variation in cell morphology there is variation in immunophenotype. Mature plasma cells exhibit CD38 antigen; however, lymphoid cells are typically CD19, CD20, CD22, and fmc7 positive.

Waldenstr_m_s macroglobulinemia usually affects people in the fifth to seventh decades of life and can cause symptoms due to tumor infiltration (marrow, lymph nodes, and/or spleen), circulating IgM (hyperviscosity, cryoglobulinemia, and/or cold agglutinin hemolytic anemia), and tissue deposition of IgM (neuropathy, glomerular disease, and/or amyloidosis).

Hyperviscosity syndrome: With hyperviscosity syndrome, patients may have visual symptoms, dizziness, cardiopulmonary symptoms, decreased consciousness, and a bleeding diathesis. Neuropathy is usually due to an IgM antibody reacting with a myelin-associated glycoprotein (MAG).

Therapy for hyperviscosity: consists of plasmaphereses followed by chemotherapy to control the malignant proliferation. Patients with poor performance and elderly patients unable to tolerate chemotherapy may be maintained with periodic plasmapheresis.

Treatment: Alkylating agents in combination with steroids or purine analogs remain the mainstay of therapy. Alkylating agents alone or in combination with steroids effect a 50% reduction in paraprotein in about half the patients and the median survival is around 5 years. The purine analogs fludarabine (Fludara) and 2-CdA (cladribine [Leustatin]) elicit a more rapid response with a response rate of more than 75% observed in small series of patients. Preliminary results of a large, US multi-institution evaluation of fludarabine reported partial responses in only 33% of patients.

Purine analog therapy may result in significant myelosupression in later cycles of therapy and prolonged immunosupression with increased opportunistic infections. Purine analogs are effective salvage options in patients refractory to or relapsing following alkylator therapy. Patients refractory to one purine analog are rarely salvaged by a different purine analog. Patients with resistant relapse are less likely to benefit (response rate, 18%) and should be considered for more intensive intervention, including high-dose therapy.

Other treatment options: Rituximab, an anti-CD20 monoclonal antibody, is effective in Walden_s_trms macroglobulinemia because the CD20 antigen is usually present on the lymphoid cell component of macroglobulinemia. Preliminary results indicate that about 30% of previously treated patients (refractory or relapsing off therapy) may benefit from rituximab.

High-dose therapy with autologous bone marrow or blood stem-cell rescue has been effective in achieving 50% reduction in paraprotein in almost all patients in small pilot trials.

Amyloidosis

Amyloidosis occurs in 10% of patients with multiple myeloma. This infiltrative process results from organ deposition of amyloid fibrils, which consist of the NH2 terminal amino acid residues of the variable portion of the light-chain immunoglobulin molecule. The abnormal protein is produced by clonal plasma cells.

Clinical features: include the nephrotic syndrome, cardiomyopathy, hepatomegaly, neuropathy, macroglossia, carpal tunnel syndrome, and periorbital purpura.

Laboratory features: Serum and urine immunofixation studies show a monoclonal immunoglobulin in approximately 80% of patients. The light chain is more frequently of l than k type. Diagnosis can be made by the presence of apple-green birefringence on polarized light examination of subcutaneous fat aspirates stained with Congo red.

Treatment: Survival is highly variable but is short in patients with cardiomyopathy, renal failure, hepatomegaly, or significant weight loss. Approximately 20% of patients may benefit from MP therapy given for at least 1 year.

Encouraging results with high-dose therapy have been reported. Patients with multiorgan or symptomatic cardiac involvement have excess treatment-related mortality with this approach. Use of high-dose therapy in patients with amyloidosis needs further study in larger numbers of patients.

POEMS Syndrome

Clinical features and course: The POEMS syndrome is a rare plasma cell dyscrasia that presents with peripheral, usually sensorimotor, neuropathy. An IgA l monoclonal gammopathy is most common, and bone lesions, noted in nearly all patients, are usually osteosclerotic.

Other features include hyperpigmentation, hypertrichosis, thickened skin, papilledema, lymphadenopathy, peripheral edema, hepatomegaly, splenomegaly, and hypothyroidism. Diabetes mellitus is not part of this syndrome.

Compared with patients with symptomatic myeloma, individuals with the

POEMS syndrome are younger (median age, 51 years) and live longer (median, 8 years). The clinical course is commonly characterized by progressive neuropathy.

Treatment: Plasmapheresis does not appear to be of benefit, and patients are often treated similarly to those with myeloma.

Heavy-chain Diseases

Heavy-chain diseases are plasma cell dyscrasias characterized by the production of heavy-chain immunoglobulin molecules (IgG, IgA, IgM) that lack light chains.

α Heavy-chain: disease results from lymphocyte and plasma cell infiltration of the mesenteric nodes and small bowel, and has features of malabsorption, such as diarrhea, weight loss, abdominal pain, edema, and nail clubbing. The heavy-chain molecule may be detected in serum, jejunal secretions, and urine.

γ Heavy-chain disease: Patients with g heavy-chain disease may present with fever, weakness, lymphadenopathy, hepatosplenomegaly, and involvement of Waldeyer's ring. Eosinophilia, leukopenia, and thrombocytopenia are common. Treatment with regimens similar to those used for non-Hodgkin's lymphoma may be effective.

μ Heavy-chain disease: is seen exclusively in patients with chronic lymphocytic leukemia (CLL). Vacuolated plasma cells are common in the marrow, and many patients have k light chains in the urine. Therapy is similar to that used for CLL

ACUTE LEUKEMIAS

Hematopoietic malignancies account for only 6-8% of new cancer diagnosed annually. In the year 2001, an estimated 31,500 new cases of leukemia will be diagnosed, and 21,500 deaths will be attributable to leukemias of all types. The total age-adjusted incidence of leukemia, including both acute and chronic forms, is 9.6 per 100,000 population; the incidence of acute lymphoblastic leukemia (ALL) is 1.5 per 100,000, while that of acute myelogenous leukemia (AML) is 2.7 per 100,000.

Epidemiology

Gender The incidence of both ALL and AML is slightly higher in males than in females.

Age: Age-specific incidences of AML are similar to those of other solid tumors of adults, with an exponential rise after age 40 years. With regard to ALL, 60% of cases are seen in children, with a peak incidence in the first 5 years of life, and a subsequent drop in incidence until age 60, when a second peak emerges.

Race and ethnicity: The incidence of acute leukemia is slightly higher in populations of European descent. Also, a recent report from the University of Southern California indicates that acute promyelocytic leukemia (APL) is more common in Hispanic populations than in other ethnic groups.

Etiology and Risk Factors

There is wide diversity in the behavior of the various subsets of acute leukemias. Thus, it is unlikely that there is one common etiology for these aberrant cellular proliferations. There are, however, some accepted risk factors for leukemogenesis:

Chemical exposure: Increased incidence of AML and myelodysplasia (preleukemia) has been reported in persons with prolonged exposure to benzene and petroleum products. The interval between exposure and onset of leukemia is long (10-30 years). Chromosomal damage is common.

Pesticide exposure also has been linked to some forms of AML. The incidence of AML is beginning to rise in developing countries as industrialization and pollution increase.

Other environmental exposures: Exposure to hair dyes, smoking, and nonionic radiation may also increase the risk of leukemia.

Prior chemotherapy or radiation: Use of alkylating agents, such as cyclophosphamide (Cytoxan, Neosar) and melphalan (Alkeran), in the treatment lymphomas, myeloma, breast and ovarian cancers has been associated with the development of AML, usually within 3-5 years of exposure and often preceded by a myelodysplastic phase. Cytogenetic abnormalities, particularly monosomy 5, 7, 11, and 17, are common. Concurrent radiation exposure slightly increases the risk of leukemogenesis posed by alkylating agents.

Topoisomerase II inhibitors (etoposide, teniposide [Vumon], doxorubicin and its derivatives, and mitoxantrone [Novantrone]), used to treat ALL, myeloma, testicular cancer, and sarcomas, have also been implicated in leukemogenesis. These agents, in contrast to alkylators, are associated with a short latency period without antecedent myelodysplasia, and with cytogenetic abnormalities involving 11q23 or 21q22 in the malignant clone.

Genetic disorders: An increased incidence of AML is seen in patients with Down?s syndrome, Bloom?s syndrome, or Fanconi's anemia, as well as individuals with ataxia-telangiectasia or Wiskott-Aldrich syndrome. In identical twins below the age of 10, if one child develops leukemia (usually ALL), there is a 20% chance that the other twin will develop leukemia within a year; subsequently, the risk falls off rapidly and joins that of nonidentical siblings, which is three to five times that of the general population.

Signs and Symptoms

Effects on hematopoiesis: Leukemia manifests symptomatically by its impact on normal hematopoiesis. Thus, easy fatigability, bruising or bleeding from mucosal surfaces, fever, and persistent infection are all reflections of the anemia, thrombocytopenia, and decrease in functional neutrophils associated with marrow replacement by malignant cells. Bone pain is common in children with ALL (occurring in 40-50%) but is less common in adults with acute leukemias (5-10%).

WBC elevation and pancytopenia Whereas a marked elevation in WBC counts is the classic hallmark of leukemia, pancytopenia is more common, particularly in patients of all ages with ALL or in elderly patients with AML, who may have had preexisting marrow dysfunction (myelodysplasia). Only 10% of newly diagnosed patients with either AML or ALL present with leukocyte counts > 100,000/?L. These patients, however, constitute a poor-prognostic group and are at increased risk of CNS disease, tumor lysis syndrome, and leukostasis due to impedance of blood flow from intravascular clumping of blasts, which are "stickier" than mature myeloid or lymphoid cells.

Leukostasis may manifest as an alteration in mental status; intermittent or persistent cranial nerve palsies, particularly those involving extraocular muscles; priapism; dyspnea; or pleuritic chest pain, due to small leukemic emboli in the pulmonary vasculature.

Physical findings: in AML are usually minimal. Pallor, increased ecchymoses or petechiae, retinal hemorrhages, gingival hypertrophy, and cutaneous involvement are more common with monocytic (M4 or M5) variants of AML.

Hepatosplenomegaly and lymphadenopathy Mild hepatosplenomegaly and lymphadenopathy are seen in many cases, particularly in childhood ALL. Massive hepatosplenomegaly occurs infrequently and should raise the suspicion of a leukemia evolving from a prior hematologic disorder, such as chronic myelogenous leukemia (CML) or myelodysplasia. Mediastinal adenopathy is seen in 80% of cases of T-cell ALL, is less common in other ALLs, and is rare in AML.

Visceral involvement is also rare, occurring as an initial manifestation of AML in < 5% of cases, but it may be more frequent during subsequent relapses. These focal collections of blasts, called chloromas or granulocytic sarcomas, can present as soft-tissue masses, infiltrative lesions of the small bowel and mesentery, or obstructing lesions of the hepatobiliary or genitourinary systems.

CNS involvement is uncommon at presentation in adult AML (< 1%) and adult ALL (3-5%). In most instances, CNS involvement is detected by screening lumbar puncture in high-risk patients who are asymptomatic at the time of the puncture. Symptoms, when they do occur, include headache, diplopia, cranial nerve palsies, radicular pain, and/or weakness in a particular nerve root distribution. CNS involvement usually is restricted to leptomeninges; parenchymal mass lesions are uncommon.

Testicular involvement Like the CNS, the testes appear to be a "sanctuary" site for isolated relapses in pediatric but not adult ALL. Signs of testicular involvement include painless, asymmetrical enlargement.

Metabolic effects: of acute leukemia relate primarily to the rate of cell death.

Hyperuricemia with possible interstitial or ureteral obstruction is seen predominantly in AML with moderate leukocytosis; this may be exacerbated by a rapid response to chemotherapy and the "tumor lysis syndrome" (hyperuricemia with renal insufficiency, acidosis, hyperphosphatemia, and hypocalcemia) that may occur within the first 24-48 hours after initiating chemotherapy. To prevent this complication, all patients should receive allopurinol and urine alkalinization before marrow-ablative chemotherapy is initiated.

Coagulopathies: can also complicate the hemostatic defects associated with thrombocytopenia. Disseminated intravascular coagulation (DIC) is most often seen in APL (French-American British [FAB] subtype M3) due to release of procoagulants from the abnormal primary granules, which activate the coagulation cascade, leading to decreased factors II, V, VIII, and X, and fibrinogen, as well as rapid platelet consumption. Lysozyme released from monoblasts in M4 and M5 subtypes of AML can also trigger the clotting cascade. Finally, DIC can occur following asparaginase (Elspar) chemotherapy for ALL.

Diagnosis

Abnormalities on the CBC raise the possibility of leukemia. The diagnosis is substantiated pathologically by a bone marrow examination.

All patients should have cytochemistry, immunophenotyping by fluorescence-activated cell sorting (FACS) using monoclonal antibodies directed at leukemia-specific antigens, and cytogenetic analysis of the marrow or peripheral blood blasts at diagnosis. Other tests used to evaluate metabolic abnormalities (electrolytes, creatinine, and liver function tests) and coagulopathies are also needed at diagnosis. A lumbar puncture should be performed at diagnosis in all pediatric patients with ALL and in all patients with neurologic symptoms regardless of age and pathology.

Pathology and Cytogenetics

Acute leukemias are comprised of a group of clonal disorders of maturation at an early phase of hematopoietic differentiation. Morphology and cytochemical stains designed to detect intracellular myeloperoxidase or esterases have been the traditional methods used to divide acute leukemias into either myeloid or lymphoid in derivation.

Coupling these traditional methods with cytogenetic analysis and highly specific monoclonal antibodies directed against cell-surface antigens has led to the detection of new prognostic factors and has provided an approach to detect minimal residual disease.

In 1997, a panel of hematopathologists met to update the FAB classification of hematologic malignancies, which had been based on morphology. They proposed a new classification, incorporating immunophenotyping, cytogenetics, and clinical disease features, that has been adopted by the World Health Organization (WHO).

Myeloid Leukemias

The new WHO classification retains the morphologic subgroups of the FAB system, but has created new categories which recognize the importance of certain cytogenetic translocations as predictors of response to therapy. In this category are: AML with t(8;21) (q22,q22), AML with abnormal eosinophils = inv(16) (p13q22) or t(16;16) (p13;q11), AML with 11q23 (MLL) abnormalities and acute promyelocytic leukemia t(15;17) (q22;q11-12).

The WHO classification also attempts to deal with the evidence that in many older patients marrow dysfunction antedates the onset of acute leukemia. These myelodysplastic syndromes (MDS) are characterized by ineffective hematopoietic production and disrupted maturation of one or more cell lines. These abnormalities are often accompanied by loss of chromosomal

Table 11.2: Morphologic, immunologic, and cytogenetic classification of ALL

		Cell markers								
Category	*Karyotype*	*Tdt*	*Ia*	*CD19*	*CD10*	*Cylg*	*Slg*	*CD7*	*CD2*	*CD33*
Precursor B-cell ALL (cytogenetic subgroups)	t(9:22) = 8CR/ABL	+	+	+	–	–	–	–	–	+
	t(v:11q23): MLL rearrangements including t(4:11)	+	+	+	+	–	–	–	–	–
	t(1:9) EZA/PBX1	+	+	+	+	–	–	–	–	–
	t(12:21) ETV/CBF	+	+	+	+	–	–	–	–	–
Burkitt-cell leukema	t(8:14), t(8:22) t(2:8), 6q–	–	+	+	+	±	±	–	–	–
Precursce T-cell ALL	t or del 9p	+	–	–	–	–	–	+	–	–
T-cell ALL	t(11:14), 6q–	+	–	–	–	–	–	+	–	–

CD=...................... of differentiation; Cylt=cytoplasmic immunoglobuin; la=1 antigen; Sig=surface immunoglobulin; Tdt=.................... decinobyrkectde trabsferate

material, particularly loss of chromosomes ? or 5q? ? or 7q? and chromosomes ? or ?0. As the bone marrow becomes more dysfunctional, increasing numbers of blasts are seen in the marrow.

In the FAB classification, the demarcation line between myelodysplasia and AML was 30% marrow blasts. However, patients with 20-29% blasts (previously classified as refractory anemia with excess blasts in transformation = RAEB-t) have a biologic behavior and poor survival similar to AML. The WHO has proposed changing the demarcation between MDS and AML to 20% marrow blasts and deleting the category of RAEB-t.

The WHO system further subdivides the AML patients with dysplastic maturation into those with or without antecedent cytopenias (usually 3 months prior to diagnosis had been the arbitrary cut off point), and those with a history of prior exposure to chemotherapy agents (alkylating agents, epipodophyllotoxins or others).

Lymphoblastic Leukemias

Lymphoblastic leukemias can arise from either B-cell or T-cell progenitors that arrest at an early stage of maturation and then proliferate. Marrow involvement of > 25% lymphoblasts is used as the demarcation line between lymphoblastic lymphoma, in which the preponderance of tumor bulk is in nodal structures, and ALL. Approximately 75% of adult ALLs are B-cell in derivation and 25% are T-cell.

Precursor B-cell ALL: Most B-cell leukemias are early or "pre-B" cell, expressing CD19 and CD10 (the common acute leukemia antigen [cALLa]) but lacking surface or cytoplasmic immunoglobulin; this group of early B-cell leukemias has a more favorable prognosis than B-cell leukemias in which the cells have a more mature phenotype. Chromosomal rearrangements juxtaposing an oncogene with a promoter region are often seen in this disease category. The new WHO classification identifies these cytogenetic subgroups.

Mature B-cell ALL: The more mature B-cell ALL, or Burkitt-cell leukemia, is associated with translocations of the c-*myc* gene on chromosome 8 and the immunoglobulin heavy-chain gene on chromosome 14q32 in 80% of cases, or with the light-chain genes of chromosome 2p11 or 22q11 in the other 20%. Burkitt-cell leukemia has increased in frequency recently, as it is one of the lymphoproliferative disorders that occur in individuals infected with the human immunodeficiency virus (HIV); leukemia may appear early in the course of the HIV infection before the onset of opportunistic infections or severe T-cell deficiency

T-cell ALL: is frequently associated with translocations of T-cell receptor genes on chromosome 14q11 or chromosome 7q34 with other gene partners. T-cell ALL had been associated with a poor prognosis when treated with conventional ALL regimens but has now assumed a good risk status with more aggressive antimetabolite therapy. Precursor T-cell ALL has a poorer outcome.

Infection with human T-cell leukemia virus-1 (HTLV-1) should be looked for in T-cell ALL patients presenting with hypercalcemia and lytic bone lesions. HTLV-1 infection is endemic in southern Japan, the southern Pacific basin, the Caribbean basin, and sub-Saharan Africa. High infection rates are also seen in parts of Iran, India, and Hawaii. Recent immigrants from endemic areas retain a risk of infection similar to their point of origin. However, fewer than 0.1% of persons carrying HTLV-1 will develop T-cell leukemia.

ALL with myeloid antigen expression vs undifferentiated leukemia: A subset of patients with leukemia exhibit features of both myeloid and lymphoid differentiation. These patients were originally classified as having mixed lineage leukemia. Patients with a leukemic clone that expresses two or more ALL antigens and one myeloid antigen comprise 20% of adult ALL cases. While expression of myeloid antigen is considered to be a poor-risk feature in children, it does not constitute a distinct poor-risk feature in adults

Immunophenotyping has also helped define a group of patients with undifferentiated myeloid leukemia (M0) who previously were likely to be treated as if they had ALL. These leukemias have a very primitive morphology and lack myeloperoxidase. On immunophenotyping, they express at least one early myeloid antigen, usually CD13 or CD 33, and no T-or B-cell markers. Based on immunophenotyping, undifferentiated leukemias are treated in the same manner as myeloid malignancies.

ALL prognostic factors

Cytogenetic abnormalities have a significant impact on the prognosis of ALL. Approximately half of ALL patients have cytogenetic abnormalities; these usually take the form of translocations of genetic information, rather than deletions of genetic material, which are seen more commonly in AML.

Philadelphia chromosome: The most ominous cytogenetic abnormality in ALL is the translocation of the *abl* gene from chromosome 9 to the breakpoint cluster region (BCR) on chromosome 22, forming a new gene product (BCR-ABL) with tyrosine kinase activity. This translocation, referred to as the Philadelphia chromosome (Ph+), is found in 95% of cases of chronic myelogenous leukemia (CML) and in 20-30% of newly diagnosed adult ALL patients.

The fusion protein produced by the *bcr/abl* translocation in Ph+ ALL (p190) differs from the product seen in CML (p210); the P190 product is a smaller protein than the p210 product and has higher tyrosine kinase activity. Use of PCR techniques that target only the p210 product will underestimate the incidence of Ph+ ALL by 50% or more.

Although patients with Ph+ ALL may attain a morphologic remission with conventional chemotherapy (82%), almost all such patients will have persistent molecular evidence of disease. Patients who do achieve a molecular remission have a longer remission duration than those who continue to express p190 or p210 activity (30 vs 12 months).

Other translocations Translocations involving the mixed lineage leukemia (MLL) gene at 11q23 are partnered with several other chromosomes, including 4q21, 9q22, and 19q13. Translocations involving 11q23 are frequently seen in secondary leukemias, particularly those arising after chemotherapy with etoposide or teniposide. Although most of these translocations are associated with AML, ALL has also arisen in this setting. All the 11q23 translocations, as well as the more common (1;19) translocation, are associated with poorer outcomes when compared with similar immunophenotypes coupled with normal cytogenetics.

Treatment

Treatment of All

Although 70-80% of pediatric patients with ALL can anticipate a long-term remission or cure of their disease with combination chemotherapy, the overall long-term disease-free survival rate for adults with ALL is 35-50%. Poorer outcomes in adults are attributed to a higher incidence of unfavorable cytogenetic abnormalities [t(9;22), t(8;14), or t(4;11)] or coexpression of myeloid antigens, as well as to higher WBC counts at diagnosis.

Adults also have poorer tolerance for some of the chemotherapeutic agents used in treatment, such as asparaginase, as well as higher rates of infection and comorbid disease, all of which result in a higher incidence of end-organ toxicity and treatment delays.

Induction Therapy

The initial goal of therapy is to rapidly reduce the leukemic burden to a level undetectable by conventional methods of light microscopy and flow cytometry, a state that is deemed a "complete remission" (CR).

The addition of an anthracycline to the standard pediatric leukemia induction regimen of vincristine, prednisone, and asparaginase increased the CR rate in adults from 50-60% to 70-80% in several series. The addition of cyclophosphamide or cytarabine (Ara-C) to these agents produced additional toxicity without any substantive increase in CR rates in unselected patients. In a recent CALGB study, the use of cytokines, ie, granulocyte colony-stimulating factor (G-CSF, filgrastim [Neupogen]), during induction in patients over 60 years of age reduced treatment-related mortality from 31 to 5% when compared with placebo-treated controls.

T-cell ALL There is some evidence that patients with T-cell ALL may benefit from early treatment with Ara-C and cyclophosphamide. Pharmacologic studies show high levels of Ara-C triphosphate accumulation in T lymphoblasts and synergy between cyclophosphamide and Ara-C in cell lines of T-cell malignancies.

Mature B-cell ALL Patients with the more mature B-cell ALL (Burkitt-cell leukemia) experienced an improvement in survival when high doses of cyclophosphamide, methotrexate, and Ara-C were incorporated early in the treatment course. The probability of leukemia-free survival improved from 35% with standard ALL induction to 60-70% with these newer regimens.

Consolidation Therapy

As yet, no randomized trials have compared these regimens. However, in sequential studies from Memorial Sloan-Kettering and the BFM group, as well as the Linker study, use of multiple cycles of non? cross-resistant drugs for 3-8 cycles after remission followed by maintenance with methotrexate and mercaptopurine (Purinethol) resulted in overall long-term disease-free survival rates of 33-38%.

Prognostic factors for relapse The BFM trials have found the following factors to be associated with a poor outcome in ALL patients: time to CR > 4 weeks, age > 35 years, WBC count > 30,000/?L, and null-cell ALL (non-T, non-cALLa). Burkitt-cell leukemia patients were not included in this analysis. Patients with no risk factors had a 62% 5-year disease-free survival, whereas disease-free survival for those with one, two, and three risk factors fell to 33%, 22%, and 11%, respectively. Only 27% of patients over age 15 years fell into the good-risk group.

Prognostic factors in a recent CALGB report included WBC > 30,000/?L, age > 60 years, absence of a mediastinal mass (i.e., a non?T-cell ALL), and poor-risk cytogenetics, such as Ph positivity or t(4;11). Rates of survival at 3 years were 64%, 49%, 21%, and 0% for patients with one, two, three, and four risk factors, respectively.

Molecular techniques, such as PCR amplification of leukemia-specific sequences of RNA or DNA, have been used in research settings to reveal residual leukemia cells. These sensitive techniques can detect the persistence of cells with the leukemic phenotype at a sensitivity of 1 cell in 10^4 normal cells in patients who are deemed to be in CR by conventional techniques. In two pediatric studies, detection of leukemia-specific gene rearrangements (? 1 cell in 10^4 normal cells) 5-6 months after initiation of treatment was associated with a high relapse rate.

High-risk patients: While the BFM regimen is now standard therapy for good-prognosis patients, high-risk patients are being selected for dose-intensive therapies, including high-dose Ara-C ([cytarabine], HDAC) and methotrexate or etoposide; high-dose methotrexate and asparaginase.

Investigators at M. D. Anderson have reported on a regimen which alternates 4 cycles of fractionated high-dose cyclophosphamide, vincristine, doxorubicin, dexamethasone with 4 cycles of HDAC and high-dose methotrexate. When the regimen was used as salvage therapy for relapsed ALL, it produced a CR rate of 44%. When this regimen was used as initial therapy, the CR rate was 91% (with a median remission duration of 34 months), and the 5-year disease-free survival rate was 38%.

Transplantation Recent series have reported a disease-free survival rate of 55-60% for "high-risk" ALL patients undergoing transplantation during first CR. When treated with conventional-dose chemotherapy, patients with Ph+ ALL have a disease-free survival rate of < 10% regardless of other risk factors and a median time to relapse of 12 months; these patients should be referred for allogeneic or matched-unrelated-donor (MUD) transplantation expeditiously upon attaining a CR. Allogeneic transplantation has produced a 68% long-term disease-free survival rate in patients with Ph+ ALL who received a transplant during first CR.

CNS Prophylaxis

The incidence of CNS relapse is much higher in patients with ALL than in those with AML; among pediatric ALL patients who did not receive adequate CNS therapy, the rate of CNS relapse was 20% in the first year.

Patients with ALL require preemptive therapy for occult CNS disease with either (1) intrathecal methotrexate, Ara-C combined with cranial irradiation (2) or with high-dose systemic Ara-C or methotrexate combined with intrathecal therapy.

Maintenance Therapy

Adult patients: In adults, the benefit of maintenance therapy is unknown. In low-risk adults, who have an outcome more similar to the pediatric population, maintenance therapy would appear to be justified. In individuals who are positive for the Philadelphia chromosome or who have mature B-cell ALL, it is unlikely that maintenance therapy has any effect. In other high-risk adult populations, more than half of patients relapse while on maintenance therapy, indicating the need for other strategies to eradicate minimal residual disease.

Treatment of Relapse

Treatment of relapsed adult ALL is a major challenge. Since most protocols for initial treatment incorporate 6-11 agents with different cytotoxic mechanisms, a selection process for drug resistance has occurred. The overall remission (CR) rates are 30-40%, with a median remission duration of 6 months.

Salvage strategies: include reinduction with the initial regimen in patients with late relapse or high dose antimetabolites (cytarabine [Ara-C] or methotrexate [see hyperCVAD regimen]) in those who relapse early. Recent experimental approaches include monoclonal antibodies directed against leukemia-specific antigens conjugated to either radionuclides or toxins, tyrosine kinase inhibitors, allogeneic or autologous transplantation, or new agents.

TREATMENT OF AML

Induction Therapy

Ara-C and the anthracyclines have been the mainstays of initial therapy for AML since the 1970s. Idarubicin (Idamycin) is beginning to replace the older daunorubicin as the anthracycline of choice to pair with Ara-C.

Idarubicin, which attains higher intracellular drug concentration and longer retention, has shown superior response rates and response durations, as well as better overall survival, when compared with daunorubicin (Daun) in younger (? 60 years old) patients.

Both mitoxantrone and etoposide have significant antileukemic activity in relapsed or refractory leukemia, achieving remission rates of 30-40%. However, a recent phase III trial compared daunorubicin (Cerubidine, DNR) plus standard Ara-C (D+A) to mitoxantrone plus etoposide (M+E) in newly diagnosed AML patients ? 56 years. The CR rates were 44% for D+A and 33% for M+E, with a median survival of 8 months and 6 months, respectively. There does not appear to be a clinical advantage to early use of M+E in older patients.

Increased dose intensity: Two recent large cooperative trials showed no difference in the rate of CR when HDAC was compared with standard doses.

In the Australian Leukemia Study Group (ALSG) trial, which randomized 301 patients under age 60 to receive either HDAC or standard 7-day infusional Ara-C combined with daunorubicin and etoposide, the CR rates were 71% and 74%, respectively. For patients who achieved a CR, remission duration was 45 months with HDAC vs 12 months with standard Ara-C. The 5-year disease-free survival rate was also significantly better in patients given HDAC than in those treated with standard-dose Ara-C (48% vs 25%), but overall survival was not statistically different, due to the higher number of deaths during induction in patients in the HDAC arm and the lack of effective salvage therapy for these patients.

In a Southwest Oncology Group (SWOG) protocol comparing HDAC (2 g/m^2 q12h ? 12 doses) plus daunorubicin with the standard 7-day Ara-C infusion plus daunorubicin, the CR rates for patients under age 50 were 55% and 58%, respectively. For patients who achieved a CR and who received 1 cycle of consolidation with the same Ara-C dose schedule as they received for induction, the relapse-free survival rate was 32% vs 22% in favor of HDAC (*P* = .05). However, many patients who achieved a CR with HDAC did not receive consolidation therapy.

Dose intensity may be more important to achieving or maintaining remission in different subcategories of leukemia. In the SWOG trial, patients treated with standard-dose Ara-C who expressed the CD34 antigen had a lower CR rate than CD34-negative patients (36% vs 62%). HDAC, in contrast, produced a higher CR rate in CD34-positive patients. There was a strong correlation between CD34 expression and expression of the multidrug resistance (MDR1) gene product, suggesting that higher dose intensity may help overcome drug resistance.

Prognostic factors: Cytogenetics and immunophenotyping for leukemia-associated antigens have helped define risk groups. In a large CALGB trial, patients with translocations 15,17 [t(15;17)] or 8,21 [t(8;21)] or inversion 16 [inv(16)] had a higher CR rate and longer median remission duration, while patients with monosomy 5 or 7 (?, ?q, or ?) or trisomy 8 (+8) had a significantly lower CR rate and short remission duration. Patients with normal karyotypes or other cytogenetic abnormalities had an intermediate prognosis.

Poor-prognosis cytogenetic abnormalities, antecedent myelodysplasia, and MDR_1 expression are found more frequently in older (> 60 years old) patients, which may account for the lower CR rates seen in this age group (40-60%) compared to their younger counterparts (60-80%). Cytogenetic abnormalities, age, myelodysplasia, and high tumor burden (as evidenced by WBC count > 50,000/?L) are adverse factors both for attaining and maintaining remission. Remission rates are also lower in patients whose blasts express CD34+ or have high expression of the MDR1 gene. Strategies for clinical trials based on prognostic indicators for outcome are currently being developed.

Therapy-related AML: has a particularly poor prognosis. At best, only 50% of patients will achieve a remission, usually of brief duration (median, 5 months), despite the use of aggressive drug combinations. Allogeneic or unrelated-donor transplantation appears to offer the only curative option in these patients, achieving a 3-year disease-free survival rate of 25% in two recent studies of allogeneic transplantation.

GM-CSF: A recent Eastern Cooperative Oncology Group (ECOG) study showed that granulocyte-macrophage colony-stimulating factor (GM-CSF, sargramostim [Leukine]), used following completion of induction chemotherapy in older patients (55-70 years old), shortened the duration of neutropenia by 6 days and, thus, decreased treatment-related mortality, leading to both an improved CR rate and longer survival. The FDA approved GM-CSF for use in this setting. However, other trials using different cytokines in younger patients have not shown a survival benefit.

Consolidation Therapy

Once remission of AML is attained, consolidation chemotherapy is required to achieve a durable remission or cure.

Increased dose intensity In a CALGB study, 596 patients in CR were assigned to receive 4 courses of post-remission Ara-C in one of three dosages: 100 mg/m^2 as a continuous infusion for 5 days, 400 mg/m^2 as a continuous infusion for 5 days, or 3 g/m^2 as a 3-hour infusion every 12 hours on days 1, 3, and 5. For patients ? 60 years old, the percentage of patients in CR at 4 years was significantly higher in the HDAC group (44%) than in either the 400-mg/m^2 or 100-mg/m^2 group (29% and 24%, respectively). For patients > 60 years old, consolidation dose intensity had no impact on disease-free survival, with all groups plateauing at a rate of 16% by 2 years.

Other approaches to consolidation include 1-3 cycles of consolidation followed by autologous or allogeneic BMT. Both of these approaches also tend to be limited to patients < 60 years old and have produced long-term disease-free survival rates of 45-60% in several studies. Long-term disease-free survival is strongly influenced by cytogenetic abnormalities present at diagnosis.

CNS Prophylaxis

Routine CNS prophylaxis is recommended only for adult AML patients at high risk of CNS recurrences; ie, patients with WBC count > 50,000/mL at presentation or those with myelomonocytic or monocytic AML (FAB M4 or M5). Patients receiving HDAC (? 7.2 g/m^2) for induction or consolidation achieve therapeutic drug levels in the CSF, obviating intrathecal therapy. Patients given conventional Ara-C doses may be treated with intrathecal methotrexate (12 mg IT) or Ara-C (30 mg IT). Both agents are combined with hydrocortisone (30 mg IT) for patients with active CNS disease.

TREATMENT OF REFRACTORY OR RELAPSED AML

Patients who do not respond to initial therapy or who relapse within 6 months of attaining a CR, as well as those with antecedent myelodysplasia or therapy-related AML, are considered to have relatively resistant disease.

Efforts to overcome drug resistance have focused on: (1) HDAC-containing regimens, (2) new agents, (3) targeted therapy using leukemia-specific MoAbs antibodies conjugated with radionuclides or toxins, and (4) nonchemotherapeutic agents to block the drug efflux pump associated with MDR_1 gene expression.

HDAC: High doses of Ara-C (2-3 g/m^2 for 8-12 doses) paired with mitoxantrone, etoposide, methotrexate, or fludarabine (Fludara) have produced short-lived CRs in 40-60% of relapsed AML patients. Response rates were higher in patients who had received standard-dose Ara-C for induction and patients with relapsed leukemia than in those in whom induction therapy had failed. Median remission durations were 4-6 months.

New agents: Combinations of mitoxantrone and etoposide produce a 40-50% CR rate in populations at high risk of relapse, again with a median remission duration of 4-6 months. Combinations of intermediate-dose Ara-C (1 g/m^2/d for 6 days) with mitoxantrone and etoposide produced CR rates of 79% in relapsed patients and 46% in those who did not respond to induction or had AML evolving from myelodysplastic syndrome, with a median CR duration of 8 months.

Topotecan in combination with Ara-C has been reported to produce a CR in 35-70% of patients with high grade myelodysplasia (RAEB or refrac-tory anemia with excess blasts in transformation [RAEB-t]) and AML.

Nucleoside analogs, such as cladribine (2-CdA [Leustatin]) and fludarabine, showed activity in pediatric AML. A recent British trial reported a 61% CR rate for a combination of fludarabine, Ara-C, G-CSF, and idarubicin, with a median CR duration of 7 months.

Targeted therapy: Gemtuzumab ozogamicin (Mylotarg), an anti-CD33 antibody conjugated with calicheamicin, has recently been approved for the treatment of relapsed AML in older patients. In the preliminary phase II trials, 43% of AML patients who relapsed after a CR duration of more than 6 months achieved clearance of marrow and peripheral blood blasts when treated with gemtuzumab. Treatment-related toxicity was low; the only infusional side effects were fever and chills and slow platelet plus granulocyte recovery (? 5 weeks). Liver function abnormalities have also been reported in 25-30% of patients.

Radiolabeled anti-CD33 immunoconjugates have also been used as part of the preparatory regimen for allogeneic marrow transplantation.

Multidrug resistance (MDR) modification: Cyclosporine (Neoral, Sandimmune) is a potent inhibitor of p-glycoprotein?mediated drug efflux. A SWOG trial compared HDAC, 3 g/m^2/d ?5 d, followed by daunorubicin, 45 mg/m^2/d as a continuous infusion on days 6-8, either alone (arm 1) or together with cyclosporine, 16 mg/m^2/d as a continuous infusion on days 6-8 (arm 2) in 226 patients with relapsed or refractory AML. While the CR rates were similar for arms 1 and 2 (33% vs 40%), the relapse-free survival rates favored patients treated with the MDR modifier (10% for arm 1 vs 73% for arm 2 at 3 years; $P = .03$). The overall survival rate was also superior (6% for arm 1 vs 20% for arm 2 at 3 years; $P = .03$) (List AF, Kopecky KJ, Willman CL, et al: Blood 92:312a [abstract], 1998). Trials substituting the cyclosporine analog PSC-833 (Amdray) have not demonstrated a significant improvement in CR rate or survival.

Transplantation: Although none of the options discussed above currently offers more than a 10-15% chance of long-term disease-free survival, they do provide temporary cytoreduction sufficient to permit further high-dose treatment strategies, such as marrow transplantation using sibling, unrelated-donor, or purged autologous marrow. Allogeneic marrow transplantation achieves a 30-40% disease-free survival rate at 5 years in patients transplanted during first relapse or second remission. Autologous BMT also has curative potential for patients beyond first CR, with most large series reporting disease-free survival rates of 30-35%.

Currently, new methods of marrow purging and post-transplant immune stimulation are being explored as methods for decreasing relapse-related mortality.

TREATMENT OF APL

APL: represents a uniquely homogeneous subset of AML defined by its cytogenetic abnormality, t(15;17), which results in fusion of the retinoic acid receptor (RAR) a-gene on chromosome 17 with the promyelocytic leukemia (PML) gene on chromosome 15. This abnormality yields an RAR-a?PML fusion protein, detectable by polymerase chain reaction (PCR) techniques, which is useful for both diagnosis and evaluation of minimal residual disease. Most (80%) patients with APL have characteristic hypergranular blasts, and lab evidence of DIC is present in 70-90% of patients at diagnosis or shortly after.

Because of the unique biology and specific clinical features of APL, coupled with a molecular abnormality that suggested a new therapeutic approach, induction and consolidation regimens for APL differ from strategies used for other FAB types.

Although low-dose heparin (5-15 U/kg/h) and factor replacement are used as supportive adjuncts during chemotherapy, hemorrhagic events contribute 10-15% excess mortality during induction chemotherapy of APL compared to other AML subtypes. Standard-dose Ara-C and daunorubicin produce CR rates of 70-80% and disease-free survival rates of 40-50%.

Initial Treatment of APL

Three large studies have shown that all-trans-retinoic acid (ATRA [Vesanoid]) in combination with anthracycline-based chemotherapy results in an improved long-term disease-free survival. The recent European APL trial compared sequential ATRA followed by chemotherapy to concomitant ATRA plus chemotherapy. Patients achieving CR received 2 cycles of consolidation and then were randomized to receive: (a) intermittent ATRA (2 weeks every 3 months for 2 years), (b) low-dose oral chemotherapy (6 mercaptopurine + MTX for 2 years),

(c) both, or d) observation. The CR rate in both induction arms was 92%. However, relapse rates were 6% for the ATRA plus chemotherapy arm vs 16% for ATRA followed by chemotherapy (P = .04).

Two hundred eighty-nine patients were randomized for maintenance treatment. Relapse rates at 2 years were 30% for patients who received no maintenance, 18% for patients receiving ATRA maintenance alone, 14% for chemotherapy without ATRA, and 7% for patients receiving chemotherapy plus ATRA. Overall survival was significantly better in patients receiving maintenance chemotherapy with or without ATRA for 2 years.

All-Trans-retinoic Acid

Involvement of the RAR-a gene in the pathogenesis of APL suggested the use of retinoids as therapy. The HL60 (APL) cell line can be induced to differentiate in culture with ATRA, and a 1988 study from Shanghai showed CR rates of 85% with this retinoid. ATRA offers the advantages of a shorter neutropenic period (2 weeks) and slightly faster resolution of DIC (4 vs 7 days), as compared with standard chemotherapy with Ara-C and daunorubicin. Normalization of marrow morphology and cytogenetics requires 30-60 days with ATRA.

Retinoic acid syndrome: Difficulties with ATRA therapy include short remission durations (median, 3-5 months) when used as a single agent, and development of the "retinoic acid syndrome" in approximately 25% of patients. Symptoms of this syndrome are fever, respiratory distress with pulmonary infiltrates or pleural effusions, and cardiovascular collapse. While these symptoms most often correlate with leukocytosis (WBC count > 10,000/mL), many patients develop symptoms with counts between 5,000 and 10,000/mL.

Treatment of this syndrome involves temporary discontinuation of ATRA, use of high-dose steroids, and initiation of either hydroxyurea or conventional Ara-C/daunorubicin chemotherapy to control leukocytosis.

Temporary pseudotumor cerebri: is another fairly common (10%) side effect of ATRA.

ATRA vs standard induction chemotherapy: The Italian "AIDA" study combined ATRA with idarubicin for induction. The CR rate was 95%, with only 5% mortality during induction, suggesting that Ara-C is not required to achieve remission.

NEW AGENTS IN THE TREATMENT OF APL

Arsenic trioxide (Trisenox) as a single agent has produced complete responses in 40 of 47 (83%) patients with relapsed APL and 8 of 11 (73%) patients with newly diagnosed APL. Relapsed patients who received arsenic alone have a median relapse-free survival of 10 months; those who received arsenic and chemotherapy have a 70% relapse-free survival at 2 years.

Liver injury was the major dose-limiting toxicity. Patients with relapsed disease (30%) had mild transaminitis, but newly diagnosed patients (66%) had moderate to severe liver dysfunction, including two deaths from liver failure.

The US intergroup APL trial is incorporating arsenic trioxide consolidation therapy for APL in first CR. Patients are randomized to receive either 2 cycles of daunorubicin plus ATRA or 2 cycles of arsenic trioxide followed by 2 cycles of daunorubicin plus ATRA.

Monitoring response to therapy: Reverse-transcriptase (RTPCR) for the PML/RAR-a fusion protein can be used to follow response to therapy. The marker clears slowly, with many patients still positive following induction. However, patients with persistence of PML/RAR-a at the end of consolidation are at high risk of relapse, as are those with reemergence of the marker following a period without detectable protein.

CHRONIC LEUKEMIAS

There are 2 main types of chronic leukaemia called CLL and CML (or CGL). Another less common type of chronic leukaemia is hairy cell leukaemia. The risk factors for all these conditions are slightly different.

The two commonest types of chronic leukaemia are:

- Chronic myeloid leukaemia (CML) and
- Chronic lymphocytic leukaemia (CLL)

The difference between them is the type of white blood cell that has become cancerous. In CLL the abnormal cells develop from the lymphoid blood stem cells. The cancerous white blood cells are B lymphocytes, also called B cells.

In CML, the abnormal cells develop from the myeloid blood stem cells. So the cancerous white blood cells are myelocytes. These cells are sometimes called granulocytes. So you may hear this type of leukaemia called chronic granulocytic leukaemia or CGL. ('Myeloid is pronounced 'my-el-oyd' and granulocytic 'gran-you-low-sit-ik'.)

Prolymphocytic Leukaemia and Richter's Syndrome

In about 1 in 10 people with CLL, the disease changes into another type of leukaemia called prolymphocytic leukaemia. Sometimes prolymphocytic leukaemia is diagnosed in people who have not had CLL.

Advanced CLL can sometimes develop into a cancer of the lymphatic system (a lymphoma). This is called Richter's syndrome.

Hairy Cell Leukaemia

This type of chronic leukaemia is rarer than CLL or CML. The leukaemia cells have projections that look like hairs on their surfaces. These can be seen under a microscope and give this type of leukaemia its name.

Large Granular Lymphocytic Leukaemia

This is a rare condition that is similar to CLL. There are 2 different types of lymphocyte blood cells – B cells and T cells. The white blood cells affected in CLL are B cells. The white blood cells affected in LGLL are T cells. This rare leukaemia tends to be diagnosed in younger people than CLL and is more common in women than men.

Although they are all similar diseases in many ways, these different types of chronic leukaemia all behave differently from one another.

CML

The common risk factors for CML are

- Age–CML is commonest between the ages of 40 and 60
- Gender–it is slightly more common in men
- Radiation-atomic bomb survivors had an increased risk of leukaemia and if you have had radiotherapy for another cancer in the past, this could increase your risk of developing CML
- Contact with a chemical called benzene for some years may increase CML risk

Electromagnetic fields are often talked about as a possible risk factor but probably do not increase leukaemia risk. We are all exposed to electromagnetic radiation. It is all around us. There has been some research that suggested this might by a risk factor for leukaemia. But no increase in risk of either CML or CLL has ever been found in adults who are exposed to the normal background levels people generally experience in their own homes. Statistically, there is a small increased risk for children exposed to the highest end of the normal home levels. But researchers are fairly sure this is a blip. They can't find a way that electromagnetic radiation could cause leukaemia. It certainly isn't responsible for most cases of leukaemia.

There may be a genetic factor in CML. Most people diagnosed with it are found to have an abnormal chromosome This is called the 'Philadelphia chromosome'. It is caused by some of the DNA from chromosome no. 9 getting stuck onto chromosome no. 22. This is called a translocation and is a known type of genetic abnormality. The *Philadelphia chromosome* causes the cell to make a protein which encourages the leukaemic cells to grow and multiply. It is this chromosome change that causes CML. We do know that it is not inherited and you can't pass it on to your children.

Benzene is one of the chemicals in petrol. It is also a solvent used in the rubber industry.

Hairy Cell Leukaemia

The common risk factors for hairy cell leukaemia (HCL) are:

- Age-HCL tends to be more common after the age of 30 with the commonest age for diagnosis being around 50
- Gender–4 times as many men are diagnosed with this type of leukaemia as women.

CLL

The common risk factors for CLL are:

- Age–it is much more common to get CLL if you are older. It is commonest in those over 60 and is very rare under 40.
- Gender–men are twice as likely to develop CLL as women
- Family history of CLL–there may be a greater risk if it runs in your family (one relative with a disease does not mean there is a family history)

Electromagnetic fields are unlikely to be a risk factor for CLL.

Screening

Screening means testing people for the early stages of a disease, before they show any signs of having it.

Before screening for any type of cancer can be carried out, doctors must have an accurate test to use. The test must be reliable in picking up cancers that are there. And it must not give a positive result in people who do not have cancer. Or for groups of people who are known to be at a particularly high risk. The aim of screening is to diagnose cancer

- At an early stage
- Before symptoms start
- When it is easier to treat
- When it is more likely to be curable

There is no screening programme for chronic leukaemia. If screening was to be introduced for chronic leukaemia, the test would have to be simple, quick and not too expensive. Leukaemia is not a common condition. It would probably be most cost effective to screen people who are thought to be at higher risk. There are no easily identifiable risk groups for chronic leukamaemia that we know of.

About 1 in 4 people with chronic leukaemia won't have any symptoms at all. Their chronic leukaemia may be diagnosed because they have a routine blood test for something else. In chronic leukaemia symptoms tend to be mild at first and get worse slowly.

Many symptoms are vague. You may feel as if you had the flu. Some common symptoms are listed below. Remember that many of these symptoms are more likely to be caused by other illnesses. Chronic leukaemia may cause

- Infections that will not get better
- Swollen lymph glands
- Abdominal discomfort from an enlarged spleen
- Bleeding or bruising
- Tiredness from a shortage of red blood cells (anaemia)
- Bone pain
- Night sweats
- Fever
- Weight loss
- Headaches and visual disturbances

One has a tendency to get infections because the white blood cells, which usually fight infection, are abnormal and do not work properly. The other symptoms are mainly caused by the unusually large numbers of white blood cells in your circulation.

The extra white blood cells can clog up the lymph nodes and spleen, causing them to swell. The spleen is an organ on the left of your body, just under your ribs. If it becomes enlarged, it can be uncomfortable or painful.

The extra white blood cells take up space in the bone marrow. There is not enough room for platelets to be made. These normally help to clot the blood, so you may have nosebleeds, unexplained bruising or unusually heavy periods.

The lack of space in the bone marrow also interferes with the production of red blood cells. These normally help to carry oxygen around the body. The extra white blood cells in the bone marrow increase the pressure inside the bones and can cause bone pain.

If the patient has a very high white blood cell count, the extra cells can clog the smallest blood vessels in the eyes and brain. This causes headaches and eye problems in some people with chronic leukaemia.

If signs and symptoms suggest a person may have leukemia, the doctor will need to check samples of blood and bone marrow in order to be certain of this diagnosis. Other tissue and cell samples may also be taken in order to guide treatment.

Blood cell counts and blood cell examination: These tests recognize changes in the numbers of different blood cell types and in the appearance of these cells under the microscope. Most patients with chronic leukemia have too many white cells in their blood, not enough red blood cells, and not enough blood platelets. Even though these findings suggest leukemia, usually the disease cannot be accurately diagnosed without testing a sample of bone marrow cells.

Blood chemistry tests: These tests measure the amount of certain chemicals in their blood but are not used to diagnose leukemia. In patients already known to have leukemia, these tests help detect liver or kidney problems due to damage caused by the spread of leukemic cells or to the side effects of certain chemotherapy drugs.

These tests also help determine whether treatment is needed to correct abnormally low or high blood levels of certain minerals.

Bone marrow tests: The bone marrow sample is taken from the pelvis. The patient lies on the stomach and the doctor feels the bones at the top of the buttocks. The area is cleaned with a special soap. Prior to the bone marrow test, your doctor will inject a local anesthetic, usually lidocaine, into the back of the pelvic bone about an inch or two from the middle of your back. This will cause some very brief stinging. When this has had a few moments to take effect, the doctor will make a small cut so he or she can insert a needle (the needle is about half as wide as a pencil and has a handle on one end that the doctor holds while he or she moves it through your bone). The biopsy needle is moved through the bone with a twisting motion. In bone marrow aspiration, a syringe is used to suck out a small amount of liquid bone marrow (about 1 teaspoon). Sometimes the needle going into the bone is painful, but it only lasts a short time. The sucking out is often painful or at least uncomfortable for a brief moment. Usually this is followed by a bone marrow biopsy in the same area. The doctor will carefully move the needle further into the bone marrow to collect a second sample of bone marrow called a core biopsy. This contains a small solid piece of bone and marrow (about 1/16 inch in diameter and ½ inch long) is removed with a slightly larger needle. You may also feel some pressure as the doctor removes the marrow specimen. After the needle is pulled out, this solid sample is pushed out with a wire so that it can be examined under a microscope. You will have pressure held against your buttock at the biopsy site for a few minutes and a pressure dressing applied. These bone marrow tests are used to diagnosis leukemia and later, to tell if the leukemia is responding to therapy.

Excisional lymph node biopsy: A surgeon cuts through the skin to remove the entire lymph node. If the node is near the skin surface, this is a simple operation that can be done with local anesthesia (numbing medication), but if the node is inside the chest or abdomen, general anesthesia (the patient is asleep) is used. This procedure is important in diagnosing lymphomas, but is only rarely used to diagnose chronic lymphocytic leukemia.

Lumbar puncture: A doctor places a small needle into the spinal cavity in the lower back (below the level of the spinal cord) to withdraw some cerebrospinal fluid (CSF), to look for leukemia cells. This procedure is not a routine test for patients with chronic leukemia and is only done if the patient is suspected of having leukemia cells in their brain and or spinal cord.

Laboratory Tests Used to Diagnose and Classify Leukemia

Routine microscopic exam: All of the samples (bone marrow, lymph node tissue, blood and cerebrospinal fluid) are examined under a microscope. The samples are usually examined by a pathologist and are often reviewed by the patient's hematologist/oncologist The doctors will look at the size and shape of the cells and whether they contain granules (microscopic collections of enzymes and other chemicals that help some types of white blood cells fight infections).

Based on a cell's size, shape, and granules, doctors can classify bone marrow cells into specific types. An important element of this cell classification is whether the cell appears mature (resembles normal cells of circulating blood, that can fight infections and are no longer able to reproduce) or immature (lacks features of normal circulating blood cells, not effective in fighting infections, and are able to reproduce). The most immature cells are called blasts.

Another important feature of bone marrow samples is its cellularity. Normal bone marrow contains hematopoietic (blood-forming) cells and fat cells. Marrow with too many blood-forming cells is said to be hypercellular. If too few of these cells are found, the marrow is called hypocellular.

Cytochemistry: After cells from the sample are placed on glass microscope slides, they are exposed to chemical stains (dyes) that are attracted or react with to only some types of leukemia cells. These stains cause a color change that can be seen only under a microscope. The leukocyte alkaline phosphatase (LAP) test is particularly useful in distinguishing CML from other types of leukemia and benign blood conditions.

Flow cytometry: This test is sometimes used to examine the cells from bone marrow, lymph nodes and blood samples. It is very accurate in determining the exact type of leukemia. A sample of cells is treated with special antibodies and passed in front of a laser beam. Each antibody sticks only to certain types of leukemia cells. If the sample contains those cells, the laser will cause them to give off light that is measured and analyzed by a computer. This test is often helpful with classification of acute leukemias but is not needed for most chronic leukemia patients.

Immunocytochemistry: As in flow cytometry, cells from the bone marrow aspiration or biopsy sample are treated with special antibodies. But instead of using a laser and computer, the sample is treated so that certain types of cells change color. The color change can be seen only under a microscope. Like flow cytometry, it is sometimes helpful in determining the exact type of an acute leukemia, but is not necessary in most cases of chronic leukemia.

Cytogenetics: Normal human cells contain 46 chromosomes, pieces of DNA and protein that control cell growth and metabolism. In certain types of leukemia, part of one chromosome may be attached to part of a different chromosome. This change, called a translocation, can usually be seen under a microscope. Recognizing these translocations helps in identifying certain types of CLL and CML and is important in determining the patient's prognosis (the outlook for chances of survival) and in choosing the most suitable treatment.

Over 90% of CML patients have a translocation between chromosomes 9 and 22 present in their leukemic cells. This chromosome change is called the Philadelphia chromosome and was named by the doctors from that city who first noticed the translocation. This was the first translocation discovered that is consistently found in a specific type of cancer. This translocation is not only a useful feature in helping to identify this type of cancer, it has an important role in making the cells cancerous, and studies of the regions of DNA affected by the translocation have provided much information about genes that cause cancer.

Some types of leukemia have an abnormal number of chromosomes. For example, cells in 10 to 20 percent of patients with CLL have three copies of chromosome 12, instead of the usual two copies and about 25 percent have a deletion in chromosome 13.

Cytogenetic testing looks at chromosomal abnormalities. The testing usually takes around 3 weeks, because the leukemic cells must grow in laboratory dishes for a couple of weeks before their chromosomes are ready to be viewed under the microscope. The results of cytogenetic testing are written in a shorthand form that describes which chromosome changes are present.

- A translocation, written as t(9:22), for example, means a part of chromosome 9 is now located on chromosome 22, and part of chromosome 22 is now attached to chromosome 9.
- An inversion, written as inv 16 for example, means that part of the chromosome 16 is upside down and is now in reverse order but is still attached to the chromosome it originated from.
- A deletion, written as-7, for example indicates part of chromosome 7 has been lost.
- An addition, +8 for example, happens when all or part of a chromosome has been duplicated, and too many copies of it are found within the cell.

Molecular genetic studies: Certain substances, called antigen receptors, occur on the surface of lymphocytes. Normal lymphoid tissue contains cells with many different antigen receptors, which help the body respond to infection. Lymphocytic leukemias (such as CLL), however, start from a single abnormal lymphocyte, so all leukemic cells in a patient have the same antigen receptor. Laboratory tests of the DNA that contains information on each cell's antigen receptors are a very sensitive way to diagnose CLL. Because different subtypes of CLL cells have different antigen receptor features, this test is sometimes helpful in CLL classification. However, the test is not necessary in most cases.

DNA tests of leukemia cells can find most translocations that can be seen under a microscope in cytogenetic tests. DNA tests can also find some translocations involving parts of chromosomes too small to be seen with usual cytogenetic testing under a microscope. This sophisticated testing is not needed in most cases of chronic leukemia, but it is sometimes helpful in classifying CML. Between 5 and 10% of CML cases do not have the Philadelphia chromosome on cytogenetic testing. In over half of these Philadelphia chromosome-negative cases, the translocation involving chromosomes 9 and 22 can be identified by a DNA test called polymerase chain reaction (PCR). Information about these translocations may be useful in predicting response to treatment. These tests are also useful after treatment in finding small numbers of remaining leukemia cells that may be missed under a microscope.

Imaging Studies

Imaging studies are ways of producing pictures of the inside of the body. There are several imaging studies that might be done in people with leukemia.

X-rays: During the course of diagnosis and evaluation of a person with leukemia, a chest X-ray and a bone scan are often obtained. These may show a mass in the chest, or evidence of leukemia in the bones or rarely in the joints.

Computed tomography (CT) scan: This is a special kind of X-ray in which the beam moves around the body, taking images from different angles. The images are then combined by a computer to produce a detailed cross-sectional picture of the inside of the body. CT scans are not often used in leukemia, but they can show involvement of lymph nodes in the chest or in the back of the abdomen. Involvement of these areas can occur in CLL.

Magnetic resonance imaging (MRI): This procedure uses powerful magnets and radio waves to produce computer-generated pictures of internal organs. The pictures look very similar to a CT scan, but are more detailed. This scan may be used when there is concern about leukemia involving the brain.

Ultrasound: This test uses sound waves to produce images of internal organs. The test can distinguish solid from fluid-filled masses. It can help to show whether the kidneys, liver, or spleen have been affected by leukemia.

TREATMENT

Adult chronic leukemia is not a single disease. It is really a group of related diseases, and it is important to remember that different types of chronic leukemia vary in their prognosis and response to treatment. Treatment options for each patient are based on the type of leukemia, its stage, and certain prognostic features.

Treatment of Chronic Myelogenous Leukemia

Treatment options for people with CML depend on their phase of the disease (chronic, accelerated, or blast phase), their age, other prognostic factors, and the availability of a stem cell donor with matching tissue type.

Chronic Phase CML

High-dose chemotherapy and total body irradiation (TBI), followed by stem cell transplantation (SCT) is the most effective treatment for CML and the best chance for curing this disease. This is particularly true for people with high Sokal scores. The side effects of SCT are very serious and can be fatal. This treatment is not recommended for older patients who are less able to tolerate the side effects and are more likely to die of treatment-related complications. Some oncologists consider only patients younger than 60 for SCT. Others limit this treatment to those under age 55 or even under age 50, while some oncologists consider patients as old as 70 years old. Close relatives with the same tissue type as the patient are the best source of stem cell transplantation. The 5-year survival rate for patients who receive transplants from matched relatives is between 50% and 66%. The rate for matched unrelated donor transplants is about 33%. For either type of transplant, the survival rate is better for younger patients and those with other favorable prognostic features.

The 5-year survival rate refers to the percent of patients who live at least 5 years after their cancer is diagnosed. Many of these patients live much longer than 5 years after diagnosis, and 5-year rates are used to produce a standard way of discussing prognosis. Five-year relative survival rates exclude from the calculations patients dying of other diseases, and are considered to be a more accurate way to describe the prognosis for patients with a particular type and stage of cancer. Of course, 5-year survival rates are based on patients diagnosed and initially treated more than 5 years ago. Improvements in treatment often result in a more favorable outlook for recently diagnosed patients.

For patients who cannot receive a stem cell transplant (because of age or lack of a suitable donor) interferon-alpha is the most effective option. Interferon is sometimes combined with chemotherapy drugs such as hydroxyurea or cytarabine (ARA-C). The 5-year survival rate for patients with chronic phase CML treated with interferon is about 66%. A small number of patients who are treated with interferon appear to be cured by the treatment.

If a patient's CML does not respond to interferon or if this treatment is stopped because of severe side effects, chemotherapy is the next option. Hydroxyurea is used most often. It has been found to be more effective than an older drug called busulfan (myleran). The 5-year survival rate for chronic phase CML patients treated initially with chemotherapy is about 50%. The outlook is less favorable if chemotherapy is given after interferon therapy was not successful.

If CML returns after stem cell transplantation, treatment options include interferon, chemotherapy, or donor lymphocyte infusion (DLI). For DLI, the patient receives a transfusion of lymphocytes from the same person who donated their stem cells. In some patients, DLI strengthens their immune system's attack against the leukemia cells.

Splenectomy (an operation to remove the spleen) is an option when spread of CML to the spleen causes it to grow large enough to cause symptoms.

Accelerated Phase CML

The treatment options for accelerated phase CML are similar to those for patients with chronic phase CML. But patients with accelerated phase CML are less likely to have a long remission (disease-free period) after treatment. About 15% of patients with accelerated phase CML are alive several years after stem cell transplantation. Interferon is much less effective in this phase. About 20% of patients have some response to chemotherapy but their remission is usually shorter then 6 months.

Blast Phase CML

Most patients with blast phase CML have leukemia cells that resemble cells of acute myeloid leukemia (AML) and are particularly resistant to the chemotherapy drugs generally used for AML. A minority of patients have blast cells that resemble cells of acute lymphoblastic leukemia (ALL). These cells are more sensitive to chemotherapy drugs such as vincristine, prednisone, and doxorubicin.

Allogeneic stem cell transplantation (from a donor) is rarely successful treatment for blast phase CML and the long-term survival rate is less then 10%. Autologous transplantation of stem cells taken from the patient during the chronic phase may return the patient to the chronic phase. This may extend survival and relieve symptoms for a period of months to several years.

Palliative treatment (intended to relieve symptoms rather than a cure) is an important part of treating patients with blast phase CML. Radiation therapy can reduce pain from areas of bone involvement with leukemia. Chemotherapy may relieve some symptoms for a few months.

Clinical trials of new chemotherapy combinations and biological or immunological therapies are important options.

CML Affecting the Brain and Spinal Cord

Symptoms of CML which has spread to the nervous system can be relieved in many cases by chemotherapy injected into the spinal fluid or by radiation therapy to the brain.

Chronic Lymphocytic Leukemia

Treatment options for people with chronic lymphocytic leukemia (CLL) vary greatly, depending on the disease stage and if the leukemia is causing any symptoms.

Low risk-CLL (Rai Stage 0): The prognosis for people with stage 0 CLL is very good with an average survival of nearly 15 years. Most of these patients are over age 60, and no curative treatment is currently available. The usual practice is to give no immediate treatment. Careful and frequent follow-up exams are recommended and treatment should be considered if there is evidence of progression of the leukemia or if the patient later develops bothersome symptoms. More than half of patients with low-risk CLL live at least 14 years after being diagnosed.

Intermediate-risk CLL (Rai Stage I and II): Patients with intermediate-risk CLL who do not have any symptoms may not need immediate treatment. Like those patients with low-risk CLL, they are followed later for signs of progression and onset of new symptoms. Half the people in this category live over 7 years.

The usual treatment for intermediate-risk CLL that is causing symptoms is chemotherapy with chlorambucil. Cyclophosphamide, may be substituted if chlorambucil causes side effects. Combinations of drugs have been also tried but have not been better than chlorambucil alone. Fludarabine is a chemotherapy drug that has been very useful in CLL. Oncologists usually reserve fludarabine for CLL that has recurred after treatment with other drugs. Recently, however, many are using fludarabine as the first treatment, particularly in younger people.

If enlargement of the spleen or lymph nodes in one region of the body is the only problem, localized treatment with low-dose radiation therapy is often used. Splenectomy (surgery to remove the spleen) is another option if enlargement of this organ causes symptoms. If very high numbers of leukemia cells are interfering with normal circulation, leukapheresis is used before chemotherapy. Leukapheresis involves passing the blood through a special machine that removes white blood cells (including leukemia cells) and returns the rest of the blood cells and plasma to the patient. The benefit of this treatment is immediate but temporary. Leukapheresis is useful because chemotherapy may not affect the number of cells until a few days after the first dose.

Clinical trials of interferons and other drugs that boost the immune system's response to the leukemia as well as trials of new chemotherapy drugs are an option for patients with intermediate-risk CLL.

High-risk CLL: As with intermediate-risk CLL, the usual treatment is chemotherapy with chlorambucil or cyclophosphamide, or fludarabine in younger patients, or when CLL persists (does not respond to treatment) or recurs after chlorambucil or cyclophosphamide treatment.

If enlargement of the spleen causes symptoms, surgical removal or radiation therapy (TBI) of the spleen may be helpful.

If several lymphoid tissue regions are affected, total body irradiation therapy is an option.

High-dose chemotherapy and total body irradiation with stem cell transplantation is being studied in clinical trials. Clinical trials of immunotherapy drugs, including interferon, and new chemotherapy drugs are currently being conducted.

The average survival time after diagnosis for patients with high-risk CLL is about 4 years.

Treatment of other complications of CLL: Sometimes CLL alters a patient's immune system in a way that causes it to attack his or her own red blood cells (immunohemolytic anemia) or blood platelets (immune-mediated thrombocytopenia). These conditions are treated with corticosteroid drugs such as prednisone, which is taken by mouth.

One of the most serious complications of CLL is transformation of the leukemia to a high-grade or aggressive non-Hodgkin's lymphoma. This is called Richter Syndrome or Richter Transformation. If this occurs, patients receive treatment for lymphoma. Refer to the American Cancer Society's document "Non-Hodgkin's Lymphoma (Adult)" for more information.

Patients with CLL rarely will have their leukemia transform into the acute form of lymphocytic leukemia.

Treatment of Hairy Cell Leukemia (HCL)

Patients without symptoms are not given any treatment, but do have careful follow-up exams every few months to check for progression and appearance of new symptoms. Some patients with hairy cell leukemia (HCL) live for many years without having any symptoms or receiving any treatment.

Patients with discomfort because of a very enlarged spleen (caused by leukemia cells growing in the spleen) may have that organ surgically removed. This operation is called a splenectomy and was once the main treatment for HCL patients with complications due to low blood cell counts, such as fatigue, frequent infections, and easy bleeding or bruising. Oncologists now recommend chemotherapy for HCL patients with low blood cell counts. The usual treatment is 2-chlorodeoxyadenosine (2-CDA). Pentostatin or interferon is sometimes used, especially if the cancer becomes resistant to 2-CDA. High-dose chemotherapy followed by stem cell transplantation (SCT) is being studied in clinical trials as an option for young patients whose HCL has not responded to other treatments.

The average survival time after diagnosis for HCL patients who receive no treatment is about 5 years. Splenectomy improves this figure to about 7 years. The average survival time for patients treated with chemotherapy is much better, and over 80% are alive and without evidence of leukemia 3 years after treatment. Because most of these chemotherapy drugs used for HCL are relatively new, the exact survival times are not yet known.

Patients without symptoms are not given any treatment, but do have careful follow-up exams every few months to check for progression and appearance of new symptoms. Some patients with hairy cell leukemia (HCL) live for many years without having any symptoms or receiving any treatment.

Patients with discomfort because of a very enlarged spleen (caused by leukemia cells growing in the spleen) may have that organ surgically removed. This operation is called a splenectomy and was once the main treatment for HCL patients with complications due to low blood cell counts, such as fatigue, frequent infections, and easy bleeding or bruising. Oncologists now recommend chemotherapy for HCL patients with low blood cell counts. The usual treatment is 2-chlorodeoxyadenosine (2-CDA). Pentostatin or interferon is sometimes used, especially if the cancer becomes resistant to 2-CDA. High-dose chemotherapy followed by stem cell transplantation (SCT) is being studied in clinical trials as an option for young patients whose HCL has not responded to other treatments.

The average survival time after diagnosis for HCL patients who receive no treatment is about 5 years. Splenectomy improves this figure to about 7 years. The average survival time for patients treated with chemotherapy is much better, and over 80% are alive and without evidence of leukemia 3 years after treatment. Because most of these chemotherapy drugs used for HCL are relatively new, the exact survival times are not yet known.

LYMPHOMAS

There are 2 main types of lymphomas. Hodgkin's lymphoma (also known as Hodgkin lymphoma, Hodgkin disease, or Hodgkin's disease) is named after Dr. Thomas Hodgkin, who first described it as a new disease in 1832. All other types of lymphoma are called non-Hodgkin lymphomas.

These 2 types of lymphoma can usually be distinguished from each other by examining the cancerous tissue under a microscope. In some cases, more tests to identify specific chemical components of the lymphoma cells or tests of the cells' DNA may be needed.

Non-Hodgkin Lymphoma

Non-Hodgkin lymphoma (non-Hodgkin's lymphoma, NHL) is cancer that starts in lymphoid tissue (also called lymphatic tissue), part of the lymphatic system. The lymphatic system is important for filtering bacteria and cancer cells and carrying fluid from the limbs and internal organs back into the blood.

Classification of Non-Hodgkin Lymphoma

The classification of non-Hodgkin lymphoma seems quite confusing (even for many doctors) because there are so many types and because several different systems of classification have been developed. The most recent system is the *Revised European-American Lymphoma/World Health Organization (REAL/WHO)* classification.

The reason for the changes in classification is that the old systems of classifying lymphomas by their appearance alone no longer worked. Modern science had discovered many chemical and genetic characteristics that identified lymphoma cells better than did their appearance. As we learn more about genes in humans, the genetic changes in lymphomas will play a larger role in classification, and new systems will be developed.

REAL/WHO system: The REAL/WHO system not only uses the appearance of the lymphoma cells for classification but also uses genetic features (chromosome defects) of the cells and their chemistry. Mostly the chemistry is evaluated by the presence of proteins on the surface of the cells. This overview classifies the most common lymphomas according to whether they are B-cell or T-cell lymphomas and lists them by how common they are.

B-Cell Lymphomas

Diffuse large B-cell lymphoma (DLBCL): This kind makes up about 31% of all lymphomas. The cells are large when viewed under the microscope. This is a fast growing lymphoma.

The usual symptoms are a quickly growing mass in the body or in a lymph node that you can feel. Although this lymphoma usually starts in lymph nodes, it can grow in other areas such as the intestines, bone, and the brain or spinal cord.

About one-third of these lymphomas are confined to one part of the body (localized). When it is localized this type of lymphoma is considered to be more curable than when it has spread to other parts of the body.

DLBCL can affect any age group but occurs mostly in older people. The average age is in the mid-60s. About 40% to 50% of people with this lymphoma are cured with therapy.

Follicular lymphoma: About 22% of all lymphomas are follicular lymphomas. The name *follicular* is used because the cells tend to grow in a circular, or nodular, pattern in lymph nodes. This is a slow growing lymphoma.

Most of the time this lymphoma arises in many lymph node sites in the body, as well as in the bone marrow.

The average age for people with this lymphoma is about 60. It is rare in very young people. In advanced stages, it is not considered curable by standard treatment. But it is slow growing, and the 5-year survival rate (the percentage of people surviving at least 5 years) is around 60% to 70%. Over time, many follicular lymphomas change (transform) into a fast growing diffuse B-cell lymphoma.

Chronic lymphocytic leukemia (CLL)/ small lymphocytic lymphoma (SLL): These related diseases account for 7% of all lymphomas. In both kinds, the same type of cell, the small lymphocyte, is involved. The only difference is in where the cancer occurs. In CLL it is mostly in the blood, whereas it is mainly in the lymph nodes in lymphoma. Both are slow growing diseases, although CLL, which is much more common, tends to be slower.

CLL and SLL are not considered curable with standard treatments. But depending on the stage and growth rate of the disease, patients can live well over 10 years with this lymphoma. Occasionally over time these slow growing lymphomas transform into a more aggressive type of lymphoma.

Mantle cell lymphoma: About 6% of lymphomas are this kind. The cells are small to medium in size. It is usually widespread when it is diagnosed, involving lymph nodes, bone marrow, and, very often, the spleen.

Men are most often affected. The average age of patients is about 63. Although this is not a very fast growing lymphoma, only 20% of patients survive at least 5 years.

Extranodal marginal zone B-cell lymphomas-mucosa-associated lymphoid tissue (MALT) lymphomas: These account for about 8% of lymphomas. The cells are small.

Most MALT lymphomas arise in the stomach and are thought to stem from an infection by the bacteria *Helicobacter pylori*. Other possible sites are lung, skin, thyroid, salivary gland, and tissues surrounding the eye. Usually it is confined to the area where it began and is not widespread.

The average age for patients with this lymphoma is about 60. It is a slow growing lymphoma and is often curable in its early stages.

Nodal marginal zone B-cell lymphoma: This kind accounts for about 2% of lymphomas. The cells are small. Mostly lymph nodes are involved, although the cells can also sometimes be found in the bone marrow.

This is a slow growing lymphoma, and many patients are cured if they are diagnosed in the early stages.

Splenic marginal zone B-cell lymphoma: This is a rare lymphoma. The cells are small. Most often the lymphoma is found only in the spleen and bone marrow.

Patients are often elderly and male and suffer from fatigue and discomfort caused by an enlarged spleen. Because the disease is slow growing, treatment may not be necessary unless the symptoms become troublesome.

Primary mediastinal B-cell lymphoma: This type accounts for about 2% of all lymphomas. The cells are large. This lymphoma starts in the mediastinum (the area around the heart and behind the chest bone). It usually is localized at the beginning. It rarely involves the bone marrow. It can cause trouble breathing because it often presses into the air passages leading into the lung. It can also block the superior vena cava (the large vein that returns blood to the heart from the arms and head). This can cause the arms and face to swell.

About two-thirds of people with this lymphoma are women. Most are young, in their 30s. It is a fast growing lymphoma, but it is treatable. About half of patients can be cured.

Burkitt's lymphoma: This type (also known as Burkitt lymphoma) makes up about 2% of all lymphomas. It is named after the doctor who first described this disease in African children and young adults. The cells are medium sized. Another kind of lymphoma, called Burkitt's-like lymphoma, has slightly larger cells. Because this second kind of lymphoma is hard to tell apart from Burkitt's lymphoma, the REAL/WHO classification combines them.

This is a very fast growing lymphoma. In the African variety, it often starts as tumors of the jaws or other facial bones. In the more common types seen in the U.S., the lymphoma usually starts in the abdomen, where it forms a large tumor mass. It can also spread to the brain and spinal fluid.

Close to 90% of patients are male, and the average age is about 30. Although this is a fast growing lymphoma, about half of patients are cured by aggressive chemotherapy.

Lymphoplasmocytic lymphoma (Waldenstrom's macroglobulinemia): This kind is not common, accounting for 1% of lymphomas. The cells are small and found mainly in the bone marrow, lymph nodes, and spleen. It is slow growing. Most of the time the lymphoma cells produce an antibody called a macroglobulin, immunoglobulin M (IgM), which is a very large protein. This antibody circulates in the blood and causes it to thicken, leading to the symptoms typical of this disease.

Symptoms caused by high IgM levels include weakness, fatigue, problems with vision (due to poor circulation in blood vessels in the back of the eyes), a tendency to bleed easily, and neurological problems (such as headache, dizziness, and confusion) caused by poor blood flow within the brain. High blood IgM levels can also damage some organs, such as the kidneys.

Although this lymphoma is not curable, most patients live longer than 5 years.

For more information, see the ACS document "Waldenstrom's Macroglobulinemia."

Hairy cell leukemia: This lymphoma is rare-about 500 people in the U.S. are diagnosed with this type each year. The typical cell is small with projections around it that have a hair-like appearance. It typically is found in the bone marrow and spleen and circulating in the blood. It is slow growing, and some patients never need treatment. An enlarging spleen or dropping blood counts because of bone marrow replacement by lymphoma are the usual reasons to begin treatment. Patients are older in general.

Primary central nervous system (CNS) lymphoma: This lymphoma usually involves the brain (called primary brain lymphoma), but it also can be found in the spinal cord and in tissues around the spinal cord and the eye. Over time, it becomes widespread in the central nervous system. Although this was a rare tumor in the past, it has become more common in patients with acquired immune deficiency syndrome (AIDS). Most people develop headache and confusion. They can also have vision problems and, rarely, paralysis.

The outlook for people with this condition is poor. But about 30% of people can live at least 5 years with modern therapy.

T-Cell Lymphomas

Precursor T-lymphoblastic lymphoma/leukemia: This disease can be considered either a lymphoma or leukemia. The distinction depends on whether more or less than 25% of bone marrow cells are lymphoma cells. Leukemias have more than 25% involvement; lymphomas have less. Usually there is a mass of lymphoma in the mediastinum (the area around the heart and behind the chest bone).

About 2% of all lymphomas fall into this category. Patients are most often (75%) men, and their average age is about 25. The typical cell is small to middle sized. The lymphoma is fast growing, but if it hasn't spread to the bone marrow when it is first diagnosed, the chance of cure with chemotherapy is quite good. Once it involves the bone marrow, only 20% of patients can be cured.

Peripheral T-cell lymphomas: There are several kinds of peripheral T-cell lymphomas, which, in total, account for about 7% of all lymphomas.

Cutaneous T-cell lymphoma (mycosis fungoides, Sezary syndrome): This T-cell lymphoma starts in the skin. It is rare, making up less than 1% of all lymphomas. Most patients are in their 50s or 60s.

This lymphoma usually begins as patchy, scaly, red lesions on the skin. They then progress to more solid, raised tumors that can become bigger and mushroom-like (so first named *mycosis fungoides*). In time, the lymphoma can invade lymph nodes and then organs like the liver and spleen. The growth rate varies among patients.

In the Sezary syndrome, the lymphoma cells are found in the blood. Here the skin is involved all over instead of in patches. It usually appears thickened and very red, and it is often itchy.

Survival depends on whether the lymphoma spreads. In Sezary syndrome the lymphoma has spread all over the body through the blood. Patient survival at 5 years ranges from 58% for slow growing lymphomas to 5% for faster growing ones.

The same is true for mycosis fungoides. If only the skin contains lymphoma as patches and not tumors, few patients die of this lymphoma. But once it forms tumors and invades lymph nodes, only about half of patients survive at least 5 years. Once it invades internal organs, very few patients survive 5 years.

Angioimmunoblastic T-cell lymphoma: This lymphoma tends to occur in the lymph nodes. Patients usually have fever, weight loss, and skin rashes and often develop infections. This lymphoma progresses rapidly, with some patients getting better with steroids and/or chemotherapy. But it's not clear that anyone with this lymphoma can be cured.

Extranodal natural killer/T-cell lymphoma, nasal type: This type often involves the upper airway passages, such as the nose and upper throat, but also invades the skin and digestive tract. All ages can be affected. If the lymphoma is localized to the nasal passages, it can be cured by chemotherapy and radiotherapy. But if it is widespread, then only a few patients are cured by very aggressive chemotherapy.

Enteropathy type T-cell lymphoma: This lymphoma occurs in people with sensitivity to gluten, the main protein in wheat flour. The disease, called gluten-sensitive enteropathy, can progress to this lymphoma, which typically invades the walls of the intestines. Once it occurs, outlook is poor because of damage to the intestines.

Subcutaneous panniculitis-like T-cell lymphoma: This lymphoma invades the deepest layers of the skin, where it causes nodules to form. These are often slow growing at first and can be treated with radiation therapy. In time, they begin to grow faster. Chemotherapy can sometimes control the growth, but after a while it no longer works. This lymphoma usually cannot be cured.

Anaplastic large T/null-cell lymphoma: About 2% of lymphomas are this kind. The cells are large. It is more common in young people. It usually starts in lymph nodes and can also spread to skin. There is also a form that begins in the skin. Although this type of lymphoma appears to be a fast growing, treatment with chemotherapy often works well. Many patients with this lymphoma are cured.

Unspecified: This group has no other name. Most patients with this form are in their 60s. The lymphoma tends to be widespread and grows quickly. Cells can be small or large. Few patients survive 5 years.

The Risk Factors for Non-Hodgkin's Lymphoma

A risk factor is anything that increases a person's chance of getting a disease such as cancer. Risk factors can be classified as genetic (inherited), lifestyle-related, or environmental.

However, most patients with non-Hodgkin lymphoma have no known risk factors. It's also important to note that having one or more risk factors doesn't mean that a person will develop this cancer. Age is the greatest factor for this disease, with most cases occurring among those in their 60s.

Genetic Risk Factors

Several genetic diseases can cause children to be born with an abnormal or deficient immune system. In addition to developing serious infections due to reduced immune defenses, they also have an increased risk of developing non-Hodgkin lymphoma during childhood or as young adults. How this happens is discussed in the section "Do We Know What Causes Non-Hodgkin Lymphoma?"

Although these congenital (present at birth) immune deficiency diseases can be passed on to children, people with non-Hodgkin lymphoma who do not have these inherited diseases *do not* pass an increased risk of lymphoma to their children.

Lifestyle-Related Risk Factors

Examples of lifestyle-related risk factors for some cancers include exposing skin to strong sunlight, a diet high in fat and low in fruits and vegetables, and habits such as smoking and excessive drinking of alcohol.

Lifestyle-related factors such as these do not strongly affect a person's risk of developing non-Hodgkin lymphoma. However, being obese may increase your risk of non-Hodgkin lymphoma.

Environmental Risk Factors

Environmental risk factors are influences in our surroundings, such as radiation, chemicals, and infections.

Radiation: Survivors of atomic bombs and nuclear reactor accidents have an increased risk of developing several types of cancer, including leukemia, thyroid cancer, and non-Hodgkin lymphoma. Patients treated with radiation therapy for some other cancers have a slightly increased risk of developing non-Hodgkin lymphoma later in life. This risk is greater for patients treated with both radiation therapy and chemotherapy.

Chemicals: Some studies have suggested that chemicals such as benzene and certain herbicides and insecticides (weed-and insect-killing substances) are associated with an increased risk of non-Hodgkin lymphoma. Recent studies have found that this is not certain, and research to clarify this issue is still in progress.

Some chemotherapy drugs used to treat other cancers can increase the risk of developing leukemia or non-Hodgkin lymphoma many years later; however, a direct cause and effect relationship has not yet been definitely established. For example, patients who have been treated for Hodgkin disease have an increased risk of later developing non-Hodgkin lymphoma. This may be related to the disease itself or may be an effect of the treatment.

Immune deficiency: Patients with transplanted organs (kidney, heart, liver) and some other conditions like rheumatoid arthritis are treated with drugs that interfere with their immune system to prevent it from attacking the new organs. This effect on the immune system carries a significant risk to the patient of developing non-Hodgkin lymphoma. The exact risk depends on which drugs and at what doses they are used.

Infections: Infection with human immunodeficiency virus (HIV), also known as the AIDS virus, is an increasingly common cause of immune system deficiency. HIV infection is a risk factor for developing certain types of non-Hodgkin lymphoma.

Infection with the human T-cell leukemia/lymphoma virus (HTLV-1) increases a person's risk of developing certain types of T-cell non-Hodgkin lymphoma. This virus is most common in some parts of Japan and in the Caribbean region. In some areas of Japan, it is responsible for about half of the non-Hodgkin lymphoma cases. In the United States, it causes less than 1% of lymphomas. HTLV-1 belongs to the same family of viruses as HIV. Like HIV, it spreads through sexual intercourse and contaminated blood and can be passed to children through breast milk.

In areas of Africa where Burkitt's lymphoma is common, infection with the parasite that causes malaria and with the Epstein-Barr virus (EBV) are important risk factors for this disease. EBV is also associated with lymphomas in developed countries, particularly in patients infected with HIV.

Scientists have recently found that a type of bacteria, *Helicobacter pylori,* known to cause stomach ulcers, can also cause some lymphomas of the stomach. The body's immune reaction to this infection increases the risk of non-Hodgkin lymphoma. The most important consequence of this recent discovery is that antibiotics can be helpful in treating some patients who have already developed lymphomas of the stomach.

Although researchers have found that non-Hodgkin lymphoma is associated with a number of risk factors, most patients with non-Hodgkin lymphoma do not have any known risk factors, and the causes of their cancers are unknown.

Scientists have recently made great progress in understanding how certain changes in DNA can cause normal lymphocytes to become lymphoma cells. DNA is the chemical that carries the instructions for nearly everything our cells do. We resemble our parents because they are the source of our DNA. But DNA affects more than our outward appearance. Some genes (parts of our DNA) contain instructions for controlling when cells grow and divide.

Certain genes that speed up cell division are called *oncogenes*. Others that slow down cell division or cause cells to die at the right time are called *tumor suppressor genes*. We know that cancers can be caused by DNA mutations (defects) that turn on oncogenes or turn off tumor suppressor genes.

Some people with certain types of cancer have DNA mutations they inherited from a parent, which increased their risk for the disease. But non-Hodgkin lymphoma is not one of the cancer types often caused by these inherited mutations.

DNA mutations related to non-Hodgkin lymphoma are usually acquired after birth, rather than being inherited. Acquired mutations may result from exposure to radiation or cancer-causing chemicals, but often these mutations occur for no apparent reason. They seem to occur more often as we age, and lymphomas for the most part are a cancer of older people.

Every time a cell prepares to divide into two new cells, it must duplicate its DNA. This process is not perfect and, sometimes, copying errors occur. Fortunately, cells have repair enzymes that proofread DNA. But some errors may slip past, especially if the cells are growing rapidly.

Translocations are another type of DNA abnormality that can cause non-Hodgkin's lymphoma to develop. Human DNA is packaged in 23 pairs of chromosomes. A translocation means that DNA from one chromosome breaks off and becomes attached to a different chromosome. When this happens, oncogenes can be turned on or tumor suppressor genes can be turned off. This often occurs in cases of non-Hodgkin lymphoma. Some lymphomas classified in the REAL/WHO system are characterized by specific chromosomal defects that may lead to the development of lymphoma.

Scientists are learning much about the exact genes involved in this process and how they cause lymphoma and other cancers. This information is already being used to develop new and more accurate tests for detecting and classifying certain types of non-Hodgkin lymphoma. Hopefully, these discoveries will soon be applied to developing new treatments.

Even though researchers have found many of the key DNA changes that cause lymphoma and are beginning to understand how these changes develop in people with certain risk factors, they still do not know why most lymphomas develop in people with no apparent risk factors.

The immune system seems to play an important role in many cases of lymphoma. People with *immune deficiencies* (due to inherited conditions, drug treatment, organ transplantation, or HIV infection) have a chance of developing lymphoma that is many times that of people without an immune deficiency.

Signs and Symptoms of Non-Hodgkin Lymphoma

Non-Hodgkin lymphoma may cause many different signs and symptoms, depending its location in the body.

Non-Hodgkin lymphoma can involve easily seen or felt lymph nodes close to the *surface of the body* (such as on the sides of the neck, in the groin or underarm areas, or above the collar bone). These are often discovered by the patient, a family member, or a health care professional.

When the lymphoid tissue inside the *abdomen* is involved, the abdomen can become swollen. This may be due either to large collections of fluid or to a tumor. When lymphoma causes swelling near the intestines, the passage of feces may be blocked, which may lead to nausea or vomiting. The pressure or blockage can also cause discomfort or abdominal pain.

When lymphoma starts in the thymus or lymph nodes in the *chest*, it may irritate or compress the nearby trachea (windpipe), which can cause coughing or trouble breathing.

The *superior vena cava* (SVC) is the large vein that carries blood from the head and arms back to the heart. It passes near the thymus and lymph nodes inside the chest. Growth of lymphoma may push on this vein. This causes swelling of the head and arms known as *SVC syndrome.* This can be life threatening-patients with SVC syndrome need to be treated as soon as possible.

Lymphomas of the *stomach* often cause pain in the stomach, nausea, and reduced appetite.

Lymphomas of the *brain,* called primary brain lymphomas, can cause headache, trouble thinking and moving parts of the body, personality changes, and, sometimes, seizures.

Lymphomas of the *skin* can be seen and felt. They often appear as itchy, red to purple lumps or nodules under the skin.

In addition to symptoms and signs resulting from local effects of cancer growth, non-Hodgkin lymphoma can produce *generalized symptoms,* such as:

- Unexplained weight loss
- Fever
- Profuse sweating (enough to soak clothing), particularly at night
- Severe itchiness

Oncologists sometimes call these generalized effects *B symptoms.* The presence of B symptoms is associated with a poor outlook and is related to an increased tumor burden (more cancer cells) in some patients.

The diagnosis of lymphoma may be delayed because enlarged lymph nodes are more often caused by infections than by non-Hodgkin lymphoma. Because of this, doctors will often wait a few weeks to see if they remain large. Sometimes they will prescribe antibiotics to see if they cause the nodes to shrink.

If the node continues to grow, either a small piece of the node or, more commonly, the entire node should be removed for viewing under the microscope and for other lab tests. This procedure is called a biopsy.

An immediate biopsy may be needed if the size, texture, or location of the node or the presence of other symptoms strongly suggests cancer is present. But there is no evidence that a delay in diagnosis of a few weeks is harmful in most instances. The exception to this would be a very rapidly growing lymphoma.

Types of Biopsies Used in Diagnosis of Non-Hodgkin Lymphoma

A biopsy is the only way to diagnose non-Hodgkin lymphoma. There are several biopsy procedures, and the doctor's choice is based on the unique aspects of each person's situation.

Excisional or incisional biopsy: In this procedure, a surgeon cuts through the skin to remove either the entire node (excisional biopsy) or a small part of a large tumor (incisional biopsy). If the node is near the skin surface, this is a simple operation that can be done with local anesthesia (numbing medication). But if the node is inside the chest or abdomen, general anesthesia is used (the patient is asleep). This method almost always provides enough tissue to diagnose the exact type of non-Hodgkin lymphoma. It is preferred, if it can be done without too much discomfort to the patient.

Fine needle aspiration (FNA) biopsy: FNA uses a very thin needle and a syringe to withdraw a small amount of tissue from the tumor mass. The doctor can aim the needle while feeling an enlarged node near the surface of the body. If the tumor is deep inside the body, the doctor can guide the needle while viewing a computed tomography (CT) scan (see discussion of imaging tests later in this section).

The main advantage of FNA is that it does not require surgery. The disadvantage is that in some cases the thin needle cannot remove enough tissue for a definite diagnosis of non-Hodgkin lymphoma. However, advances in performing lab tests (discussed later in this section) and the growing experience of many doctors with FNA have improved the accuracy of this procedure. FNA is very useful in diagnosing cancers that spread to nodes from other organs and in identifying nodes swollen by infection that don't need to be removed.

Other Types of Biopsies

These procedures may be done to diagnose lymphoma, but they are more often done to help stage (determine the extent of) a lymphoma that has already been diagnosed.

Bone marrow aspiration and biopsy: These procedures are usually done at the same time. In bone marrow aspiration, a needle and syringe are used to remove small amounts of bone marrow. For bone marrow biopsy, a larger needle is used to remove a cylinder of bone and marrow, about 1/16 inch across and 1 inch long. Both samples are usually taken from marrow at the back of the hip bone after numbing the area with local anesthesia. These tests can be used for the initial diagnosis and for staging (to see how far the cancer has spread).

Lumbar puncture (spinal tap): During a lumbar puncture, a thin needle is inserted between the bones in the spine in the lower back (below the level of the spinal cord) to withdraw some cerebrospinal fluid (CSF), which is then examined for lymphoma cells.

Laboratory Tests Used to Diagnose and Classify Non-Hodgkin Lymphoma

All biopsy specimens are examined under a microscope by pathologist (a doctor with special training in recognizing cancer cells). The pathologist looks at the size and shape of the cells and how the cells are arranged in the lymph node. This may reveal not only whether or not the person has a lymphoma, but also what type of lymphoma it is.

The many specific types are sometimes grouped together into low-grade, intermediate-grade, or high-grade categories. High-grade lymphomas grow more rapidly and spread through the body quickly. Without treatment, most patients with these lymphomas would live only a short time. The term "aggressive" is also sometimes used to describe high-grade lymphomas. Most high-grade lymphomas respond well to chemotherapy, and many can be cured.

Pathologists who specialize in diagnosing lymphoma can often tell which kind of lymphoma a patient has, but sometimes this exam does not provide a definite answer, and other lab tests are needed.

Immunohistochemistry: In this test, a part of the biopsy sample is treated with special laboratory antibodies that attach to specific molecules on the cell surface. These antibodies cause color changes, which can be seen under a microscope. This test may be helpful in distinguishing different types of non-Hodgkin lymphoma from one another and from other diseases.

Flow cytometry: Some specific molecules on the surface of lymphoma cells can be detected using fluorescent antibodies. The cells being examined by this test are treated with the antibodies and passed in front of a laser beam. Each antibody sticks only to certain types of cells. If the sample contains those cells, the laser light will cause them to give off light of a different color, which is measured exactly and analyzed by a computer. This test can look at many more cells than immunohistochemistry.

Flow cytometry can help determine whether lymph node swelling is due to non-Hodgkin lymphoma, some other cancer, or a non-cancerous disease. It has also become very useful in helping doctors determine the exact type of non-Hodgkin lymphoma so that they can select the best treatment.

Cytogenetics: This technique involves using a microscope to examine cells to see if the chromosomes have any translocations (where part of one chromosome has broken off and is now attached to another chromosome), as happens in certain types of lymphoma. In addition to translocations, some lymphoma cells may have too many chromosomes.

Molecular genetic studies: Molecular tests of lymphoma cell DNA can detect translocations that are not visible under a microscope in cytogenetic tests. These tests can also detect certain genes that have been "turned on" and are contributing to the lymphoma cells abnormal growth. In the future, as we learn more about lymphomas, these may become the most useful tests for determining what kind of lymphoma is present.

Imaging Studies Used to Diagnose and Stage Non-Hodgkin Lymphoma

Imaging tests are used to find and look at tumors inside the body. These tests are an important part of staging.

Chest X-ray: An X-ray of the chest is often done to look for enlarged lymph nodes in this area.

Computed tomography (CT, CAT) scan: The CT scan is an X-ray procedure that produces detailed cross-sectional images of your body. Instead of taking one picture, as does a conventional X-ray, a CT scanner takes many pictures as it rotates around you while you are lying on a table. A computer then combines these pictures into an image of a slice of your body. The machine can create many images of the part of your body that is being studied. A CT is useful for looking for lymphoma in the abdomen, pelvis, chest, head, and neck.

After the first set of pictures is taken, you may receive an intravenous (IV) injection of a "dye" (radiocontrast agent) that helps better outline structures in your body. You may also be asked to drink 1 to 2 pints of a solution of contrast material. This helps outline the intestine so that it is not mistaken for tumors. A second set of pictures is then taken.

CT scans take longer than regular X-rays. You must lie still on a table while the part of your body to be examined is placed within the scanner, a doughnut-shaped machine that completely surrounds the Table.

You may need an IV line through which the contrast dye is injected. The injection can cause flushing. Some people are allergic and get hives or, rarely, have more serious reactions like trouble breathing or low blood pressure. Be sure to tell the doctor if you have ever had a reaction to any contrast material used for X-rays.

A newer kind of CT, known as a *spiral CT,* uses a rapid scanner that takes quicker images. This reduces the chances that body movement caused by the patient taking breaths will distort the images, and therefore can provide greater detail. This type of CT scan is still relatively new, and is not yet available in all areas.

CT scans can also be used to precisely guide a biopsy needle into an enlarged lymph node deep in the body. For this procedure, called a *CT-guided needle biopsy,* the patient remains on the CT scanning table while a radiologist advances a biopsy needle toward the mass. CT scans are repeated until the doctors are sure that the needle is within the mass. A fine needle biopsy (tiny fragment of tissue) or a core needle biopsy (a thin cylinder of tissue about ½ inch long and less than 1/8 inch in diameter) sample is then removed and viewed under a microscope.

Magnetic resonance imaging (MRI) scan: MRI scans use radio waves and strong magnets instead of X-rays. The energy from the radio waves is absorbed and then released in a pattern formed by the type of tissue and by certain diseases. A computer translates the pattern of radio waves given off by the tissues into a very detailed image of parts of the body. Not only does this produce cross-sectional slices of the body like a CT scanner, it can also produce slices that are parallel with the length of your body. You may receive a contrast material just as with CT scans, but this is used less often.

MRI scans are helpful in examining the brain and spinal cord.

MRI scans are a little more uncomfortable than CT scans. First, they take longer-about an hour. Also, you have to lie inside a narrow tube, which can upset people with claustrophobia. The machine also makes a thumping noise, so some places may provide earplugs or headphones with music to block this out.

Positron emission tomography (PET) scan: PET scans use glucose (a form of sugar) that contains a slightly radioactive atom. The glucose solution is injected into a vein and travels throughout the body. Cancer cells absorb high amounts of the radioactive sugar because of their high rate of metabolism. A special camera can then detect the radioactivity.

PET is useful to look for lymphoma throughout your body. A PET scan can be more helpful than several different X-rays because it scans your whole body. It can also tell if an enlarged lymph node contains lymphoma or is benign.

PET is also used after treatment in helping decide whether an enlarged lymph node still contains lymphoma or is merely scar tissue. Although this test is relatively new, it is becoming widely used to examine people with lymphomas.

Gallium scan: During this procedure, the radiologist injects slightly radioactive gallium into a vein. It is attracted to areas of lymphatics in the body. A special camera can then detect the radioactivity, showing the location of the gallium. These tests can find tumors that might be non-Hodgkin lymphoma in bones and other organs.

The gallium scan will not detect most indolent (slow growing) lymphomas but will recognize most aggressive (fast growing) lymphomas. It was used before PET scans were available, and can still be useful in finding lymphoma deposits that the PET scan may miss. It is also useful in separating infectious abscesses from lymphomas when the diagnosis is not clear.

Bone scan: For bone scans, a different radioactive substance is used. After it is injected, it travels to areas of the bone that are damaged. Lymphoma in bone often causes bone damage, and a bone scan will find it. But a bone scan will also pick up non-cancerous problems, such as arthritis and fractures. This test is not generally used in the early staging process for non-Hodgkin lymphoma.

Ultrasound: Ultrasound uses sound waves and their echoes to produce a picture of internal organs or masses. A small microphone-like instrument called a *transducer* emits sound waves. These waves are transmitted into the area of the body being studied and echo back. The echoes are picked up by the transducer and converted by a computer into an image that is displayed on a computer screen.

This is a very easy procedure. It uses no radiation, which is why it is often used to look at developing fetuses. To have an ultrasound examination, you simply lie on a table and a technician moves the transducer along the skin over the part of your body being examined. Usually, the skin is first lubricated with oil.

Sometimes an ultrasound is used to find masses in the abdomen. It can also detect kidneys that have become swollen because the outflow of urine has been blocked by enlarged lymph nodes.

Once non-Hodgkin lymphoma is diagnosed, tests are done to determine the stage (extent of spread) of the disease. The treatment and prognosis (the outlook for chances of survival) for a patient with non-Hodgkin lymphoma depend on both the exact type and the stage of the lymphoma. This disease tends to be widespread, although the less aggressive types may be localized.

Tests used to gather information for staging include:

- Physical examination
- Blood tests
- Imaging tests, including a chest X-ray, CT or MRI scan of the chest/abdomen/pelvis, and PET scan
- Bone marrow aspiration and biopsy (often but not always done)

- Lumbar puncture (spinal tap-this is not often done)

These tests are described in the section "How Is Non-Hodgkin Lymphoma Diagnosed?"

The staging system most often used to describe the spread of non-Hodgkin lymphoma in adults is called the *Ann Arbor staging system.* The stages are described by Roman numerals I through IV. Lymphomas that affect organs outside of the lymph system ("extranodal' organs) have "E" added to their stage (for example, stage IIE).

Stage I : Either of the following means the disease is a stage I:

The lymphoma is in a lymph node or nodes in only 1 region, such as the neck, groin, underarm, and so on.

The cancer is found only in one area of a single organ outside of the lymph system (IE).

Stage II : Either of the following means the disease is a stage II:

The lymphoma is in 2 groups of lymph nodes on the same side of (above or below) the diaphragm (the breathing muscle that aids breathing and separates the chest and abdomen). For example, this might include nodes in the underarm and neck area, but not the combination of underarm and groin nodes.

The cancer extends locally from the lymph node(s) into nearby tissue (IIE).

Stage III : Either of the following means the disease is a stage III:

The lymphoma is found in lymph node areas on both sides of (above and below) the diaphragm.

The cancer may also have extended into an area or organ next to the lymph node (IIIE), into the spleen (IIIS), or both (IIISE).

Stage IV : Any of the following means the disease is a stage IV:

The lymphoma has spread to more than 1 spot in an organ or to 2 or more organs outside of the lymph system. Cancer cells may or may not be found in nearby lymph nodes.

Cancer has spread to only 1 organ outside of the lymph system, but lymph nodes far away from that organ are involved.

The lymphoma has spread to the brain or spinal cord, liver, or bone marrow.

The letter "B" is added (stage IIIB, for example) if any B symptoms are present:

- Unexplained weight loss (more than 10% of weight)
- Soaking night sweats
- Unexplained high fever

For patients without these symptoms, the letter "A" is added to their stage.

International Prognostic Index (IPI)

This index was developed to help predict how rapidly the lymphoma would grow and how well patients would respond to treatment (or whether they would need treatment at all). Although the REAL/WHO classifications give us some idea of this, many times people with so-called low-grade lymphomas have a very fast growing disease that does not respond to treatment, while patients with high-grade lymphomas may respond very well to treatment.

The index depends on 5 factors:

- Age
- Stage of the lymphoma
- Whether or not it is in organs outside the lymph system

- Performance status (PS)-how well the person can complete normal daily activities
- Blood (serum) level of lactate dehydrogenase (LDH)-this level goes up in the presence of fast growing tumors

Good prognostic factors	*Poor prognostic factors*
Age 60 or below	Age above 60
Stage I or II	Stage III or IV
No lymphoma outside of lymph nodes	Lymphoma present outside of lymph nodes
PS: Able to function normally	PS: Needs a lot of help with daily activities
Serum LDH is normal	Serum LDH is elevated

For each poor prognostic factor, 1 point is assigned. The index divides people with lymphomas into 4 categories. The low category (0 or 1 point) means the person with lymphoma has mostly good factors (is young, has stage I disease, can still work, and so on). The highest category indicates mostly or all unfavorable factors (high stage, high LDH, bedridden, and so on). No matter what the type of lymphoma, over 75% of people in the lowest group will live longer than 5 years, whereas only 30% of people in the highest group live 5 years.

This prognostic index is important because it allows doctors to plan treatment better than they could from just the pathology report and staging information. This has become more important as new, more effective treatments have been developed that sometimes have more side effects. The index tells us whether these treatments are needed. It also provides information to patients about the outlook for their future.

TREATMENT

Treatment usually depends both on the type of lymphoma and on the extent of the disease in the body.

B-Cell Lymphomas

Diffuse large B-cell lymphoma: This lymphoma can be cured in around 40% of patients. The cure rate is much higher if the International Prognostic Index is low, and lower if the index is high.

The main treatment is chemotherapy, usually with a regimen of 4 drugs known as CHOP (cyclophosphamide, doxorubicin, vincristine and prednisone).

If the lymphoma is localized to 1 or 2 lymph node groups on the same side of the abdomen (that is, if it is *stage I or II*), radiation therapy to the lymph node areas may be added to the chemotherapy. The usual chemotherapy regimen is given anywhere from 3 to 8 months depending on the size of the lymph nodes and whether the lymphoma is growing into nearby organs.

For *stage III or IV* lymphoma, chemotherapy is the main treatment. Once again, the usual regimen is CHOP. Many doctors are now adding rituximab (Rituxan) to the chemotherapy. Studies in older patients (over 60) have shown a benefit for adding rituximab. It is not yet clear if this is true for younger patients, though.

If the lymphoma *relapses* (comes back) after treatment or is *refractory* (doesn't respond well to primary treatment), doctors will suggest another chemotherapy regimen. If the lymphoma shrinks with this, a stem cell transplant is often suggested, because otherwise the lymphoma will usually grow back. Stem cell transplants are not effective unless the lymphoma responds to chemotherapy. As of yet, they have not been shown to be better than standard treatment as the initial treatment.

New techniques for studying the gene composition of large cell lymphomas have shown there may be two types. One responds well to usual treatment and the other doesn't. Clinical trials are now in progress to find out how best to treat the type that doesn't respond.

Follicular lymphoma: This lymphoma has not been shown to be curable by any of the standard treatments. Although some new, more aggressive treatments seem to be very effective, it still isn't clear that they are better than standard treatment.

If the lymphoma is localized to 1 or 2 lymph node groups on the same side of the abdomen (*stage I or II*), it can be treated with radiation therapy to the lymph node areas. Chemotherapy is not usually recommended if the lymphoma is localized.

If the lymphoma is not localized (*stage III or IV*), then chemotherapy can be given. Radiotherapy can also be given to any large areas of lymphoma to reduce symptoms even if it is not stage I or II. Another option is observation with no treatment. This is reasonable if the lymphoma isn't very large and isn't causing symptoms, harming vital organs, or growing fast. While some patients are uncomfortable with this approach, it's important to remember that because follicular lymphoma isn't curable, the point of therapy is to control the disease for as long as possible while causing the fewest side effects.

The usual chemotherapy regimens consist of a single drug such as chlorambucil (Leukeran) or fludarabine (Fludara). Some doctors prefer combinations of cyclophosphamide (Cytoxan), vincristine (Oncovin), and prednisone. Other choices for treatment are rituximab (either alone or combined with chemotherapy) or interferon (either alone or combined with chemotherapy). The newer monoclonal antibodies, Zevalin and Bexxar, are also possible treatment options when other treatments are no longer working.

Sometimes patients with follicular lymphoma *relapse* with a large diffuse B-cell lymphoma. If this happens, then the treatment becomes the same as for that disease. If the relapse remains a follicular lymphoma, other chemotherapy drugs can be given. If the lymphoma responds to a new chemotherapy, stem cell transplant can be considered. This may help some patients, but it is best done in a clinical trial. A nonmyeloablative transplant is another option.

Chronic lymphocytic leukemia/small lymphocytic lymphoma: The treatment of chronic lymphocytic leukemia (CLL) is described in the ACS document on chronic leukemia. Treatment for small lymphocytic lymphoma (SLL) is the same as for follicular lymphoma.

Mantle cell lymphoma: Although not a rapidly growing lymphoma, this disease can be fatal and often requires intensive treatment. All stages are treated in a similar way.

Chemotherapy is an option, but no specific chemotherapy regimen has proved better than others. Rituximab is sometimes added to the chemotherapy. Many clinical trials are underway that use high-dose chemotherapy and stem cell transplantation.

Another treatment has included Zevalin. This is given in high doses and is followed by stem cell transplantation. Because there is no curative or generally accepted treatment for this lymphoma, patients should consider entering a clinical trial.

Extranodal marginal zone B-cell lymphomas-mucosa-associated lymphoid tissue (MALT) lymphomas: The most common of these, gastric lymphoma, is thought to occur as a result of an infection with *H. pylori*. Because of this, therapy for gastric lymphomas is different than for the other lymphomas in this group.

Treatment of early stage *gastric* MALT lymphomas *(stages I and II)* consists of antibiotics directed against *H. pylori* along with drugs that block acid secretion by the stomach. Usually the drugs are given for 10 to 14 days. Examination of the stomach using a flexible tube with a viewing lens (gastroscopy) is then repeated at certain intervals to see if the *H. pylori* is gone and the lymphoma has decreased in size.

Radiation therapy to the stomach or chemotherapy may be used for *stages II through IV*. They are also given for early stage disease if the symptoms are so severe that they need to be relieved before the antibiotics can take effect, which can take several weeks to months. The drugs used are the same as those used for follicular lymphoma. Single agents such as chlorambucil or fludarabine or combinations such as cyclophosphamide, vincristine, and prednisone are used.

Local radiation and single-agent chemotherapy as outlined above are the treatments for MALT lymphomas that arise in *sites other than the stomach.*

Nodal marginal zone B-cell lymphoma: This is generally a low-grade lymphoma. It is treated like follicular lymphoma with either observation or low-intensity chemotherapy. It can also transform into a high-grade large cell lymphoma, which requires more aggressive chemotherapy such as CHOP.

Splenic marginal zone B-cell lymphoma: This is also a low-grade lymphoma and is treated with either observation or low-intensity chemotherapy like follicular lymphoma.

Because the lymphoma invades and enlarges the spleen, an organ in the right upper part of the abdomen, doctors may decide to surgically remove it. This alone can lead to a long term remission of the disease. Radiation therapy is an alternative to surgery.

This lymphoma can transform into a large-cell aggressive lymphoma, which requires more intensive chemotherapy.

Primary mediastinal B-cell lymphoma: This is treated like localized diffuse large B-cell lymphoma. The main treatment is radiation to the chest mass along with about 6 courses of CHOP chemotherapy.

Burkitt's lymphoma: This is a very fast growing lymphoma that must be treated intensely. Most regimens for this disease include high doses of cyclophosphamide (Cytoxan), doxorubicin (Adriamycin), cytarabine (Cytosar), and methotrexate, along with standard doses of vincristine (Oncovin). Prednisone or dexamethasone is also used. Finally, because this lymphoma tends to invade the spinal fluid, chemotherapy with methotrexate is given into the spinal fluid. About half of all patients are cured.

Lymphoplasmocytic lymphoma (Waldenstrom's macroglobulinemia): The main treatment for this lymphoma is chemotherapy. Because this is a slow growing lymphoma, treatment does not have to be intense. The chemotherapy programs include alkylating agents such as chlorambucil or cyclophosphamide, either as single agents or combined with other drugs. Rituximab has also been successful in treating this disease. Fludarabine and 2-chlorodeoxyadenosine (2-CdA) also have been effective.

By destroying the lymphoma cells, production of abnormal IgM is reduced. (The IgM proteins make the blood unusually thick, which can reduce blood flow to vital areas of the body, such as the brain and kidneys.)

Another important treatment is called *plasmapheresis*. This removes blood through a vein and separates the blood cells from the blood plasma (liquid part of the blood). The blood cells are returned into another vein. Because plasma contains the abnormal IgM, it is discarded and replaced with a salt solution and blood proteins from donors.

Plasmapheresis is helpful in relieving symptoms of newly diagnosed patients (while chemotherapy is starting to work) and for those whose lymphoma is not controlled by chemotherapy. When patients have symptoms from these elevated levels of IgM, they need to have plasmapheresis right away to prevent complications.

Hairy cell leukemia: This is also a slow growing lymphoma that invades the spleen and lymph nodes as well as the blood. The drugs used to treat it are called pentostatin and 2-CdA. Both are equally effective. They are given intravenously for either a few months (pentostatin) or a week (2-CdA). Most patients go into remission. Only a small percentage relapse, and those that do usually can be treated successfully again. Sometimes the disease is resistant to these drugs. Rituximab has been used to treat these patients with success. Removing the spleen by surgery can also help.

T-Cell Lymphomas

Precursor T-lymphoblastic lymphoma/leukemia: This disease can occur as leukemia in both children and adults. This is discussed in the ACS documents on acute leukemia.

It is called a *lymphoma* if there are tumor masses and the number of lymphoma cells in the bone marrow is less than 25%. This is a fast growing disease and is treated with intensive chemotherapy.

Many drugs are used. These include cyclophosphamide (Cytoxan), doxorubicin (Adriamycin), vincristine (Oncovin), L-asparaginase, methotrexate, prednisone, and, sometimes, cytosine arabinoside (ara-C, Cytosar). Chemotherapy with methotrexate is also given into the spinal fluid. Some doctors will suggest high-dose chemotherapy followed by an autologous stem cell transplant after a patient goes into remission.

Peripheral T-cell lymphomas

- *Cutaneous T-cell lymphomas (mycosis fungoides, Sezary syndrome):* The treatment of these lymphomas depends on how advanced they are.
- Early disease with only patches or plaques (raised patches) of lymphoma is treated with the following skin-directed treatments:
  - o *Chemotherapy solutions or ointments* can be applied directly to the whole body surface except uninvolved face, hands, and genitals. The drugs used are either nitrogen mustard or BCNU. Sometimes steroid creams can help. The nitrogen mustard can cause redness and itching.
  - o *PUVA (psoralen ultraviolet A) light treatment* involves receiving psoralen, a light-sensitizing drug that is taken by mouth, followed by exposing the skin to a special ultraviolet light. This is done 3 times a week until the lesions regress and then less often. Sometimes interferon therapy is added.
  - o *Electron beam therapy* is a type of external radiation. It is different from standard radiation therapy because the beam is made of electrons and does not penetrate but only treats the skin. This can be aimed at specific lesions or the whole skin. The major side effect is moderate sunburn.
  - o *Bexarotene (Targretin)* a new topical skin gel, is also useful in some instances. This is a vitamin A-like compound.

More advanced disease that is either forming tumors or is invading the whole skin surface is treated with:

- *Electron beam therapy to the whole skin*
- *Electron beam therapy combined with PUVA*
- *Photopheresis* is a treatment like PUVA except that instead of the skin being treated, the blood is treated. First the patient receives psoralen. Then blood is removed through a vein in the arm and circulated through an apheresis machine, where the white blood cells are separated out. These are treated with the special ultraviolet light and are returned to the body through another vein along with the red blood cells.

If the skin lymphoma has spread to lymph nodes or other organs, chemotherapy is usually needed. Drugs used include doxorubicin, cyclophosphamide, methotrexate, bleomycin, and prednisone (alone or in combination). Nucleoside analogs (pentostatin, 2-CdA, or fludarabine) and interferon are sometimes used. Biological therapies using newer man-made molecules such as denileukin diftitox (Ontak) or the monoclonal antibody alemtuzumab (Campath) are other treatment options. In this situation, a clinical trial may be the best option.

Angioimmunoblastic T-cell lymphoma: This type is often treated with corticosteroids (such as prednisone or dexamethasone) alone. This treatment can reduce fever and stop the weight loss. The effect is temporary, however. Usually some form of chemotherapy is needed. But even chemotherapy is not completely successful, and remissions are usually short.

Extranodal natural killer/T-cell lymphoma, nasal type: Because this lymphoma is often confined to the nasal passages, it can be treated with radiation therapy. However, this is usually not enough, and chemotherapy is often added. A typical chemotherapy regimen is CHOP. If the lymphoma has spread, the chemotherapy is more intense. Multiple drugs are used at high doses, and stem cell transplantation may be added.

Enteropathy type T-cell lymphoma: The only effective treatment is prevention. This lymphoma develops from hypersensitivity to gluten. If the symptoms of this hypersensitivity are recognized early, then a gluten-free diet will help prevent the lymphoma from developing. Otherwise, there is no accepted treatment, although a clinical trial of chemotherapy may be suggested.

Subcutaneous panniculitis-like T-cell lymphoma: This type of lymphoma responds poorly to chemotherapy. Radiation therapy is useful to relieve symptoms.

Anaplastic large T/null-cell lymphoma: This lymphoma is treated like diffuse B-cell lymphoma with CHOP or similar regimens. Response rates are high, and results are excellent.

Unspecified: These lymphomas are treated the same way as diffuse large B-cell lymphomas. Chemotherapy with CHOP or other combinations is used. The outlook is not as good as in diffuse B-cell lymphoma. Stem cell transplants may be recommended as part of the treatment.

Primary central nervous system (CNS) lymphoma: This is a special class of lymphoma because it begins in the brain or spinal cord. This type usually develops in people with immune system problems caused by AIDS or side effects of drugs given to prevent rejection of transplanted organs.

Patients often respond temporarily to prednisone or to radiation therapy, but recurrence within a year or two is common. High doses of methotrexate have been shown to be effective. The patient's general condition and seriousness of the underlying immune system problems affect the outlook, which is usually poor.

HODGKIN'S DISEASE

Hodgkin's disease (also called Hodgkin's lymphoma) is a type of cancer that starts in lymphatic tissue. Hodgkin's disease is named after Dr Thomas Hodgkin who first recognized it in 1832.

A risk factor is anything that increases a person's chance of getting a disease such as cancer. Different cancers have different risk factors. Scientists have found a few risk factors that may make a person more likely to get Hodgkin's disease. There seems to be a slightly higher risk of Hodgkin's disease among people who have had infectious mononucleosis.

Some people who have reduced immune systems, for example, those with AIDS, and organ transplant patients, are also at a higher risk of Hodgkin's disease.

Unlike many other types of cancer, Hodgkin's disease does not seem to be caused by something wrong with a person's genes or their diet or even something in the environment. Even if someone does have one or more risk factors for Hodgkin's disease, it's impossible to know for sure how much that risk factor contributed to causing the cancer. For the most part, we can say that no major risk factors for Hodgkin's disease have yet been found.

Since we do not know what causes Hodgkin's disease, it is not possible to prevent the disease. A great deal of research is under way to try to find the cause of this cancer.

Symptoms of Hodgkin's Disease

There are no screening tests to find Hodgkin's disease early, and some people with the disease have no symptoms at all. When they do occur, symptoms can include enlarged, painless lymph nodes. But in most people, especially children, enlarged lymph nodes are caused by an infection or other illness and not cancer. If you (or your child) have lymph nodes over an inch in size and no recent infection, it is best to have them checked by the doctor.

Other symptoms of Hodgkin's disease can be caused by the swelling of lymph nodes inside the chest, creating pressure on the windpipe. These symptoms can include coughing or shortness of breath. Some people have fever, drenching night sweats, or weight loss. The fever can come and go over periods of several days or weeks.

Itching, tiredness, and decreased appetite are other symptoms that can occur. If you or you child have these symptoms, talk to your doctor right away. And remember, there are often reasons for these symptoms other than cancer.

Tests to Diagnose Hodgkin's Disease

If there is any reason to think that a person has Hodgkin's disease, the doctor will want to conduct certain tests. The first step would be a complete medical history and thorough physical exam to see whether there is an infection. During the exam, the doctor will pay special attention to the lymph nodes. Since it is so common for people, especially children, to have swollen lymph nodes the doctor will probably prescribe antibiotics first to see if the lymph nodes shrink. If they do not, then more testing will be done.

The only way to know for sure whether a person has Hodgkin's disease is to do a biopsy, that is, an examination of a tissue sample under the microscope. There are several different kinds of biopsies, and the doctor will choose the one best suited for the patient. The goal is to obtain enough tissue to make a diagnosis as quickly as possible with the fewest side effects.

Some biopsies involve cutting through the skin to remove an entire node or a small part of a large tumor. In another type of biopsy, the doctor uses a thin needle to remove a small amount of fluid and tiny bits of tissue from the tumor.

Staging

Staging is the process of finding out how far the cancer has spread. This is very important because the treatment and the outlook for recovery depend on the stage of the cancer.

The staging system for Hodgkin's disease is called the *Ann Arbor Staging Classification*. This system has four stages, labeled stage I through stage IV (1-4). In general, the lower the number, the less the cancer has spread. A higher number, such as Stage IV, means a more serious cancer.

After a biopsy has confirmed that Hodgkin's disease is present, the next step is clinical staging. This consists of taking the patient's medical history, doing a physical exam, and then doing several kinds of imaging studies. Imaging studies such as CT (computed tomography) and MRI (magnetic resonance imaging) are used to create pictures of the inside of the body. They can help show the size and shape of lumps or tumors that might be cancerous.

For many people, the results of the clinical staging are all that are needed to plan their treatment. Others, however, require another step called pathological staging. In this process, the doctor performs an operation called a laparotomy, checking inside the abdomen to see if any of the organs contain cancer. Small pieces of tissue are removed and looked at under a microscope to see if Hodgkin's disease is present. The spleen is also usually removed at this time.

Survival Rates by Stage of Hodgkin's Disease

The 5-year survival rate refers to the percent of patients who live at least 5 years after their cancer is treated. Many of these patients live longer than 5 years. Five-year relative survival rates are seen as more accurate because they do not include statistics for people who die of causes other than their cancer. Since these figures go back 5 years, results for people diagnosed recently can be even better since treatments are always improving.

Stage	*5-year relative survival rate*
I	90% to 95%
II	90% to 95%
III	85% to 90%
IV	about 80%

In recent years, much progress has been made in treating Hodgkin's disease. For nearly all patients, complete cure is the goal of treatment, and about 90% of patients are cured with chemotherapy or radiation therapy.

After Hodgkin's disease is staged, the doctor will discuss treatment choices with you. It is important to take time and think about all the choices. Some factors to consider include you (or your child's) overall health and the type and stage of the disease. Be sure that you understand all the risks and side effects before making a decision.

The two main methods of treating Hodgkin's disease are chemotherapy, the use of cancer-killing drugs, and radiation therapy, the use of high-energy X-rays to kill cancer cells and shrink tumors. Sometimes one treatment is used and sometimes both.

Bone marrow transplantation, discussed later, is used for certain people. For the most part, surgery plays little role in the treatment of Hodgkin's disease.

Chemotherapy

Chemotherapy refers to the use of drugs to kill cancer cells. Usually the drugs are given into a vein or by mouth. Once the drugs enter the bloodstream, they spread throughout the body. Several drugs are given at the same time.

Although the drugs kill cancer cells, they also damage normal cells, causing side effects. The exact side effects depend on the type and dose of drugs used and the length of time they are taken, but they can include hair loss, mouth sores, greater chance of infection, easy bruising or bleeding, fatigue, loss of appetite, nausea, and vomiting. These side effects are temporary and go away after treatment is finished.

If you have side effects, your cancer care team can suggest steps to ease their impact. For example, other drugs can be given along with the chemotherapy to prevent or reduce nausea and vomiting.

In addition, some of these drugs can have side effects that occur long after treatment is finished. These can affect a person's heart, lungs, growth, and ability to have children. There is also a risk of developing a second type of cancer. It's important to discuss these possible side effects with the doctor before treatment begins.

Radiation Therapy

Radiation therapy is the use of high-energy X-rays to destroy cancer cells. When radiation therapy is given for Hodgkin's disease, it usually involves a focused beam of radiation, given from a machine outside the body. This is known as external beam radiation.

Radiation therapy is often given after three to four courses of chemotherapy. Radiation therapy can produce some serious side effects including damage to nearby healthy tissue. Other problems can include skin changes similar to sunburn, tiredness, upset stomach, and loose bowels. There can be long-term side effects as well. To reduce the risk of side effects, doctors are careful to give the exact dose needed and to aim the beam so it hits only the cancer.

Bone Marrow Transplantation

Sometimes Hodgkin's disease stops responding to standard treatment. In those cases, another type of treatment might be offered as part of a clinical trial (see below) or outside of a clinical trial.

In one approach, the patient's own bone marrow is removed and stored. Then very high doses of chemotherapy (with or without radiation therapy) are given to the patient to kill the cancer. These high doses will destroy bone marrow, too. So, after the treatment, the stored marrow is given back to the patient through a vein. The bone marrow cells enter the bloodstream and return to the bone, replacing the marrow and making new red and white blood cells.

Another type of transplant is called peripheral blood stem cell transplant (PBSCT). For this treatment, a machine removes the patient's blood a little at a time. Only the stem cells—immature cells from which all blood cells develop—are removed. The rest of the blood is returned to the body. This process usually takes a few hours. The stem cells are then frozen until they are returned to the patient after treatment is finished.

Doctors are finding that it is better to do these procedures earlier rather than later in the course of the disease. If the first set of treatments doesn't completely get rid of the cancer, many doctors would recommend transplantation right away. On the other hand, if a patient's disease comes back after it had gone away for a long time, most doctors would favor a second course of standard treatment before doing transplantation.

Hodgkin's Disease in Children

Although the treatment for Hodgkin's disease is generally the same for adults and children, there are some differences. If the child is more mature, the treatment is often the same as that given to adults. But if the child's body is still growing, then the doctor is more likely to use chemotherapy instead of radiation therapy because the latter can affect bone and muscle growth. The goal of treatment for children is to cure the child without causing long-term problems. Cure rates for children can reach 85 to 100%, even with advanced disease. This topic is dealt with more generosity in the "PAEDITRIC ONCOLOGY SECTION".

Twelve

Lung Cancer

Lung cancer is an uncontrolled growth of abnormal cells in one or both of the lungs.

The body is made up of different types of cells that normally divide and multiply in an orderly way. These new cells replace older cells. This process of cell birth and renewal occurs constantly in the body.

Cancer, also known as a *malignant* growth, occurs when:

- Some cells in the body begin to multiply in an uncontrolled manner
- The body's natural defenses, such as certain parts of the immune system, cannot stop the uncontrolled cell division.
- These abnormal cells become greater and greater in number, and come together to form a tumor, which is a cellular growth that forms a progressively enlarging mass. A tumor is benign-that is, not a cancer-unless it tends to invade surrounding tissues and organs, in which case it is malignant or cancerous.

Cancerous tumors grow out of control and can invade, replace, and destroy normal cells near the tumor. In some cases, cancer cells spread to other areas of the body.

Lung cancer generally takes many years to develop even though damage to the lungs may occur shortly after a person is exposed to cancer-causing substances.

Different Types Of Lung Cancer

There are different types of cells in the lung, of varying size, for the different functions of the lung. This has resulted in the classification of two main types of lung cancer:

- Cancer developing from the smaller cells in the lung is known as *small-cell lung cancer*.
- Other types of cancers in the lung are known as *non-small-cell lung cancer*.
- Some lung cancers are a mixture of both types and are generally called *mixed-small-cell/large-cell cancer*.

The different types of lung cancers tend to grow and spread differently and are therefore not treated in the same way.

- Non-small-cell lung cancer is the more common type, accounting for about 80% of lung cancers. It is this more common type of lung cancer that grows and spreads more slowly.
- This less common type of cancer, small-cell cancer, is the type that grows more quickly and has a greater chance of spreading to other parts of the body.

Since the more common non-small cell group of cells in the lung are themselves made up of differing kinds of cells, three distinct types of non-small cell lung cancer are recognized. They are:

- *Squamous cell carcinoma*, found usually in the central part of the lung.

- *Adenocarcinoma*, mostly occurring in the outer part of the lung.
- *Undifferentiated carcinoma*, which can occur anywhere in the lung.

People with adenocarcinoma have a more favorable outlook. Undifferentiated carcinoma is the least common and has the poorer prognosis.

In general, the choice of treatment and the chances of recovery from lung cancer following treatment will depend on:

- How advanced the cancer is at the time of diagnosis
- How healthy the person generally is

Recognizing The Symptoms

The symptoms that may suggest lung cancer are similar to symptoms of other lung conditions that may not be as serious as lung cancer.

The main symptoms suggesting lung cancer are:

- Coughing up blood
- Coughing that does not seem to improve and gets worse with time

Other symptoms may include:

- Chest pain
- Shortness of breath
- Recurrent episodes of pneumonia
- Weight loss
- Feeling tired

Weight loss and feeling tired can be symptoms of cancer in general.

Facts About Lung Cancer

- Over 80% of all lung cancers are caused directly by smoking.
- Stopping smoking can reduce the risk for developing lung cancer.
- Lung cancer is more common in men; they are 25% more likely to develop lung cancer.
- When initially diagnosed, only about 15% of lung cancers are found to still be in the early stage, while 85% have already spread locally or to more distant sites in the body.
- The five-year survival rate is approximately 50% in those cases when the cancer is still in the early stage when first diagnosed-but only 15% of lung cancers are discovered this early.
- In the USA, in 1998, there were about 171,500 new cases of lung cancer, accounting for 14% of all cancer diagnoses.
- In the USA in 1998, 28% of all cancer deaths were due to lung cancer.
- Since 1987, more women have died each year of lung cancer than breast cancer.

The most common cause of lung cancer is smoking.

Smoking causes lung cancer because there are substances within tobacco that are known to cause cancer. These substances are known as carcinogens (which means "cancer-causing agents"), and it is these carcinogens that cause the actual damage to the cells in the lungs. A cell that is damaged may become cancerous over a period of time.

One cannot predict which smoker is at greater risk of developing lung cancer. In general, though, a smoker's chances of developing cancer depends on:

- The age that the person began smoking
- How long the person has smoked
- How many cigarettes per day the person smokes

Passive smoking-breathing in someone else's smoke-may also increase the risk for developing lung cancer.

There are other causes of lung cancer not related to smoking. People who smoke and who also are exposed to these other causes have an even higher risk for lung cancer.

These other causes include:

- Exposure to cancer-causing agents through a person's job. This includes exposure to asbestos, either in the mining or construction industries. Inhaled asbestos particles may remain in the lungs, damaging lung cells. It also includes exposure to certain industrial substances like coal products, vinyl chloride, nickel chromate, arsenic, and exposure to some organic chemicals like chloromethyl ethers.

- Exposure to radiation, either through one's occupation or for medical reasons, such as repeated X-rays.
- Radon gas, which occurs naturally in rocks and soil in certain areas, may cause lung damage and may eventually result in lung cancer if it seeps into your home. The presence of radon in the home can be measured using an inexpensive kit that can be purchased at department or hardware stores.

Research suggests that some people are more at risk for developing cancer if their body is not as easily able to deal with certain cancer-causing chemicals. This inability to neutralize cancer-causing chemicals is believed to be inherited.

Researchers also believe that in some people, when they come into contact with certain cancer-causing agents, their immune system, instead of neutralizing them, will actually make these agents more aggressive within the body. Such people, therefore, would be more sensitive to tobacco smoke and chemicals known to cause cancer.

DIAGNOSIS

- Ask about your medical history
- Perform a physical examination
- Order specialized medical tests

Medical tests that may be performed include:

- *Chest X-ray:* This is the first and basic test that will be ordered.
- *CT scan:* This is a highly specialized X-ray with computer-generated images showing slices of the lung.
- *Sputum test:* This is the examination under a microscopy of a sample of the mucus you cough up. If an abnormality seen on an X-ray is suggestive of cancer, a sputum test may be ordered.
- *Biopsy:* This is the removal of a sample of tissue from the body to be examined under a microscopy. A biopsy is the only way that the doctor can be absolutely certain that lung cancer is present. A physician who specializes in tissue analysis (a pathologist) can then see what type of cell is causing the growth and whether or not it is a cancerous cell.

There are different ways in which a biopsy of the lung may be obtained.

- *Needle aspiration:* While you are sedated, a doctor will insert a needle through your chest directly into the growth and, guided by X-rays, will remove a sample of tissue. Alternatively, the needle may be pushed only as far as the envelope of tissue that surrounds the lungs, removing fluid from this layer to check for the presence of cancer cells.
- *Bronchoscopy:* In this procedure, which is more common than needle aspiration, a doctor passes a narrow, flexible, well-lit tube, called a bronchoscope, into your lungs while you are under sedation. The bronchoscope is passed through either your mouth or nose directly into your windpipe, and the doctor is able to see the air passages inside the lungs. The biopsy of any suspicious part of the lung can be performed through this tube.

Rarely, even after all the above medical tests, the diagnosis may still be unclear. In this case, a major operation exposing the lung may be needed. This procedure is known as a *thoracotomy*.

Bone metastases are a common complication of lung cancer. Others cancers that metastasize to bone include multiple myeloma, breast, prostate, kidney, and thyroid cancer.

Metastases are cancer cells that have spread from their site of origin to another location in the body. Cancer cells can spread, or metastasize, through the blood and lymph systems. A cancer cell may break away from the original location in the body and travel in one of these systems until it gets lodged in a small vessel in another area of the body. Once there, the cell grows and divides, thereby establishing cancer in that new tissue. Metastases are not new or different cancers; the cancer cells in the new location are the same as the original cancer, only in a different location.

Bone is one of the most common locations in the body to which cancer metastasizes. Bone metastases usually occur by way of the blood stream. Cancer may also spread to bone by erosion from the adjacent cancer, though this occurs less frequently than spread by the blood stream.

Bone metastases result in lesions, or injury to the bone tissue. There are two types of lesions: lytic lesions, which destroy bone material, and blastic lesions, which fill up bone with extra cells. Normal bone is constantly being remodeled, or broken down and rebuilt. Cancer cells that have spread to the bone disrupt the balance between the activity of osteoclasts (cells that break down bone) and osteoblasts (cells that build bone).

The damage caused by bone metastases may make the bone more susceptible to complications such as pain or fractures. Another more serious complication of bone metastases is the risk of hypercalcemia. Hypercalcemia is an increased level of calcium in the blood and can be a medical emergency.

Bone metastases generally occur in the central parts of the skeleton, although they may be found anywhere in the skeletal system. Common sites for bone metastases are the back, pelvis, upper leg, ribs, upper arm, and skull. More than 90% of all metastases are found in these locations.

Radiography, including bone scan, X-ray, and skeletal survey, remains the best method for characterizing bone metastases. Currently, there are no blood tests for bone metastases.

Bone Scan: The presence of bone metastases is usually evaluated by performing a type of X-ray called a bone scan. In this test, low level radioactive particles are injected into a vein. They circulate through the body and are selectively picked up by the bones. A high concentration of these radioactive particles indicates the presence of rapidly growing cancer cells.

X-ray: Because bone scans can reveal other conditions such as arthritis or infection, a positive scan is usually followed up with a regular X-ray. When enough of the healthy bone in any area is worn away by metastatic lesions, the damaged area will show up as a dark spot on the X-ray. Metastatic lesions look like holes in the bones.

Skeletal survey: In order to diagnose blastic lesions, or lesions where extra bone has built up, a skeletal survey may be utilized. This is a form of X-ray. Normally an X-ray is selective for a particular area of concern, but with a skeletal survey, all areas are imaged.

Other: Occasionally, a more costly radiological procedure may be used to assess bone metastases, such as a computed axial tomography (CAT) scan or a magnetic resonance imaging (MRI) scan.

The treatment of lung cancer depends on its type and extent. Therefore, the doctor must obtain specific information before suggesting a treatment. The doctor will need to know:

- The type of lung cancer the patient has-whether small-cell lung cancer or non-small-cell lung cancer
- The size of the growth
- Exactly where in the lung it is
- Whether the cancer has spread, and, if so, how far

Obtaining all this information is known as *staging the cancer*. "Staging" is a method that has been developed to describe the extent of cancer growth. Staging helps to predict:

- How an individual is expected to fare over time
- The chances that the cancer will come back (recur)

Staging allows the physician to customize cancer treatment. In general, the lower the stage the better the person's prognosis (expected outcome).

Lung cancer is "staged" by information that is obtained from the *biopsy* and the results of the various imaging studies, such as chest X-ray or CT scan. The physician uses all available findings to determine the stage that best describes the person's condition.

Tests performed for staging may include:

- *CT scan or MRI scan or both:* Computerized images are obtained from both of these tests, which allows the lung to be seen in thin slices, clearly showing the extent of any growth within the lung. These tests may also be performed on other parts of the body if there is suspicion that the growth may have spread to other parts of the body.
- Other scanning techniques include various forms of *radionucleid scanning and bone scans.* These tests can help detect whether the cancer has spread to other organs in the body or to the bones. A low dose of harmless radioactive substance is injected into a vein, and as it travels around the body a specialized scanning machine is able to record radioactivity levels throughout the body. Since the uptake of the radioactive material is different in areas of the body affected by cancer, these areas are readily identified.
- A further specialized test called *mediastinoscopy* may be offered. This procedure is done while a patient is under general anesthesia. A narrow telescope, to which a camera may be attached, is introduced into the front of the chest through a small incision, or sometimes through a small incision in the neck. A sample of tissue can then be removed from the lymph nodes and other nearby tissue.

Understanding Lung Cancer "Staging"

"Staging" is a method that has been developed to describe the extent of the cancer growth, based on the results of biopsy and other investigations. This information helps to predict how an individual will fare over time. Staging a cancer also allows a physician to customize the cancer treatment to a particular individual.

In lung cancer patients, staging methods are used for non-small-cell lung cancers, which account for about 80% of all cancers.

The *TNM cancer staging system* is defined as:

- T (for tumor)
- N (for lymph nodes)
- M (for metastasis, or spread of the cancer)

T refers to the size of the tumor itself:

- TX and T0-Cancer cells have been found in sputum or lung tissue but cannot be seen.
- Tis-Carcinoma in situ, which means cells are cancerous but the growth does not show evidence of spreading.
- T1-The tumor is small, still contained in the lung, and has not reached the main airway.
- T2-The tumor has one or more of the following characterists: it is larger than 3 cm; it involves the main airway; it is close to the windpipe; it has invaded the membrane covering the lung; it has damaged or inflamed the lung tissue but has not affected the entire lung.
- T3-The tumor has invaded the chest wall, diaphragm, membrane covering organs in the chest, or the outer wall of the membrane around the heart, and/or it has affected the entire lung.
- T4-The tumor has invaded the area between the lungs, heart, major blood vessels of the heart, trachea, esophagus, or spine, and/or separate tumors are present in the same lung lobe, and/or cancer is present in fluid between the membrane covering the lung and the lung (pleural effusion).

N refers to whether the cancer has reached the lymph nodes:

- N0-Lymph nodes are cancer-free.
- N1-Cancer has spread to nearest lymph nodes around the airways.

- N2-Cancer has spread to lymph nodes in the middle of the chest that are adjacent to the affected lung.
- N3-Cancer has spread to lymph nodes in the middle of the chest that are adjacent to the opposite lung, to lymph nodes in nearby or opposite muscle tissue, or to lymph nodes above the collar bone.

M refers to metastasis, or spread of the cancer:

- M0-Metastasis has not occurred.
- M1-Cancer has spread to distant locations within the body.

  This information is compiled to determine a staging category for the cancer. In general, the lower the staging category, the better the expected outcome.

- *Stage I*-The cancer growth is confined to the lung and is surrounded by normal lung tissue.
- *Stage II*-The cancer has spread to the nearby lymph nodes (these are structures that drain lymph fluid from the lungs).
- *Stage III*-The cancer has now spread outside of the lung, to the chest wall or to the *diaphragm* muscle beneath the lungs, or to the lymph nodes on the other side of the chest, or to the lymph nodes in the neck. Stage III is divided into *Stage IIIa,* implying that the cancer may still be removed by surgery, and *Stage IIIb*, in which the cancer cannot be removed by surgery.
- *Stage IV*-The cancer has broken away from the original cancer growth and has spread beyond the lungs to other parts of the body. This is known as *metastasis* of the cancer.

Treatment Options

The treatment of lung cancer will usually consist of a combination of therapies, rather than a single therapy, which may result in a better outcome. The different treatment modalities include:

- *Chemotherapy:* This involves the use of medications that are able to kill cancer cells. Chemotherapy may be selected as the major treatment to kill the cancer cells, or as a treatment to kill any remaining cancer cells once a tumor has been surgically removed. It also can be used to treat a cancer growth elsewhere in the body.

  Chemotherapy drugs are mainly given through a catheter, which is a thin tube that is placed into a large vein. The catheter may be left in place for the duration of the treatment or removed after each treatment session. A number of chemotherapy drugs are available as a pill.
- *Radiation therapy:* Radiation therapy involves the use of high-dose X-rays to destroy the cancer cells or make the growths smaller. It is also used after surgery to destroy any remaining cancer cells. Radiation therapy can be directed precisely to those areas in the body to where cancer has spread, such as the bones, brain, or spine.
- *Surgery:* Depending on the "stage" of the cancer, a number of surgical options are available. A *wedge resection* involves removing a small part of the lung in which the growth is located. Alternatively, a whole lobe of the lung may be removed, in a procedure is known as a *lobectomy*. On occasions, it may be necessary to remove the entire lung; this procedure is called a *pneumonectomy*.
- *Photodynamic therapy:* Photodynamic therapy is a newer treatment, used more often during clinical trials. It involves the use of a laser light aimed at the cancerous growth, which activates a chemical that has been injected into the blood stream and is absorbed and held for a period of time by cancer cells (while normal cells release the chemical quickly). The chemical, activated by the laser, then kills the cancer cells.

- *Other experimental therapies:* This includes immunotherapy, which uses drugs to boost a person's immune system to fight cancer. It also includes gene therapy, which involves methods to attack genetic mutations that are causing the cancer. Under investigation are angiogenesis inhibitors, which are agents that inhibit the formation of new blood vessels that are critical to the spread of cancer.

Thirteen

Skin Tumors and Related Cancer

Ephelide

These are small, benign evenly pigmented macules occurring on light-exposed sites. Freckles consist of malanocytes which have produced an abnormally large amount of melanin but have not increased in number. They are more common in redheads of Celtic origin.

Sun avoidance is the best therapy since light-exposure is stimulating.

Melanotic Naevi

These localised collections of melanocytes are extremely common and usually first appear during childhood. They increase during adolescence and may decrease in the elderly. Histological changes may occur during puberty and pregnancy. Most people have 5-20 melanocytic naevi. Many are acquired; some are inherited.

The importance of pigmented naevi lies in the identification of those with potential for malignant change-for example, include enlargement, altered pigmentation-increased or decreased-asymmetry, irregularity of the surface or edge, inflammation, bleeding, ulceration, itch or nodularity.

Excision is indicated if malignant transformation is suggested or for cosmetic reasons. However, less than 30% of melanomas arise from pre-existing naevi.

Pathological Classification

- Junctional-the naevus remain in contact with the overlying epidermis. They are usually flat, may be hairy, and often present at or before puberty.
- Compound-there are additional cells in the underlying dermis. They are usually slightly raised and moderately pigmented. Often, they develop in early adulthood.
- Intradermal-the naevus is entirely within the dermis. They are relatively pale because of masking from overlying epidermis which is normal. They may be elevated.

Progression is usually from junctional to intradermal. In time, the naevus cells mature to resemble neural tissue.

Clinical Classification

- Acquired/banal
- Congenital including bathing trunk naevus
- Dysplastic
- Blue
- Spitz
- Halo

Spitz Naevi (Spitzoid)

This is a rare, benign, reddish-brown naevus seen in juveniles. Cytological examination of this naevus reveals characteristics consistent with malignant melanoma although the architecture is regular.

Granuloma Telangiectaticum

This is a chronic inflammatory lesion of the dermal layer of the skin that occurs as the result of minor penetrating foreign bodies eg thorns, splinters. The lesion develops over a period of about one week. However, it does not often spontaneously regress.

Histologically, a lesion consists of a mass of granulation tissue that contains numerous polymorphs.

Common sites are the feet and hands, also the lips and gums. The lesions are reddish-blue, solitary, fleshy nodules-and may be polypoid. Surface ulceration is common and may make clinical differentiation from an amelanotic malignant melanoma difficult.

The lesions should be treated by excision and the base of the lesions curetted. Histological analysis of the excised lesion should be sent for confirmation of the diagnosis.

Haemangioma of the Skin

A cutaneous haemangioma is a benign tumour made up of newly-formed blood vessels in the skin.

Different types of haemangioma are recognised:

- Capillary naevus
- Port-wine stain
- Vin rose patch
- Cavernous haemangioma-strawberry naevus
- Cherry angioma-Campbell de Morgan's spot
- Telangiectasia

Port-wine Stain

Port-wine stains are present at birth. They consist of an endothelial cell lining containing capillary vessels. The most common sites are the face and neck. There is no natural regression of the lesion with age. This condition is associated with Sturge-Weber syndrome and Klippel-Trenaunay-Weber syndrome.

Management is by camouflage of the lesions, for example with makeup. Laser therapy may be available at specialist centres.

Klippel-Trelaunay-Weber Syndrome

Klippel-Trelaunay-Weber syndrome is a vascular malformation characterised by local overgrowth of soft tissue and bone in an extremity, or of a more extensive area. It is rare.

Presentation is variable, but major features include:

- Dilated, varicose veins-often in large vessels running down the lateral side of the leg
- Cutaneous angiomata and port wine stains-most extensive over the trunk and extremities; always present

Some cases show marked osteoporosis in the involved extremity. There may be syndactylism or polydactylism.

The heart is normal and the Branham's bradycardic respone test negative. It may resemble Robertson's giant limb.

Dermatofibroma

Histiocytomas are tumours arising from primitive mesenchymal cells which occur predominantly in soft tissues, most often in relation to skeletal muscle. They contain macrophages or histiocytes.

These tumours generally occur in adults and are most common on the legs of young to middle-aged women.

The benign fibrous histiocytomas occur predominantly in the skin. These benign tumours are named depending on the predominant pattern and location:

- The most common form of fibrous histiocytoma is the dermatofibroma
- Other forms of benign fibrous histiocytoma are fibroxanthomas, histiocytomas, xantho-

granulomas, sclerosing haemangiomas, and giant cell tumours of tendon sheath

Malignant Fibrous Histiocytoma

Malignant fibrous histiocytomas are tumours arising from primitive mesenchymal cells which occur predominantly in soft tissues, most often in relation to skeletal muscle. Like benign fibrous histiocytomas, they are composed of a mixture of cells resembling myofibroblasts, fibroblasts, histiocytes, primitive mesenchymal cells, and cells having intermediate or mixed features.

- Malignant fibrous histiocytomas account for 20-30% of soft tissue sarcomas
- They affect all age groups, with a peak incidence in the seventh decade. The incidence is slightly higher in males
- Sites of origin of malignant fibrous histiocytomas
  - o lower extremities (approx. 50%)
  - o upper extremeties (approx. 20%)
  - o abdominal cavity including retroperitoneum (approx. 20%)
- Majority arise in relation to skeletal muscle; occasionally they involve the deep fascia or less often the subcutaneous tissue; the osseous tumours occur more commonly around the knee

Clinical Features

The histiocytoma generally arises from a site of trauma e.g. an insect bite.

Initially the lesion develops as a firm papule or a button-like tumour. Lesions may be slightly tender and their size may vary slightly over time.

The rapid growth and brown pigmentation of the lesion may cause it to be confused with a melanoma.

Fibrous histiocytomas tend to dimple inward upon lateral compression. This feature is useful in distinguishing them from nodular melanomas which tend to protrude outward upon lateral compression.

Papilloma

A papilloma is a benign tumour caused by overgrowth of all elements of the skin. They comprise a core of connective tissue and blood vessels with a lining of skin epithelium.

Papillomas can occur at any age but are more common in the elderly. They vary in size but are usually less than 1 cm in diameter. They tend to be pedunculated and are smooth, soft, solid and of any shape. They are frequently observed about the face and the neck but may arise anywhere. They are frequently multiple. There may be surface ulceration due to trauma.

Treatment is by excision.

Seborrhoeic Keratosis

These are benign flat, raised, or pedunculated lesions, varying in colour from yellow to dark brown. They are more usual on the trunk and increase in incidence from 40 years onwards. There may be a familial tendency for widespread forms. They are not infective.

Histological examination reveals that these lesions are a localised proliferation of the basal layer of the epidermis. Often there is hyperkeratosis in the surface crypts. These lesions may be known as basal cell papillomas because of their cells of origin but are not neoplastic and are not related to basal cell carcinomas.

Treatment is rarely necessary. If required, superficial cryotherapy is usually adequate.

There are several subtypes of seborrhoeic keratosis distinguishable by clinical or histological features:

- Common seborrhoeic keratosis
- Reticulated seborrhoeic keratosis
- Atucco keratosis
- Melanocanthoma
- Clonal seborrhoeic keratosis
- Irritated seborrhoeic keratosis
- Seborrheic keratosis with squamous atypia
- Dermatosa papulosa nigra

Warts

These are benign tumours of the epidermis induced by inoculation of specific papova viruses.

If the immune system is compromised they can present major problems to cure.

Types of Warts

- Common warts-verruca vulgaris
- Periungual warts-often painful; cryotherapy used to ablate with care as damage to nail matrix can occur
- Plantar warts-verruca plantaris
- Plane warts-small, flat, flesh coloured lesions often on the dorsum of the hands.
- Filiform-digitate-warts-usually single and found on the scalp and face. They are composed of a small cluster of spikes or fingerlike projections.
- Genital warts: these are transmitted by sexual contact and are usually seen in teenagers and young adults.

Spontaneous resolution may occur in 3 months.

30% resolve in 6 months; 66% will resolve spontaneously within 2 years.

If the wart develops a slightly blackened centre it is about to disappear.

Clinical Features

Characterized by multiple, hyperkeratotic, raised nodules which may develop in clusters. The warts may be resistant to treatment. Viral warts may enlarge during pregnancy. Also they may be large and persistent if the patient has a coexistent malignancy eg leukaemia. Cervical carcinoma may be predisposed by certain forms of genital warts.

Management

Typically warts are benign infections that may persist for months, or even years, and then finally spontaneously resolve.

Each lesion has to be treated individually because there are no systemic agents that are effective against warts.

If there are only a small number of warts then they may be treated with techniques such as curettage, diathermy or excision.

Cryotherapy is successful for many types of warts. It is often administered at 2-4 weekly intervals until all warts have resolved. The cure rate is little higher than topical treatment.

Depending on the site and type of wart, consider:

- Keratolytic agents, e.g. salicylic acid
- Caustics, e.g. silver nitrate
- Irritants, e.g. podophyllin, but not in pregnancy

In theory, lactic acid will increase the effectiveness of each of these.

For mosaic and multiple foot warts, consider the use of a 3% formalin solution as a foot soak.

For more stubborn lesions:

- DNCB (dinitrochlorobenzene)
- Bleomycin injection
- Photodynamic therapy with 5-aminolaevulinic acid

PREMALIGNANT CONDITIONS

Bowen's Disease

This is an intraepithelial carcinoma, or carcinoma in situ, most commonly seen on the legs, although it can occur on any part of the skin, including the vulva.

In this condition there are features of malignant change within squamous cells e.g. excess and abnormal mitotic figures, and lack of squamous differentiation; however there is an intact basal membrane.

These changes may occur in about one third of cases of chronic vulvitis.

Clinically this condition is characterized by a slowly expanding pink, scaly plaque that has a sharply defined border. The lesion may be covered with crusts, which when removed reveal an oozy, papilliferous surface.

This condition is potentially invasive and may be treated, either by excision, cryotherapy or by the use of topical cytotoxic agents e.g. 5-fluorouracil.

Recurrences may occur, and might be due to extension of the carcinoma in situ in the adnexal structures, which were not affected by treatment.

Keratoacanthoma

Keratoacanthoma is a rapidly growing epidermal tumour that resembles squamous cell carcinoma both clinically and histologically. It is believed to arise from hair follicles. There is little evidence that keratocanthoma has malignant potential but it may mimic histological features of squamous cell carcinoma.

Trauma, viral infection, sun exposure, and chronic exposure to tar, pitch and petroleum have all been implicated as aetiologic agents.

Surgical excision is thought to produce less scarring than leaving the lesion to resolve spontaneously.

Marjolin's Ulcer

A Marjolin's ulcer is a squamous carcinoma which develops in a chronic scar such as a long-standing ulcer or osteomyelitic sinus.

The condition was first described in 1828 by the french surgeon Jean Nicolas Marjolin. It is characterised by:

- Slow growth-the scar is relatively avascular
- Painless-the scar is devoid of nerve fibres
- Absence of secondary deposits in regional lymph nodes-as the lymphatics have been destroyed. However, if the ulcer invades normal tissue surrounding the scar, it will advance at normal rates and most likely involve lymphatics.

Paget's Disease of the Nipple

Paget's disease of the nipple is a presentation of breast cancer that invariably, is associated with ductal carcinoma in situ (DCIS) or invasive carcinoma in the underlying breast. Typically, it presents as a unilateral red, bleeding, eczematous lesion of the nipple which is eventually eroded.

This condition occurs in approximately 1 in 50 breast cancers, and is most frequent among middle-aged and elderly women.

About 40% of cases present with a palpable lump, a relatively late stage.

Rarely Paget's disease may affect other apocrine gland-bearing areas such as the vulva.

Pathology

Histologic examination of the nipple reveals multiple Paget cells:

- Clear
- Sited among the basal epidermal cells
- Typical ballooned appearance
- Pale cytoplasm
- Prominent nuclei
- Nucleus surrounded by halo-accumulation of intracellular mucopolysaccharide

At the skin, the epidermis is invaded. The underlying dermis contains an inflammatory infiltrate.

In the vast majority of cases, careful study of the breast reveals an associated DCIS or invasive carcinoma.

A popular theory is that Paget's disease results from invasion of the nipple by malignant cells spreading down the ducts from the associated breast tumour.

Other theories propose that the Paget cells arise in the nipple from local epidermal cells, and that the concurrence of DCIS and nipple malignant cells are due to common carcinogenic influences.

Clinical Features

Classically, the condition is unilateral. The earliest symptoms are those of itching, tingling and discomfort.

Later, a small patch of redness or roughening is evident on the nipple that progresses to frank erosion with red granulation tissue and bleeding. The areola is often affected. There may be a palpable lump.

Changes occur slowly. It may take 4-5 years for the nipple to be fully eroded.

Less commonly, Paget's disease is characterised by a dry, red, scaly rash that spreads widely to involve much of the breast.

Management and Prognosis

Management is concentrated on detecting and treating any associated malignancy.

Total mastectomy with axillary dissection may be preferable in older patients as it is rapid and reliable. In those who wish to avoid mastectomy, radiotherapy alone or after cone excision of the nipple, areola and underlying ducts may be offered.

Wide local excision without radiotherapy is unsatisfactory; it is associated with a 50% recurrence rate. Adjuvant therapy is indicated only for established invasive carcinoma.

Paget's disease with associated intraduct carcinoma only and no palpable lump, has an excellent prognosis, with a cure rate approaching 100%.

Senile Keratoses

- Most common premalignant skin condition
- Characterized by multifocal scaly, hyperpigmented or scaly lesions, usually brown with a scaly base
- Histologically they are characterised by marked thickening of the keratin layer (hyperkeratosis) and the prickle cell layer (acanthosis). There may be a variable degree of dysplastic change and abnormal mitotic activity. However the basal layer remains intact

Note-1: There is debate whether actinic keratoses are premalignant conditions or alternatively early-stage squamous cell carcinoma (SCC).

Clinical Features

- Patients are middle-aged or elderly:
  - o more common in outdoor workers e.g. fishermen
  - o more common in fair-skinned people who live in tropical or sub-tropical regions e.g. Southern USA & Australia
- Lesions found on sun-exposed parts e.g. face, neck, hands
- Lesions are generally flat, well-demarcated, brown (sometimes red), crusty or scaly lesions
- The skin lesions bleed easily with minor trauma
- Typically patients give a history of a lesion that loses its scale but then recurs

Management

- Established lesions:
  - o physical treatment e.g. cryotherapy, curettage, local excision
  - o topical treatment options include: topical cytotoxic preparations (e.g. 5-fluorouracil), topical retinoids, salicylic acid in emulsifying ointment, topical diclofenac gel
  - o systemic treatment may be indicated for extensive or resistant lesions e.g. systemic retinoids
- Screening-for other skin lesions that are more common in patients with marked sunshine exposure e.g. squamous cell carcinoma, basal cell carcinoma, melanomas
- Prophylaxis-sun avoidance-e.g. sunscreens such as 4% mexenone.

MALIGNANT CONDITIONS

Basal Cell Carcinoma of the Skin

This is a locally invasive carcinoma of the basal layer of the epidermis. It almost never metastasizes but it may kill by local invasion.

Epidemiology

- This is the commonest skin cancer

- Usually affects the middle aged or elderly
- The highest incidence is among Caucasians in tropical and sub-tropical regions
- Incidence is related to sunlight exposure
- Males are more commonly affected (M:F approximately 2:1)-this reflects their greater occupational and recreational exposure to sunlight.

Aetiology

The development of a basal cell carcinoma appears to be mainly related to sunlight exposure.

Lesions occur in exposed areas of the skin (75% occur in the head and neck), and the incidence is increased in parts of the world with increased sunlight. Similarly there is an increased incidence in Caucasians, whose skin is perhaps least protected against the harmful affects of the sun.

Basal cell carcinomas may also arise in association with Gorlin's syndrome. Patients with this condition appear to have a great tendency to develop basal cell epitheliomata.

Clinical Features

- Usually affects middle aged or elderly
- Common sites are in scar tissue and sun damaged skin on the face, in a region above a line drawn between the corner of the mouth and the lobe of the ear
- The initial lesion is a small pearly-white nodule with visible (telangiectatic) blood vessels; early lesions may bleed and ulcerate and then heal again
- A red nodule forms which expands to leave a characteristic rolled edge with central ulceration ('rodent ulcer')
- 30% multiple
- Invasion is usually local. Metastasis is rare-metastatic rate is 0.0028%

Treatment

Treatment is by surgery, local radiotherapy, cryo-therapy, or curretage.

Curettage and cautery with histology is only adequate for small lesions.

Systemic chemotherapy is ineffective, though topical 5-Fluorouracil cream may be helpful, particularly for multiple tumours.

Recurrence is common (0.15-15%) but it is easily dealt with.

Prognosis

The prognosis for a patient with basal cell carcinoma is very good as about 90% will be cured:

- Metastases is less than 1%
- Recurrence rate similar with surgery and radio-therapy 0.1-15%

Squamous Cell Carcinoma of the Skin

Squamous cell carcinoma (SCC) is a malignant tumour of the epidermis in which the cells, if differentiated, show keratin formation.

Development of squamous cell carcinoma of the skin is associated with excessive sunlight exposure, exposure to chemical carcinogens such as coal tar products, chronic irritation, and in patients with immunosuppression.

There is an increased frequency in persons with non- pigmented skin. It is less common than basal cell carcinoma (BCC), with an incidence ratio of BCC:SCC of 4:1.

Histology is required to discriminate the lesions-usually nodular and kerotic-from basal cell carcinoma and solar keratosis.

Aetiology

- Exposure to ultraviolet light:
  - o usually occurs in fair-skinned, elderly people
  - o may develop from pre-existing solar keratosis
- Chronic exposure to industrial carcinogens
  - o arsenic, chromium compounds
  - o ionising radiation

- o soot (carcinoma of the scrotum in chimney sweeps),
- o also tar, pitch, oils
- Chronic inflammation (Marjolin's ulcer):
  - o margins of osteomyelitic sinuses
  - o margins of long-standing ulcers
  - o lupus vulgaris
- Genetic predisposition:
  - o xeroderma pigmentosum
  - o albinism
- Premalignant conditions:
  - o Bowen's disease
  - o leukoplakia
  - o erythroplasia of Queyrat
- Immunosuppression e.g. renal transplant patients

Epidemiology

- Incidence is estimated at 9000-10,000 per annum in England and Wales
- Squamous cell carcinoma (SCC) is rare in patients under 60 years of age unless immunosuppressed
- Commonest locations for SCCs:
  - o both sexes-back of hands, face
  - o men-scalp and ears
  - o women-lower legs
- Risk factors
  - o lifetime excessive sun exposure
  - o multiple actinic keratoses
  - o poor tanning ability
  - o fair skin
  - o transplant recipients

Differential Diagnosis

The differential diagnosis of squamous cell carcinoma is:

- Basal cell carcinoma
- Keratocanthoma
- Malignant melanoma
- Solar keratosis
- Pyogenic granuloma
- Infected seborrheic wart

Clinical Features

Often lesions develop on sun-exposed skin.

Characteristically a rapidly expanding painless, ulcerated nodule rolled indurated margin. Often the lesion may have a cauliflower-like appearance with areas of bleeding, ulceration or serous exudation.

About 55% of lesions occur in the head and neck region. About 25% of lesions occur on the hands and arms.

Metastatic spread may occur via local draining lymph nodes and beyond.

Management

If the tumour is localised and well differentiated, e.g. producing keratin pearls, then there is an approximate 90% cure rate via excisional surgery. There is also an excellent prognosis for treatment of these lesions with radiotherapy.

Large, poorly differentiated lesions have a greater tendency to infiltrate extensively and to cause vascular invasion. Treatment of these lesions may be surgical removal of the primary lesion, or surgery combined with radiotherapy, or radiotherapy as the only treatment method.

Cytotoxic chemotherapy may be used for disseminated disease.

These patients are usually reviewed annually for about 5 years after successful management.

Malignant Melanoma

A melanoma is a malignant tumour of epidermal melanocytes. It accounts for less than 1% of all cancers, though its incidence is increasing.

It is more common in people with non-pigmented skin who have been exposed to excessive sunlight, especially if sunburn ensues.

Spread occurs via superficial lymphatics to give satellite lesions, to regional lymph nodes via deep lymphatics, and via haematogenous spread to the lung, liver and brain. Haematogenous spread usually follows lymphatic.

Different clinico-pathologic types are recognised. The lesions may exhibit a range of colours and uniformity, and often may bleed and ulcerate. Some malignant melanomas are amelanotic. It may cause pigmented lesions in the mouth.

Epidemiology

Of note in the epidemiology of malignant melanoma:

- The incidence has doubled every ten years in recent times
- Occurs mainly in fair-skinned people of northern European-Celtic-origin. Incidence in this group has increased considerably over the last two decades.
- Highest incidence in western and northern Australia, e.g. Queensland 33/100,000
- Very common disease in albinos
- Predisposed by dysplastic naevus syndrome
- Incidence is non-linearly related to sun exposure-short intense periods of exposure are more common in melanotic patients. Cumulative sun exposure may be more relevant in lentigo maligna melanoma.
- Peak age of incidence is from 35-55 years; very rare before puberty
- Sex:
  - o females affected twice more often than males UK but incidence in other parts of world is equal
  - o lower leg is the most common site in females but in males, the trunk is most affected. Other common sites are the head and neck.
  - o women respond better to treatment than men

Clinico-pathological Classification

Malignant melanomas undergo two growth phases-radial and vertical. Vertical invasion is a poor prognostic sign.

Different types may be recognised (Clark):

- Superficial spreading (48%)
- Nodular (23%)
- Lentigo maligna (15%)
- Acral lentiginous including periungual (6%)
- Amelanotic melanoma

Histologically and cytologically, there are several features that distinguish malignant melanomas:

- Size:
  - o most malignant melanomas are greater than 10mm in diameter
  - o most benign tumours are less than 6mm
- Symmetry: malignant lesions are usually asymmetrical with respect to cell type, extension and degree of pigmentation
- Ascent of melanocytes: malignant tumours show melanocytes travelling upwards at the lateral margins of the tumour
- Epidermal hyperplasia: commonly seen with malignant lesions
- Dermal growth:
  - o malignant melanomas vary in their cell type and architecture in different parts of the tumour
  - o benign lesions are regular in appearance and change to smaller cells within the depth of the lesion
- Cytology: with increasing malignancy, there is a wider variation in cell shape and amount of pigment contained withing the melanocyte

Superficial Spreading Melanoma

Superficial spreading melanoma is the most common malignant melanoma in both sexes comprising 67% of the total, with the average age of patients being 40 years old. Women tend to be affected more commonly on the lower leg, whilst men are affected in the upper back.

Lesions are irregular brown, black or bluish black, frequently with some intermingled inflammation. A bizarre horseshoe-shaped or crescentic lesion may occur when the tumour shows central regression with concomitant peripheral extension. Active vertical invasion manifests clinically as raised and ulcerated nodules and is a poor prognostic sign. There is significant intra-epidermal lateral extension of melanocytes over at least three rete ridges beyond the later margin of dermal spread.

Lentigo Maligna Melanoma

Lentigo maligna melanoma occurs classically in the elderly, on sun-exposed sites, and is preceded by lentigo maligna, the in situ growth phase. Lentigo maligna melanoma describes the vertical invasion of the dermis by the melanocytes and is associated clinically with the development of raised nodules within the lesion. Metastasis to lymph nodes is less common than for other malignant melanomas. Early intervention, e.g. by cryotherapy, during the lateral growth phase carries a good prognosis.

Nodular Melanoma

Nodular melanoma is the most rapidly growing and aggressive variant of malignant melanoma. It is characterized by the absence of a radial growth phase. Typically, it arises on apparently normal skin, has relatively little melanin and a rich blood supply. Ulceration is common, giving a poorer prognosis.

acral Lentiginous Melanoma

Acral lentiginous melanoma is seen on the soles and less often, the palms. It has a raised dark area surrounded by a paler macular-lentiginous-area often extending for several centimetres around the elevation.

Periungual melanoma may be regarded as a variant of acra-lentiginous melanoma. Its clinical importance is that it is often misdiagnosed. Brown pigmentation on the nail fold is suggestive of melanoma-Hutchinson's sign. Periungual warts or plantar warts are uncommon in patients over 40 years of age.

Amelanotic Melanoma

Amelanotic melanoma may occur in any of the four clinico-pathological variants. Their prognosis is poor since they are frequently recognised late. They present as erythematous papules or nodules, lacking significant pigmentation. Confusion with basal cell carcinoma, sqamous cell carcinoma and other non-pigmented skin tumours is common.

Clinical Features

The common presenting features in a cutaneous melanoma patient:

- Often history of increased sun exposure
- F>M by ratio of 2:1
- common sites include the face and neck; the lower extremities including the soles of the feet. Lesions may occur anywhere, even in the nailbeds.
- Lesions are generally black or dark brown and nodular; there may be irregularity of colour. There may be subdermal lymphatic spread and the presence of satellite lesions.
- They may bleed or ulcerate.
- They may arise from moles or lentigo maligna, or de novo. If a malignant melanoma arises from a mole or lentigo maligna, then often the area of the lesion increases and may darken or bleed. It may also become ulcerated, inflamed, become irregular in edge or depth, or itchy.
- Symptoms and signs of metastasis e.g. weight loss, dyspnoea and jaundice

Sometimes this condition may present with a non-pigmented melanoma-amelanotic melanoma.

Differential Diagnosis

A malignant melanoma must be discriminated from:

- Benign naevi
- Dermatofibroma
- Pigmented basal cell carcinoma
- Pyogenic granuloma

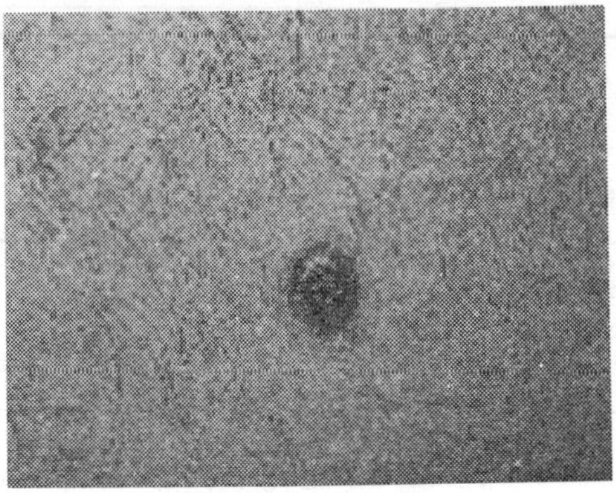

Malignant melanoma

- Kaposi's sarcoma
- Vascular malformations
- Seborrhoeic keratosis

If the lesion is gradually changing size or pigmentation, ulcerating or bleeding, then this increases the likelihood that it is a malignant melanoma.

Histology of the lesion is required for diagnosis.

Investigation

The key investigation for melanoma is excision biopsy with careful pathological analysis. Others tests may include:

- FBC
- Urine melanogens
- CXR
- LFT's
- CT scan

Management

Current management of malignant melanoma involves an initial excision biopsy and histological examination.

Following biopsy, surgery has been traditionally performed, though excision margins are controversial and influenced by functional and cosmetic considerations. Thin lesions < 0.75 mm may be treated by wide local excision, which is then directly closed. Thicker tumours >1.5 mm, however, require 3-5 cm clearance and in such cases grafting may be necessary.

Superficial spreading melanomas and nodular melanomas are radioresistant but good results have been reported from radiotherapy to lentigo maligna melanoma.

Cytotoxic agents have been disappointing although imidazole carboxamide-DTIC-and vindesine may be used.

Involved regional nodes are removed by block dissection and though prophylactic lymph node dissection is commonly practiced in the USA for thick tumours, it does not appear to improve survival and is rarely practised in the UK.

Recurrent tumours and deeply invasive ones on a limb may respond to limb perfusion. The affected limb is arterially perfused with a cytotoxic agent for example, Melphalan. Recurrence is reduced but anaemia may be a serious side effect due to penetration of the bone marrow by the cytotoxic agent.

Other therapies such as immunotherapy and hormonal therapy are currently being evaluated.

Most patients are followed up for 10 years. Patients are seen at regular intervals: 3 monthly for the first 2 years and then 6 monthly.

Prognosis

The main determinants of prognosis for malignant melanoma are the tumour thickness, measured from the overlying granular layer of the epidermis to the deepest easily identifiable tumour cells-the Breslow thickness, and the presence of ulceration of the primary tumour.

In the American Joint Committee on Cancer (AJCC) 2002 Staging system for malignant melanoma there is less significance with respect the level of invasion (Clark's levels) in prognosis. Analysis of histopathologic features of melanoma comparing Clark's level and Breslow's depth have shown that the actual tumour thickness is more predictive of outcome. However there is an instance in which Clark's level invasion continues to carry prognostic information: In patients with "thin"(<1.0 mm) melanoma, Clark's level IV or V lesion portends a worse prognosis. For this reason, pathologists need to continue to include Clark's level along with tumour thickness and ulceration in the histology report of the primary melanoma

Other Prognostic Determinants:

- Site-back, arms, neck and scalp lesions fair worse
- Pathology-worst for nodular, best for lentigo
- Sex-worse for males
- Age-worsens with age, possibly due to immunological factors or decreased motivation for treatment
- Mitotic rate-worse for higher
- Tumour volume-more accurate prognosis but difficult to perform
- Regression-associated with an unfavourable prognosis for thin tumours
- Metastasis-poor if metastasised-10% 5 year survival
- Satellites-metastases occurring at a distance of less than 50mm from the main tumour are a poor prognostic finding
- Host inflammatory response-improves prognosis
- Immunological factors-increased expression of HLA-DR correlates with worse prognosis as does the ganglioside GD2 on tumour cells.

Urgent Referral for Suspected Melanoma

Pigmented lesions on any part of the body which have one or more of the following features:

- A lesion changing shape
- A lesion growing in size
- An irregular outline to the lesion
- Changing colour of the lesion
- Mixed colour
- Inflammation
- Ulceration

Note-at the time of diagnosis, melanomas are usually 5 mm or greater, but a small number of patients with very early melanoma may have lesions of a less than 5 mm diameter.

Squamous Cell Carcinoma

- Non-healing, slowly growing lesions with significant induration on palpation (commonly on scalp, face, back of hand)-also there should be a documented expansion over a period of 1-2 months
- Patients in who squamous cell carcinoma has been diagnosed from a biopsy specimen undertaken in primary care
- Patients who are therapeutically immunosuppressed after an organ transplant have a high incidence of skin cancers particularly squamous cell carcinoma. In this situation squamous cell carcinom can be unusually aggressive and metastasize. Therefore if a transplant patient develops new or growing cutaneous lesions It is strongly recommended these patients should be referred under the two weeek standard.

Mycosis Fungoides

Mycosis fungoides is a non-Hodgkin's lymphoma that arises from CD4+ T lymphocytes.

The aetiology of mycosis fungoides is unknown, although a variety of risk factors have been proposed, including environmental factors (e.g. occupational exposure, viral infection) and genetic factors (1).

It is a cutaneous lymphoma that characteristically affects middle aged males. It usually begins as an eczematous reaction and proceeds to form plaques, tumours and fungating ulcers. Erythroderma may occur which often is highly pruritic.

Treatment is with topical steroids, topical cytotoxic agents, PUVA or radiotherapy. Visceral involvement may require systemic cytotoxic therapy, although responses are often short-lived.

Prognosis relates to extent and type of skin involvement-average survival in the early stage of this disease is at least 10-15 years (2).

Sezary syndrome is the leukaemic presentation of mycosis fungoides (3).

Clinical Features

- May present with slowly evolving scaly erythematous patches
- Sites frequently affected include the upper arms, trunk, buttocks and thighs
- There may be a slow progression and extension of the disease into plaques and eventually tumours
- The symptomatology associated with this disease is variable and ranges from being asymptomatic to severe itching
- Often the disease is initially diagnosed as eczema or psoriasis

Histology

- Various criteria for the histological diagnosis of mycosis fungoides have been proposed-the most consistent diagnostic features are the presence of epidermotropism with atypical lymphocytes (typically having a 'cerebriform' or notched nucleus) invading the epidermis and collections of atypical lymphocytes (Pautrier microabscesses) in the absence of significant spongiosis (1).

Diagnosis

- Based on correlation of clinical features with histology
- May be supplemented by molecular biology and immunohistochemistry techniques-classically mycosis fungoides expresses a CD4+-T-helper phenotype; in rare cases a CD8+ phenotype is found (this may be associated with aggressive disease and a poor prognosis)

Investigation and Staging

Routine investigations include:

- FBC, ESR
- Blood film (for Sezary cell examination)
- Biochemical profile (including lactate dehydrogenase)
- Chest X-ray

Investigations if clinically indicated include:

- Lymph node biopsy, bone marrow biopsy, CT scan (chest/abdomen/pelvis), visceral organ biopsy

Treatment

Consult expert advice.

Treatment options depend on the stage of the disease.

- Stage Ia-IIa
  - o skin directed treatment options include topical steroids, topical chemotherapy (nitrogen mustard, carmustine), phototherapy (UVA, UVB)
- Stage IIb
  - o as for Stage Ia-IIa +/- localised radiotherapy
  - o as for Stage Ia-IIa +/- biological response modifiers (retinoids/interferon)
  - o total skin electron beam therapy
  - o single or multi-agent chemotherapy
- Stage III
  - o options include:
    - § extracorporeal photochemotherapy
    - § single or multi-agent chemotherapy
    - § as for Stage Ia-IIa +/- biological response modifiers, total skin electron beam therapy, localised radiotherapy
- Stage IV
  - o options include systemic chemotherapy; radiotherapy and palliative skin directed treatment

Prognosis

- Stages Ia-IIb-median survival of 12.5 years
- Stages IIb, III, IVa-median survival of 5 years
- Stage IVb-median survival of 2.5 years

Kaposi's Sarcoma

Kaposi's sarcoma is a multicentric, malignant neoplastic vascular proliferation, characterised by the development of bluish-red nodules on the skin. Sometimes there may be widespread visceral involvement. It may metastasize to lymph nodes.

In the Classical Jewish and Mediterranean variety and the endemic African variety, Kaposi's sarcoma is an indolent condition with no significant reduction in life expectancy.

Kaposi's sarcoma may also occur in immunocompromised patients (e.g. HIV positive patients, transplant patients) and in these patients a particulary virulent, disseminated form occurs.

Epidemiology

Kaposi's sarcoma is seen more frequently in:

- Individuals with AIDS:
  - o largely restricted to homosexual and bisexual groups
  - o rare in patients who acquired HIV intravenously
- Individuals with immunosuppression for reasons other than HIV infection
- Elderly males of Jewish or Mediterranean origin-classical form
- In African populations the disease may be manifested as either the classical, locally aggressive or lymphadenopathic forms

Pathogenesis

It was previously believed that the development of AIDS-related Kaposi's sarcoma was due to the production of cytokines and HIV products in the infected individual. However careful epidemiological studies have refuted these ideas and lead to the discovery of *human herpesvirus 8 (HHV-8)*.

The discovery of HHV-8 has helped to explain the evolution of AIDS related Kaposi's sarcoma. It seems that HHV-8, which doesn't normally cause disease emerged as a pathogen during the AIDS epidemic due to sharing risk factors for transmission with HIV.

Clinical Features

The lesion or lesions of Kaposi's sarcoma may at first appear like bruises, being coloured purple and blue. However, these become slightly raised and firmer, with the colour darkening so that the lesions become purple and black. They are not usually painful or itchy though they may develop at multiple sites over the body and cause cosmetic distress.

In about 40% of cases there is gastrointestinal involvement which is usually asymptomatic, though dysphagia or obstructive symptoms may occur.

Pulmonary manifestations include pleural, parenchymal and airway lesions, and recurrent pleural effusions may occur.

There may also be liver and lymph node involvement.

Diagnosis

Once suspected, the diagnosis of Kaposi's sarcoma is made by the histology of skin or other tissue biopsy

Treatment and Prognosis

In the Classical Jewish and Mediterranean variety and the endemic African variety, Kaposi's sarcoma is an indolent condition with no significant reduction in life expectancy.

In immunosuppressed individuals, such as those with HIV infection, the tumour is more aggressive and multiple lesions may form. A third of AIDS patients who respond to treatment-detailed elsewhere-relapse later.

This condition is not generally fatal in patients with AIDS but may be an indication of increased susceptibility to opportunistic infections such as Pneumocystis carinii pneumonia. Treatment should be tailored to the needs of the individual patient.

Individuals who develop Kaposi's sarcoma whilst on immunosuppressive drugs may see their lesions regress and resolve on stopping immunosuppressive therapy.

Treatment of AIDS-related Kaposi's Sarcoma

Treatment of AIDS-related Kaposi's sarcoma should be tailored to the needs of the patient. For example, lesions causing only cosmetic symptoms may only need local treatment, whilst extensive life threatening lesions may need more agressive intervention.

- Limited intervention:
  - local therapy:
    - radiation therapy
    - liquid nitrogen
    - intralesional therapy.
- Surgery
- Alpha-interferon
- Alpha-interferon plus zidovudine
- Aggressive intervention:
  - single-agent chemotherapy: Doxorubicin, Vinblastine
  - combination chemotherapy.

Fourteen

Bone Tumors

Bone Tumors can be divided into primary and secondary. Secondary tumors can be further subdivided into:

- Metastatic tumors
- Tumors resulting from contiguous spread of adjacent soft tissue neoplasms
- Tumors representing malignant transformation of the pre-existing benign lesions.

Metastatic cancers: are the most frequent malignant tumors found in bone. They are by far more common than primary bone tumors and are characterized by the following:

- Predominant occurrence in:two age groups: adults over 40 years of age and children in the first decade of life.
- Multifocality and predilection for the hematopoietic marrow sites in the axial skeleton (vertebrae, pelvis, ribs and cranium) and proximal long bones. Metastases to long bones distal to the elbows and knees are unusual. Metastases to the small bones of the hands and feet are even rarer. Occasionally, metastases may appear as solitary lesions (particularly true for the lung, kidney and thyroid cancer).

Radiographic appearance of the metastatic tumors can be:

- Purely lytic (kidney, lung, colon, and melanoma)
- Purely blastic (prostate and breast carcinoma)
- Mixed lytic and blastic (most common appearance)

Most common malignancies producing skeletal metastases:

Adults	More than 75% of skeletal metastases originate from carcinomas of the prostate, breast, kidney, and lung. Also common are metastases from thyroid and colon cancers. And do not forget melanoma.
Children	Neuroblastoma, rhabdomyosarcoma, and retinoblastoma

Primary bone tumors are characterized by the following:

- Predominant occurrence in the first 3 decades of life, during the ages of the greatest skeletal growth activity. The commonest sites for many primary tumors, both benign and malignant, are in the distal femur and proximal tibia, the bones with the highest growth rate.
- Relatively specific radiographic presentations. In some cases, the diagnosis can be confidently made based on the radiographic features alone.
- Benign tumors are by far more common than malignant ones. Some of them are not true neoplasms, but rather represent hamartomas (e.g., osteochondroma). The most common benign tumors are osteochondroma, non-ossifying fibroma, and enchondroma.

- Some primary bone tumors are difficult to classify as benign or malignant. For example, giant cell tumor of bone is very aggressive locally but only rarely metastasizes.
- Among primary malignant neoplasms, osteosarcoma and multiple myeloma have the highest incidence, followed by chondrosarcoma and Ewing's sarcoma.

Relevant clinical information

Age group	*Most common benign lesions*	*Most common malignant tumors*
0-10	Simple bone cyst eosinophilic granuloma	Ewing's sarcoma leukemic involvement metastatic neuroblastoma
10-20	Non-ossifying fibroma fibrous dysplasia simple bone cyst aneurysmal bone cyst osteochondroma (exostosis) osteoid osteoma osteoblastoma chondroblastoma chondromyxoid fibroma	Osteosarcoma, Ewing's sarcoma, adamantinoma
20-40	Enchondroma giant cell tumor	Chondrosarcoma
40 and above	Osteoma	Metastatic tumors myeloma leukemic involvement chondrosarcoma osteosarcoma (Paget's associated) MFH chordoma

Summary

Primary osteosarcoma and Ewing's sarcoma are tumors of children and young adults. Occurrence of chondrosarcomas in children or Ewing's sarcoma in middle-aged patients is extremely unusual. In individuals older than 40 years, the commonest form of skeletal malignancy is metastatic cancer. Of the primary bone tumors in this age group, multiple myeloma and chondrosarcoma are most commonly encountered. Osteosarcomas in this age group are often secondary malignancies, which develop at the the sites of bone damage. Giant cell tumor, a locally aggressive lesion, almost exclusively occurs in skeletally mature patients, 20 to 50 years of age, with closed epiphyses. It is practically never seen in children or patients older than 60 years.

RADIOLOGICAL CORRELATION

The following imaging studies are commonly used in evaluation of bone tumors:

Plain radiograph is usually the first imaging technique for a suspected bone lesion since it is inexpensive and easily obtainable. It is also the best for assessment of general radiological features of the tumor.

Computer tomography is a method of choice when plain film assessment is difficult owing to the nature of the lesion (e.g., permeative pattern of destruction) or anatomic site (e.g., sacrum). In addition, CT is the best technique in assessment of matrix mineralization, cortical detail, and detection of the cystic and fatty lesions.

MRI is a method of choice for local staging: It is superior to CT in the definition of medullary and extracortical spread and of the relationship of the tumor to critical neurovascular structures. However, remember that the MRI appearances of the majority of bone tumors are totally non-specific. You need to examine plain films or CT films to define a neoplasm.

Bone scintigraphy is a highly sensitive but relatively non-specific technique. Its main role is in detection of suspected metastases in the whole skeleton. It may also be helpful in the detection of osteoid osteomas ("double density sign" is present in about 50% of cases and is highly suggestive of this tumor).

LOCATION

Lesions	*Most common skeletal sites*
Ewing's sarcoma, Multiple myeloma, Leukemia/lymphoma, Metastatic cancers	Hematopoietic marrow sites in the axial skeleton (vertebrae, ribs, sternum, pelvis, cranium) and proximal long bones (femur, humerus)
Non-ossifying fibroma	Metadiaphyseal regions of the tibia and distal femur *(80%)* Does not occur in the flat bones, craniofacial bones, the spine, or the small bones of the hands/feet.
Simple bone cyst	The vast majority of SBCs is found in the proximal humerus *(55%)* and proximal femur *(20%)*.
Chordoma	Base of the skull or sacrum *(90%)*
Adamantinoma	Mid-shaft of tibia *(90%)*, jaw bones
Chondroblastoma	Long bones (knee area, proximal humerus)-*70%*
Giant cell tumor	Knee area, distal radius *(65%)*
Enchondroma	Small bones of the hands and feet *(60%)*. This is in fact the commonest tumor at these sites.
Chondrosarcoma (primary, and to the less extent secondary)	Tends to develop in the axial skeleton with *25%* to *30%* occurring in the pelvic bones
Fibrous dysplasia	Femur, tibia, skull and ribs
Osteochondroma	Knee area, proximal humerus, pelvis
Osteoblastoma	*Spine (30%)*, mandible, long bones
Aneurysmal bone cyst	Any bone; common in the *spine*
Chondromyxoid fibroma	Knee area *(30%)*, pelvis, small bones of the feet
Hemangioma	***Spine***, craniofacial bones

SITE OF LONG BONE INVOLVEMENT

(Most primary bone tumors have favored sites within long bones; this may provide a clue to diagnosis).

Epiphyseal lesions: Chondroblastoma and Giant Cell Tumor (GCT) are almost invariably centered in the epiphysis. Chondroblastoma is a rare tumor seen in children and adolescents with open growth plates. GCT is the most common tumor of epiphyses in skeletally mature individuals with closed growth plates. GCT often shows metaphyseal extension.

Metaphyseal intramedullary lesions: Osteosarcoma is usually centered in the metaphysis. Chondrosarcoma and fibrosarcoma often present as metaphyseal lesions. Osteoblastoma, enchondroma, fibrous dysplasia, simple bone cyst, and aneurysmal bone cyst are common in this location.

Metaphyseal lesions centered in the cortex: Classic location for a non-ossifying fibroma (NOF). Also, a common site for osteoid osteoma.

Metaphyseal exostosis: Osteochondroma

Diaphyseal intramedullary lesions: Favored location for Ewing's sarcoma, lymphoma, myeloma. Common for fibrous dysplasia and enchondroma.

Diaphyseal lesions centered in the cortex: Adamantinoma, osteoid osteoma

Ewing's Sarcoma

Ewing's sarcoma is a malignant small cell tumour of bone, more common in males and having its highest incidence in the age group 5 to 20 years. It usually occurs in the diaphysis of long bones.

Ewing's sarcomas account for about 2% of paediatric malignancies.

It most often occurs in the femur, humerus, tibia, pelvis and ribs. Metastasis occurs early, usually to the lungs and other bones.

Ewing's sarcoma may mimic an infective process and present with localised swelling, redness, heat and fever. There may be a raised WBC and ESR. Biopsy is needed for diagnosis.

Radiology of a Ewing's tumour shows bone destruction with overlying onion-skin layers of periosteal bone formation.The medulla is more affected than the cortex. The latter may show signs of periosteal elevation.

Grossly, the tumor is gray to white in color and poorly demarcated. The consistency is soft and gray and sometimes semi-liquid especially after breaking through the cortex. Areas of hemorrhage and necrosis are common. The destruction is often greater on gross appearance than was visible on radiographs.Under the microscope, Ewing's sarcoma consists of densely packed uniform small cells in sheets. The cells have scant cytoplasm without distinct borders. The cells are two to three times as big as lymphocytes and have a single oval or round nucleus without prominent nucleoli. *The tumor spreads through Haversian canals which cause the appearance ofpermeative margins on X-ray. Glycogen is present within the cells causing a positive reaction to periodic acid-schiff (PAS) stain.* Most Ewing's sarcomas are positive with HBA-71 or 0-13 stain which is an antibody to the protein product of myc 2. The microscopic differential includes lymphoma and metastatic neuroblastoma which must be excluded by reticulin stain and urine vanillyl mandelic acid and homovanillic acid respectively. Rhabdomyosarcoma is ruled out if the specimen stains negatively with desmin, myoglobin and actin stains. A neural origin is supported by electron microscope findings of pseudorosettes. This is further supported by the common finding in Ewing's sarcoma and primitive neuroectodermal tumors of choline acetyltransferase and the translocation t(11:22)(q24;ql2). It is thought that Ewing's sarcoma with its few organelles is the poorly differentiated end of the spectrum of PNET. Neuroepithelioma is an example of well differentiated PNET and has neurosecretory granules and neuritic processes.

The differential diagnosis of Ewing's tumour includes:

- Secondary neuroblastoma
- Lymphoma
- Eosinophilic granuloma
- Osteosarcoma
- Secondary deposits e.g. of oat cell carcinoma

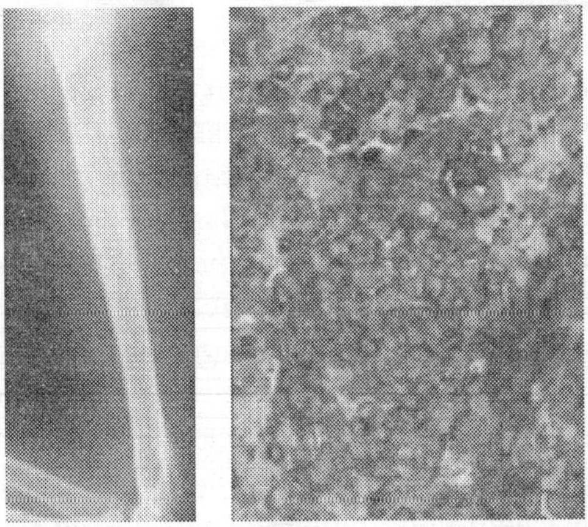

Treatment for Ewing's sarcoma includes surgery, radiation and multi-drug chemotherapy. Radiation or chemotherapy with vincristine, dactinomycin and cyclophophamide (VAC) are used preoperatively. Adjuvant chemotherapy follows surgery and decreases recurrences.i The tumor metastasizes to lungs and lymph nodes.

Poor prognostic signs include increased age, increased ESR and leukocytosis at presentation. The 5-year survival of osteosarcoma, Ewing's sarcoma, and malignant fibrous histiocytoma, now approaches 55%. In about 80% of cases patients will be suitable for some sort of limb salvage surgery and will retain the use of a functioning limb.

CHONDROBLASTOMA

Chondroblastoma is a rare, benign tumor derived from chondroblasts. It is found in the epiphysis of long bones, usually of the lower extremity. The most common site is the distal femur followed by the proximal femur, proximal humerus and proximal tibia. The tumor has a preference for males over females and the mean age of presentation is approximately 20 years old. The tumor may have behavior not normally associated with benign tumors including pulmonary metastases as well as local invasion of bone and soft tissue.

Clinically, chondroblastoma presents as pain near a joint without history of trauma. A secondary synovitis can be induced by the tumor, but pathological fracture is extremely rare.

The diagnosis of chondroblastoma can usually be made by radiograph. when the age of the patient and location of the lesion are considered. The most common site for chondroblastoma is the epiphysis. The lesion is lytic with well defined margins and can be from 1-6 cm in size. Scalloping or expansion of cortical bone may be present. Fine calcifications, either punctate or in rings, may be visible. Cysts are present about 20% of the time and both MRI and CT can define the fluid levels. CT is also useful for defining the relationship of the tumor to the joint, integrity of the cortex, and intralesional calcifications. The differential diagnosis includes enchondroma, central chondrosarcoma and aneurysmal bone cyst.

On gross examination, a chondroblastoma has a lobulated, round form and is made up of friable, soft, grayish pink tissue that may be gritty. If present, the cystic fluid is rust or straw-colored. Chondroblastoma is made up of uniform, polygonal cells that are closely packed. These primitive cells are derived from the epiphyseal cartilage plate and have abundant cytoplasm. There is little mitotic activity. A scant chondroid matrix may be superimposed by a pericellular deposit of calcification that appears like *"chicken-wire"*. The rapid proliferation of immature chondrocytes does not create lacunae or formal cartilage matrix. Giant cells are often present.

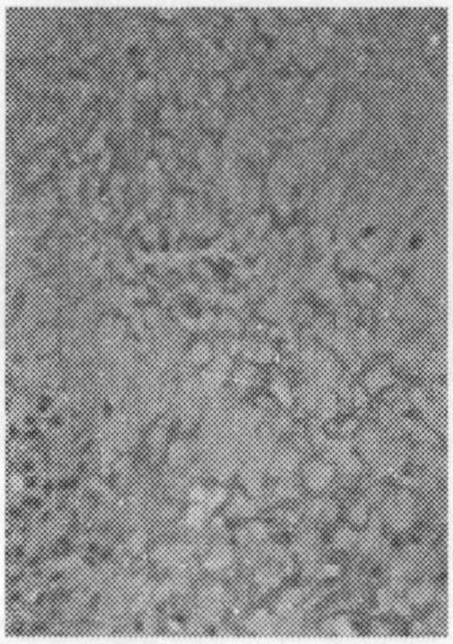

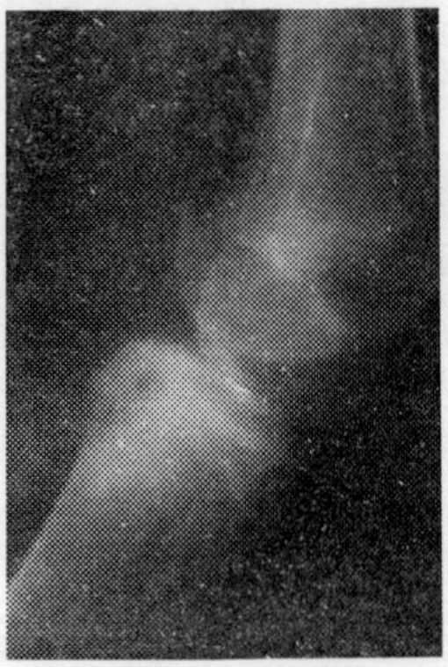

Treatment of chondroblastoma is biopsy and curettage with possible use of adjuvant liquid nitrogen or phenol, or a mechanical burr. It may be necessary to reconstruct articular surfaces due to subchondral erosion. Any joint invasion is usually secondary to previous instrumentation. All pulmonary nodules should be excised.

CHORDOMA

Chordoma is a rare malignant tumor that arises from notochord remnants. Chordomas account for 1 to 4% of all bone tumors. They occur in older adults with the highest prevalence in the fifth to seventh decade. The ratio of male to female is two to one. Due to their origin in the notochord, chordomas occur in the mid-line of the axial skeleton. One half of cases occur in the sacrococcygeal region and one third occur at the base of the skull. Other rare sites include transverse processes of vertebrae and the paranasal sinuses.

The clinical presentation depends on the location of the tumor. Sacrococcygeal tumors often present as low back pain with no characteristic pattern or time course. Sacrococcygeal tumors can also present as bowel and bladder dysfunction. Presacral tumors can sometimes be palpated on rectal exam. Sacral tumors are often large at presentation as a large volume of tumor can be accommodated within the pelvis. Anterior cervical tumors can present as dysphagia and posterior cervical tumors can cause neurological deficits. Tumors at the base of the skull may present with headaches.

On plain X-ray, chordomas appear as a solitary mid-line lesion with bony destruction. There is often an accompanying soft tissue mass. Approximately half of the time focal calcifications are present. CT and MRI scans help demonstrate the soft tissue component, calcifications and epidural extension. MRI is helpful in identifying local recurrences. Chordomas have reduced uptake on bone scan.

On gross examination, chordomas are soft, blue-gray, lobulated tumors. There are gelatinous translucent areas and often a capsule is present. The lesion often tracks along nerve roots in the sacral plexus or out the sciatic notch in planes of least resistance.

Under the microscope, the chordomas are characterized by lobules and fibrous septa. The malignant cell has eosinophilic cytoplasm. Prominent vacuoles of mucus push the nuclei to the side resulting in "physaliphorous" cells from the Greek word for bubble or drop.

During the fourth to sixth week of fetal development mesenchymal cells from individual sclerotomes merge to surround the notochord and form the vertebral bodies. The notochord normally degenerates and remnants form the nucleus pulposus of the vertebral disc. The prevailing theory is that in chordomas the notochord fails to degenerate and then undergoes malignant transformation. The major failing of this theory is that normal notochord remnants have never been observed.

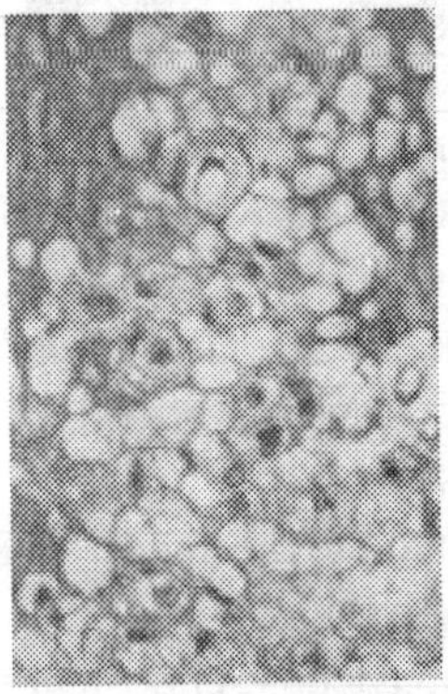

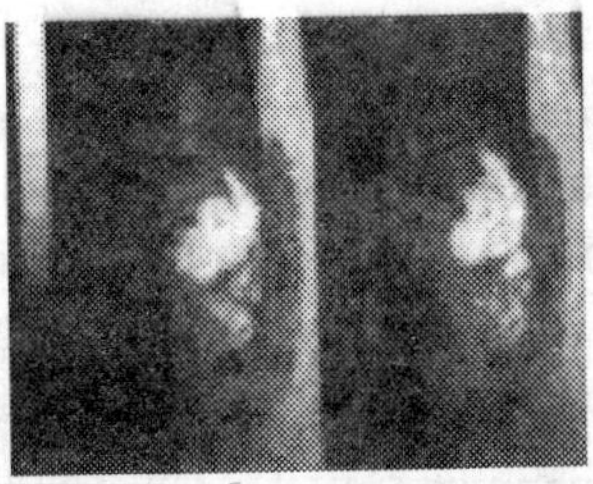

The treatment of chordomas is difficult. Wide surgical excision is desirable but rarely feasible based on the anatomic location of the tumor. With sacrococcygeal tumors, sexual function and sphincter control may be compromised after surgery. Radiation is used if complete resection is impossible. Chordomas metastasize to lymph nodes, lungs, liver and bone. Chemotherapy can be used for late stage disease.

EOSINOPHILIC GRANULOMA

Eosinophilic granuloma (EG) is a solitary, nonneoplastic proliferation of histiocytes. EG is part of a spectrum of Langerhan's cell histiocytosis, formerly known as histiocytosis X. EG is a localized lesion in bone or lung and occurs most commonly in children aged 5 to 10. It makes up 60-80% of all cases of Langerhan's cell histiocytosis and is uncommon in blacks. EG is found in the skull, mandible, spine and long bones. The male to female ratio is two to one. Letterer-Siwe disease is a fulminant systemic disease that comprises 10% of Langerhan's cell histiocytosis, occurs in children under 3 years old and is rapidly fatal. Hand-Schuller-Christian disease (HSC) is a chronic disseminated form of Langerhan' s histiocytosis and occurs in older patients. The well known triad of HSC is diabetes insipidus, exopthalmos and skull lesions. EG can convert to systemic forms of the disease.

EG is normally symptomatic. Local pain, swelling and tenderness are common and the ESR may be elevated.

The radiologic appearance of EG is non-specific and differs by location. The skull may have a lesion with sharp, punched out borders that is uneven across the inner and outer table causing a "beveled edge". Pelvic lesions are often poorly defined. Spine lesions are normally found in the vertebral body. EG is found in the diaphysis or metaphysis of long bones in the center of the medullary cavity. The lesion may cause endosteal scalloping or a periosteal reaction. Bone scan is not useful in defining EG. CT scan and MRI delineate the extent of the intramedullary and cortical penetration. The radiologic differential includes Ewing's sarcoma, osteosarcoma, metastases and osteomyelitis.

On gross examination, EG is a soft, granular or gelatinous mass. It appears gray red to brown with flecks of yellow.

Under the microscope, EG consists of sheets of Langerhan's cells. These cells are derived from the mononuclear cell and dendritic line precursors and are found in the bone marrow. The cell is identifiable under the electron microscope as the Langerhan's cell has racket shaped cytoplasmic inclusion bodies called Birbeck's granules. Also present in the lesion are varying amounts of lymphocytes, polymorphonuclear cells, eosinophils and giant cells. Early lesions have many Langerhan's cells and eosinophils. Older lesions have fewer cells and much fibrous tissue. The cause of EG is unknown and speculated to be either infection or immunological.

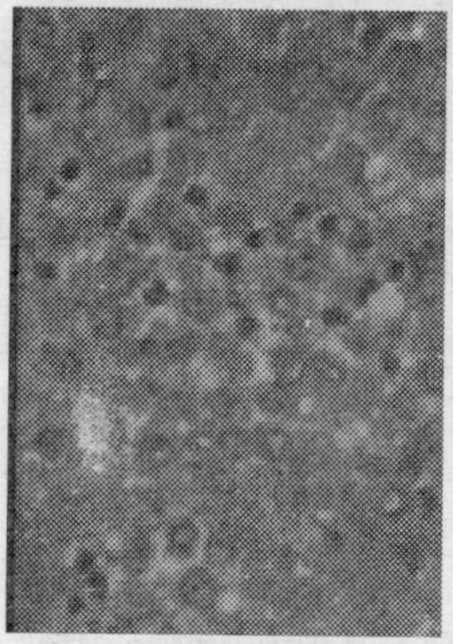

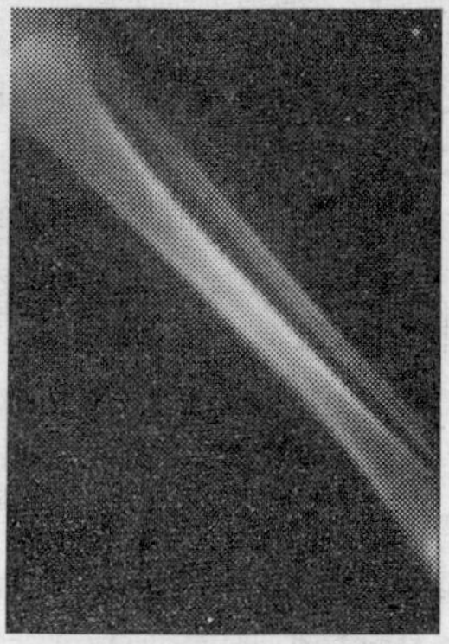

Treatment of EG depends on the form of the disease. With localized disease, often a biopsy alone is enough to incite healing. Other treatment modalities of EG include curettage, excision, steroid injection, radiation and observation. Chemotherapy is recommended for systemic disease.

CHONDROMYXOID FIBROMA

Salient Points

- Chondromyxoid fibroma (CMF) is a *rare benign tumor* with predominant occurrence in patients younger than 40 years. The peak incidence is between ages 10 and 20. It is one of two neoplasms of *incompletely differentiated cartilage*. The other neoplasm is chondroblastoma.
- *Location:* The most frequent skeletal sites are the knee area (30%), pelvis and the small bones of the feet. In the long bone, the tumor characteristically involves the metaphysis or metadiaphysis and is often seen in an eccentric position.
- Secondary cystic change in the form of aneurysmal bone cyst is not unusual.
- *Differential diagnosis* of CMF includes chondroblastoma and, more importantly, chondrosarcoma. Distinguishing features of chondroblastoma are epiphyseal location and "chiken-wire" calcifications. The diagnostic criteria for chondrosarcoma include hyaline

cartilage matrix, tumor permeation of the surrounding bone and mitotic activity. *Keep in mind that CMFs, even those showing marked cellular pleomorphism, have extremely low number of mitoses never exceeding 1 per 50 hpf.*

- *Clinical behavior:* Recurrence rate averages 15-20%. Large or recurrent lesions may be locally aggressive

Characteristic Radiological Findings

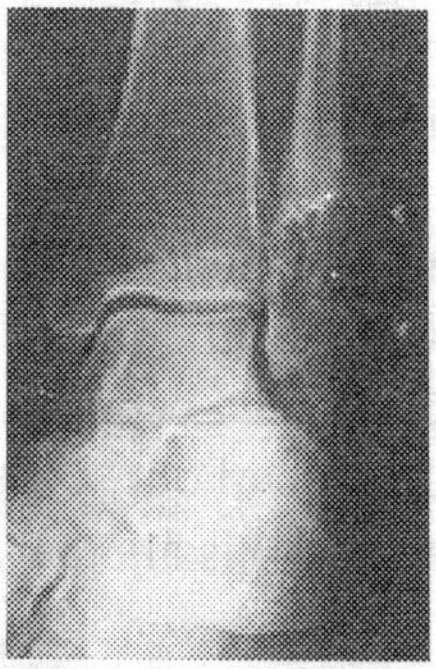

- Plain film shows a well-defined, expansile lytic lesion, which is centered at the distal fibular metaphysis and is bordered by a sclerotic rim.

  Benign nature of the lesion is suggested by its sharp demarcation from the surrounding bone, sclerotic rimming and lack of cortical disruption.

Pathological Findings

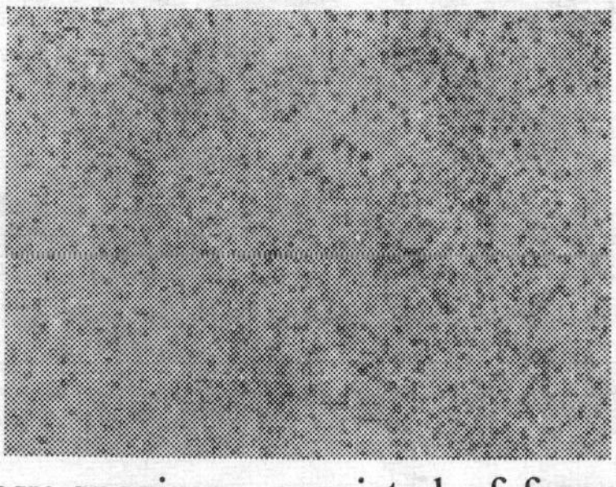

- Biopsy specimen consisted of fragments of white-gray rubbery tissue. Low power view shows a moderately cellular chondromyxoid tissue with the following *two characteristic features:*
  a. Vague lobularity caused by alternating highly cellular and less cellular areas;
  b. Increased cellularity at the periphery of the lobules.

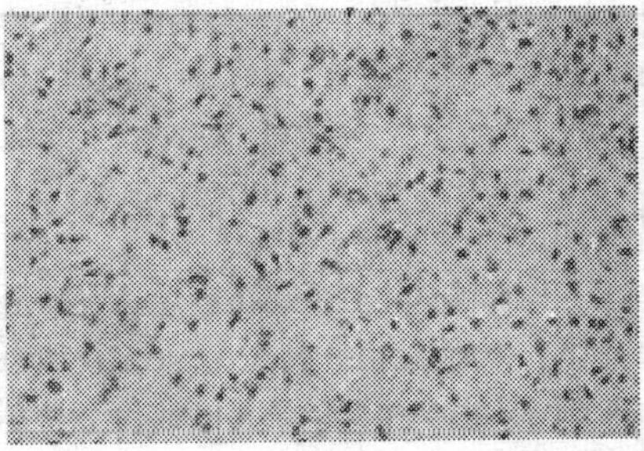

- Higher magnification view of the lobule shows mildly pleomorphic, angular and stellate cells set in bluish-pink chondromyxoid stroma. Note that the *tumor lacks true hyaline cartilage matrix* seen in enchondromas and chondrosarcomas. Another important feature is *lack of mitotic activity*

Giant Cell Tumor of Bone (GCT)

Salient Points

- Conventional GCT of bone is a *relatively common, locally aggressive neoplasm* accounting for approximately 4% of all primary bone tumors. It affects skeletally mature individuals, F > M, 20 to 50 years of age. It is extremely rare in children and patient older than 60 years. Histogenesis remains unclear. The cells of GCT have phenotypic features of both macrophage-like (CD68 positive) and osteoclastic cells (immunoreactive with tartrate-resistant acid phosphatase (TRAP), calcitonin and parathormone).
- *Location:* Most GCTs affect the long bones with the highest incidence (65%) in the distal femur, proximal tibia and distal radius. *In the long bones, the tumor is invariably centered in the epiphysis*. It can also be found in any other long bone, pelvis and sacrum, and spine (3%). GCTs of the hands and feet are very rare.
- Tumors that have radiological and morphologic features of GCT but are multifocal and/

or located in the diaphyses are unlikely to be conventional GCTs. Most often they are *"brown tumors of hyperparathyroidism"* found in patients with abnormal serum levels of calcium and phosphate.

- Certain histological features are inconsistent with the diagnosis of conventional GCT. These include marked nuclear atypia and atypical mitoses in the stromal and multinocleated giant cells, as well as the presence of neoplastic cartilage or malignant osteoid.
- Note that *in approximately 30% of cases, intravascular invasion is present.* This incidental finding does not appear to correlate with local aggressiveness or the development of pulmonary implants In a small number of patients, GCTs produce "benign", self-limited, non-invasive, pulmonary implants, which are successfully treated by surgical excision.
- Common secondary changes in GCT are hemorrhage and necrosis, fibrohistiocytic (xanthomatous) change, and aneurysmal bone cyst formation. Complications include pathologic fractures and malignant transformation (dedifferentiation).
- Clinical behavior. Conventional GCT is a locally aggressive neoplasm, which may produce bone destruction and soft tissue invasion. Local recurrences are common (25-30%) and may involve bone and/or soft tissue. *The risk of local recurrence is related to radiologic stage rather than particular histologic characteristics.* Secondary malignant transformation, a rare complication seen mostly in patients with prior irradiation, may be in the form of MFH, osteosarcoma or fibrosarcoma. *Primary de-novo malignant GCT is extremely rare* and is characterized by marked nuclear atypia of stromal cells and atypical mitoses.

Characteristic Radiological Findings

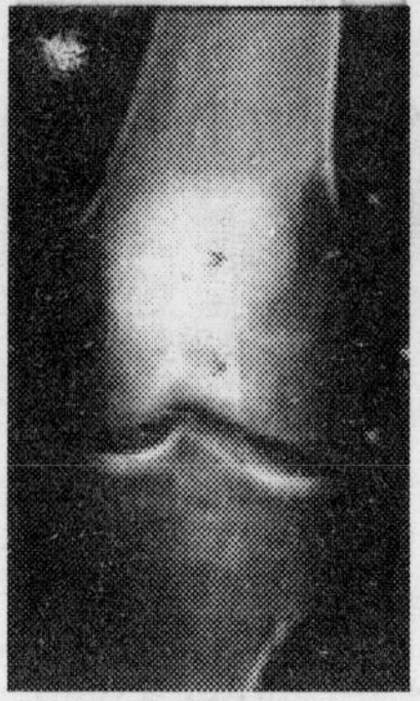

- Plain radiograph demonstrated a well defined, lytic lesion eccentrically located in the distal femoral epiphysis with subchondral and metaphyseal extension. There was associated focal thinning of the cortex.

This is a very common radiological presentation of this tumor. Note the features of a slowly growing/locally aggressive lesion: a geographic pattern of bone destruction with focal cortical erosion, and lack of a sclerotic rim. Eccentric location in the epiphysis (with or without subchondral and metaphyseal extension) is another important diagnostic clue.

Pathological Findings

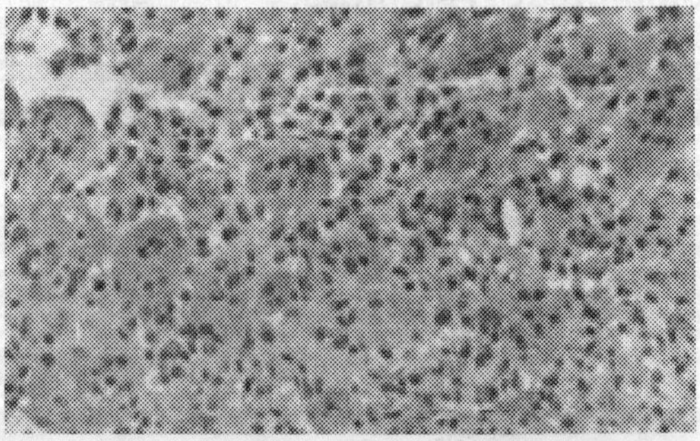

- Curettage specimen consisted of fragments of soft, hemorrhagic, tan-brown tissue with some firm areas and yellowish speckles. Microscopic examination showed a cellular lesion composed of numerous multinucleated giant cells in a background of small, ovoid, mononuclear stromal cells.

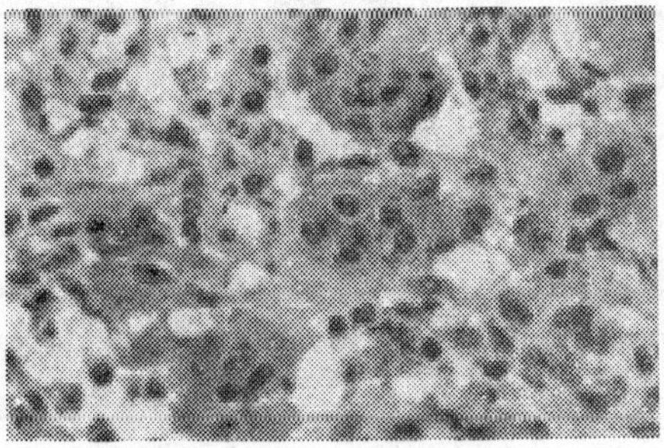

- *Stromal cells had poorly defined cytoplasmic borders and bland nuclei resembling those of giant cells.* Mitoses were easily found averaging 4 per 10 hpf. However, no atypical mitoses were identified. Multinucleated giant cells resembled osteoclasts by their centrally placed bland nuclei.

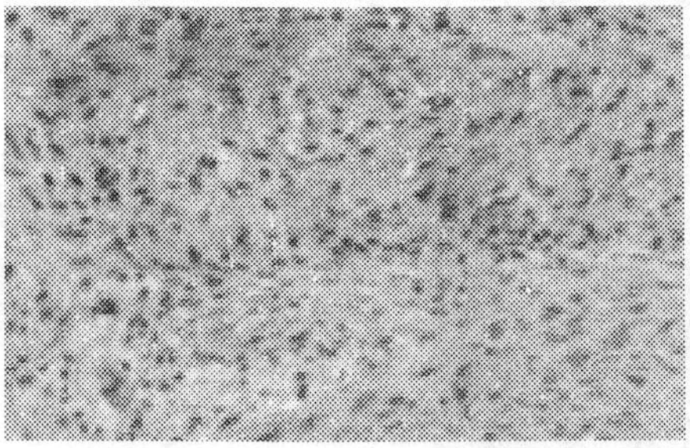

- Some areas showed prominent fibrohistiocytic changes with storiform arrangement of stromal cells and clusters of foamy histiocytes (xanthoma cells).

Salient Points

- Fibrous dysplasia is *a common benign fibro-osseous lesion*, which occurs sporadically during the period of skeletal growth (ages 10 to 25). It is a hamartoma and is characterized by the intramedullary location. There are two forms of the disease: monostotic (80% of cases) and polyostotic. Polyostotic involvement may be a part of McCune-Albright syndrome (fibrous dysplasia, patchy cutaneous pigmentation, and precocious puberty), or Mazabraud's syndrome (fibrous dysplastic lesions in close proximity to soft tissue myxomas).
- Most common locations include the long bones (femur, tibia and humerus), the ribs, craniofacial bones and pelvis. In the long bones, the lesion is found in the metaphysis or diaphysis.
- *The hallmark of fibrous dysplasia is inability of tissue at the affected site to produce mature lamellar bone.* The maturation is arrested at the level of woven bone. The difference between the two types of bone is best appreciated by using polarizing light.

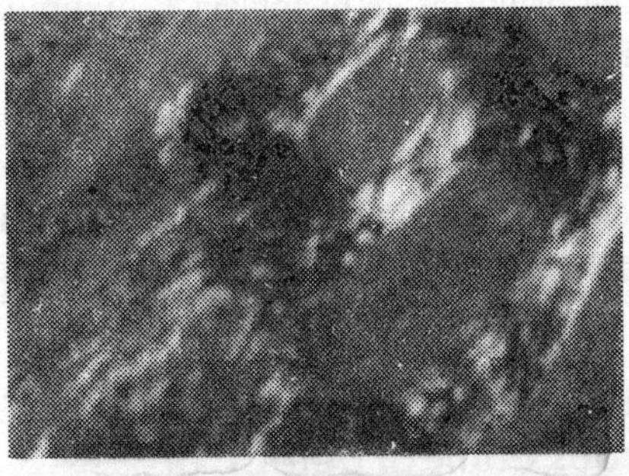

- *Woven bone (immature bone)* is characterized by random arrangement of the collagen fibers. *In adults, this type of bone is only seen in pathologic conditions such as fracture repair or bone-forming tumors.* Keep in mind that in benign conditions the bone trabeculae are surrounded by a fibrovascular stroma. In malignant tumors, those spaces are often occupied by malignant cells.

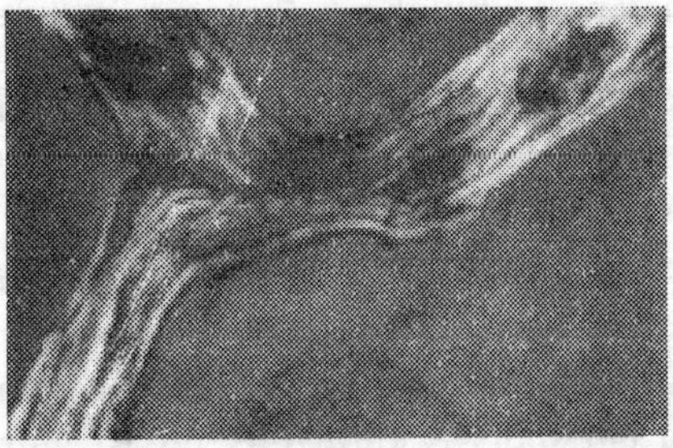

In *lamellar (mature) bone*, the collagen fibers are orderly arranged forming layers, known as *lameliae.*

- *Clinical behavior:* Pathologic fractures and bone deformities are common complications. Occasionally, lesions may show rapid enlargement due to secondary cystic changes including aneurysmal cyst formation. Malignant transformation is a rare complication (less than 1%), more common with polyostotic disease. Secondary malignancies are high-grade sarcomas (MFH, osteosarcoma, chondrosarcoma).
- *Differential diagnosis:* Two important differential diagnoses include well-differentiated intramedullary osteosarcoma and, in the tibia, osteofibrous dysplasia. Low-grade osteosarcoma is characterized by infiltrative growth pattern and mild cellular atypia. Bone spicules are often rimmed by mildly atypical osteoblasts. Osteofibrous dysplasia can be ruled out based on the intracortical location and orderly osteoblastic rimming of bone spicules.

Non-Ossifying Fibroma (NOF) (Fibrous cortical defect, or metaphyseal cortical defect)

Salient Points

- NOF is *a common, non-neoplastic, self-healing lesion occuring in skeletally immature individuals*, usually between the ages of 5 and 20 years. Small lesions are usually incidental radiological findings. The larger lesions occupying more than a half of the bone diameter may present with a pathologic fracture.
- *Location:* In most cases, NOF presents as a solitary lesion in the *metaphysis or meta-diaphysis of the long bone* at the knee (distal femur, proximal tibia or fibula), distal tibia and proximal humerus. A syndrome of multiple non-ossifying fibromas and cutaneous cafe au lait spots is known as Jaffe-Campanacci syndrome.
- For lesions that have the histologic features of NOF but occur in unusual locations such as pelvis, ribs or vertebrae, some authors use the term "benign fibrous histiocytoma". However, the designation remains controversial and is not generally accepted.
- GCT may enter your differential diagnosis. Remember, however, that it is characterized by the epiphyseal location and occurrence in adults.

Typical Clinical Presentation

An incidental finding of a bone lesion in the distal tibial meta-diaphysis of an 13-year-old male. The lesion was totally asymptomatic.

- As always, pay attention to the patient's age. The fact that the lesion did not produce symptoms and was found incidentally suggests benignancy.

Characteristic Radiological Findings

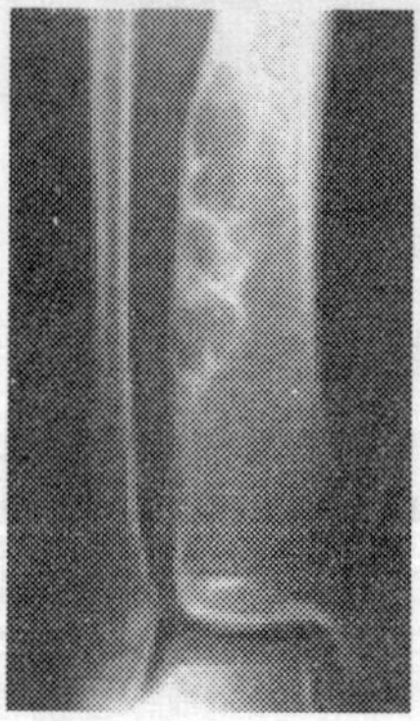

- Plain radiograph shows a sharply demarcated, lucent, loculated, *meta-diaphyseal lesion* surrounded by a rim of sclerotic bone. The lesion predominantly involves the lateral portion of the bone and produces mild cortical expansion.

Solitary Bone Cyst (SBC)

Salient Points

- Solitary bone cyst is relatively common, non-neoplastic lesion, which typically occurs in the skeletally immature patients, in the first and second decades of life (80% of cases). It is usually a unicameral cyst, which does not have an epithelial lining (hence not a true cyst) and is filled with serous fluid.
- *Location:* About 80% of cases are diagnosed in two locations: humerus and proximal femur.

In the long bone, SBC characteristically involves the metaphysis and diaphysis. Other possible skeletal sites are the ilium, talus, and calcaneus.

- *Differential diagnosis: You should be aware of the cystic nature of the lesion (ask the surgeon!*-to his eye, the lesion is a cavity filled with clear fluid) This will help you to avoid misdiagnosis of SBC as a solid lesion.
- *Clinical behavior:* SBC is a benign, slowly growing lesion with recurrence rate of approximately 15%. Pathologic fracture is a common complication. Rare cases of secondary malignancy (chondrosarcoma) have been reported

Typical Clinical Presentation

A 12-year-old boy presented with a short history of pain in his thigh.

Characteristic Radiological Findings

- Plain radiograph demonstrates a well-defined, symmetric, expansile, intramedullary lytic lesion of the proximal femur.

Above findings are common with benign, slowly growing lesions. In this case, the location and symmetric, expansile growth pattern are very important diagnostic clues. Note that there is no cortical disruption.

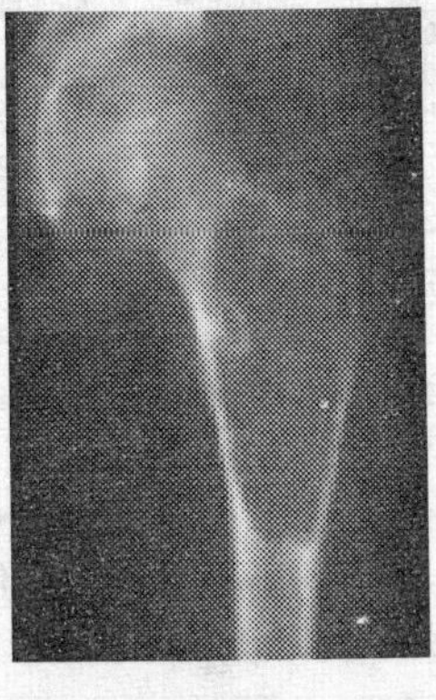

Aneurysmal Bone Cyst (ABC)

Salient Points

- Aneurysmal Bone Cyst (ABC) is a rapidly growing, locally aggressive, intramedullary, vascular lesion, which characteristically produces blowout expansion of the affected portion of the bone. ABC can be primary (de novo) or secondary. *Secondary ABC may develop in a pre-existing benign lesion such as chondroblastoma, chondromyxoid fibroma, giant cell tumor, and fibrous dysplasia, or be superimposed on a malignant tumor (osteosarcoma).*
- Although ABC can occur at any age, the majority of patients are younger than 25 years.
- ABCs are unique among bone tumors in their almost uniform skeletal distribution and ability to spread to the adjacent bones and across the joint spaces. Remember that it is a common lesion in the spine. In a long bone, ABC is usually centered in the metaphysis.
- *Differential diagnosis In diagnosis of ABC, correlation with clinical and radiological data is essential. Remember that secondary ABCs are common.* Therefore, you should examine the entire curettage specimen to search for evidence of a pre-existing lesion. The nature of that lesion, not the secondary cystic change, determines the clinical behavior. Underlying giant-cell tumor is suggested by the epiphyseal location in the knee area of a skeletally mature individual. The epiphyseal ABC in a teenager or a tarsal bone ABC suggests a chondroblastoma as an underlying lesion. Teleangiectatic variant of osteosarcoma may be extremely difficult to differentiate from an ABC, especially if the latter has "aggressive" radiological features. However, keep in mind that teleangiectatic osteosarcoma is a high-grade malignancy, and should have foci of

sarcomatous stroma with markedly atypical cells, numerous mitoses and atypical mitoses. The presence of "malignant osteoid" is another feature distinguishing osteosarcoma from a benign lesion.

Typical Clinical Presentation

A 17-year-old male presented with a slowly enlarging, painful lesion of the right clavicle.

Characteristic Radiological Findings

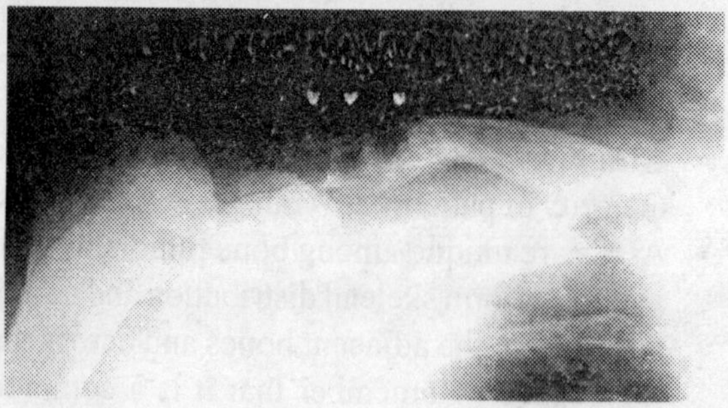

- Plain radiograph reveals a circumscribed, loculated, radiolucent lesion producing *blowout expansion* of the bone.

Salient Points

- Osteosarcoma is the most common primary sarcoma of bone. The peak incidence is in the second decade of life during the period of the most active skeletal growth. Fewer than 5% of osteosarcomas occur in children younger than 10 years (Dorfman HD, Czerniak B. Bone Tumors. 1998). In elderly, osteosarcoma is usually seen in association with a pre-existing bone disease, such as Paget's, radiation osteitis, or bone infarct. *By the time of presentation, all osteosarcomas are larger than 2 cm.*
- *Location:* In adolescents and young adults, osteosarcoma preferentially affects the most rapidly growing parts of the skeleton: the distal femur and proximal tibia (50% of cases), and the proximal humerus. Within the long bone, the metaphysis is the most common site. In elderly, osteosarcoma tends to involve the axial skeleton and the flat bones.
- *Subtypes of osteosarcoma:* Based on the location within the bone, osteosarcomas are subdivided into intarmedullary, intracortical and surface osteosarcomas. Intramedullary, or central, tumors comprise the largest group and include conventional high-grade osteosarcoma, which accounts for about 90% of all osteosarcomas, and less common types such as well-differentiated (or low-grade) osteosarcoma, chondroblastic, small cell, and teleangiectatic osteosarcoma. Based on the degree of differentiation, osteosarcomas are subclassified into high-grade and low-grade.

Pathologic diagnosis: Osteosarcoma is defined as a malignant tumor composed of neoplastic mesenchymal cells synthesizing osteoid or immature bone. However, the histologic findings can be extremely variable. For example, the tumor may appear identical to the MFH showing minimal osteoid production, or it may contain masses of malignant cartilage, or numerous giant cells. Remember that *the presence of malignant osteoid distinguishes an osteosarcoma from other sarcomas.* Mineralization distinguishes osteoid from collagen deposits.

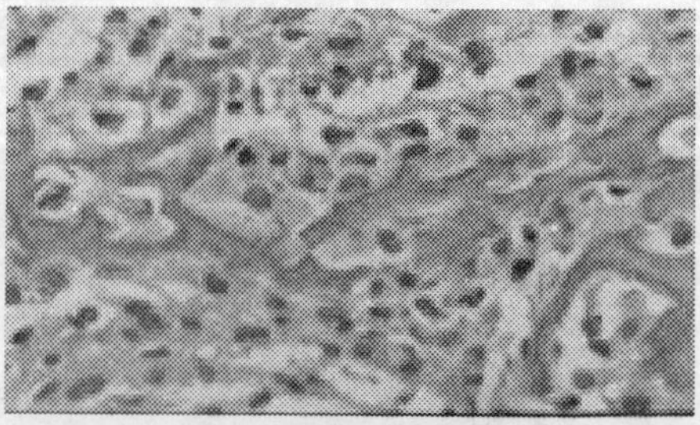

- *Malignant osteoid* is deposited either in a lace-like pattern or in the form of haphazardly arranged trabeculae of woven bone. Characteristically, the neoplastic cells fill the spaces between the osteoid deposits and often become entrapped in osteoid. This is very different from the reactive bone pattern, where the bone trabeculae are separated by a fibrovascular stroma.

- In cases of osteosarcoma, special techniques have been of little diagnostic help and used mainly to exclude other types of sarcoma.

- *Differential diagnosis*: In general, low-grade osteosarcoma should be differentiated from benign bone-producing tumors (osteoblastoma), whereas a high-grade osteosarcoma must be differentiated from other sarcomas. When you choose between benign and malignant, look for the permeative growth pattern, cellular atypia, and mitotic activity. Also, examine the spaces between the bone trabeculae. In benign tumors they are occupied by a fibrovascular stroma. In osteosarcoma, they are filled with the aggregates of malignant mesenchymal cells. The pattern of osteoid deposition is orderly in benign tumors and haphazard or lace-like in osteosarcoma. When you choose between an osteosarcoma and other types of sarcoma, look for malignant osteoid produced directly by mesenchymal cells.

- *Clinical behavior:* Conventional osteosarcoma is one of the most aggressive and highly lethal tumors. *Prognosis depends on the skeletal site of involvement, surgical stage and tumor response to pre-operative chemotherapy*. The most powerful predictor of outcome is the histologic response of the tumor to pre-operative chemotherapy. Tumor necrosis can be graded according to the following system Grade 1-0% to 50% necrosis; Grade 2-51% to 90%, Grade 3-91% to 99%, and Grade 4-100% necrosis. Data from MD Anderson Cancer Center shows that 90% and more of tumor necrosis is associated with nearly 90% 5-year disease-free survival, comparing to only 14% 5-year disease-free survival in patients with less than 90% of tumor necrosis. Metastases, usually to the lungs, bones, and liver, are extremely common. Surgical resection of solitary metastases may improve the patient's survival (similar as for Ewing's sarcoma).

Recent Advances: Abnormalities of the cell cycle regulating genes/proteins have been reported in different types of cancer. Inactivation of RB, p53, INK4A (encodes tumor supressor p16), and increased expression of CDK4 (cyclin-dependent kinase) and MDM2 have been reported in osteosarcoma.

Recent studies have shown frequent *over-expression of Her2/neu* by osteosarcoma and its correlation with a significantly worse histologic response to pre-operative chemotherapy and shorter event-free survival. Further studies are being conducted.

Recent studies have revealed the presence of SV40 (simian virus 40) genome in human malignancies (mesothelioma, osteosarcoma). It appears that SV40 integrates in human osteosarcoma DNA. Its role in the pathogenesis of osteosarcoma remains unclear.

Fifteen

Hepatocellular Carcinoma

Hepatocellular carcinomas (HCC) are also known as primary liver cancers, hepatic tumors, or hepatomas—the four terms are interchangeable.

HCC is a type of cancer that arises from hepatocytes, or specialized epithelial cells in the liver. This makes HCC different from other hepatic cancers in that HCC arises in the liver -it does not spread, or metastasize, to the liver from another part of the body.

Causes of HCC

Approximately 30 percent of HCC patients treated at UPMC Health System show no evidence of a disease that causes HCC. In other cases, however, HCC often arises after several years of cirrhosis or chronic infection with hepatitis B or C. Other diseases commonly associated with HCC include hemachromatosis and alpha-1-antitrypsin deficiency. Primary biliary cirrhosis; Budd-Chiari syndrome; and metabolic disorders, including porphyria cutanea tarda, citrullinemia, glycogen storage disease, and tyrosinemia, are occasionally associated with HCC.

In some areas of the world, HCC has a strong association with chronic exposure to toxins made by Aspergillus fungi—fungi found in grains and food products, such as peanuts.

In terms of lifestyle choices, heavy and long-term use of alcohol (ethanol) is commonly linked to development of HCC. Radiation therapy and use of cigarettes, oral contraceptives (birth control pills), or anabolic steroids are also associated with HCC.

Detection of HCC

Symptoms

Many people with HCC have no symptoms until the disease becomes advanced. Among the common symptoms of advanced HCC are:

- Abdominal (hepatic) pain (the most common symptom)
- Abdominal swelling or mass (a common symptom in children)
- Weight loss
- Decreased energy
- Fevers of unclear origin
- Feeling of fullness
- Upset or gas-filled stomach
- Reduced appetite or aversion to food
- Shoulder pain (referred pain from the liver)
- General tiredness
- An out-of-sorts mood (malaise)
- Bone pain.

Physical signs that a doctor may detect include:

- Enlargement of the liver (hepatomegaly)
- Harsh or musical sound in the abdomen
- Enlargement of the spleen (splenomegaly)

- Accumulation of fluid in the abdominal cavity (ascites).

Abnormal Test Results

At least 20 percent of HCC patients at UPMC Health System are diagnosed because of abnormal test results discovered as a result of blood tests required for routine physical or health insurance exams. Tests of people with HCC usually show what doctors call elevated liver function.

Other patients—particularly those with a known predisposing disease, such as chronic hepatitis or cirrhosis—are diagnosed because their liver function test results suddenly worsen or because they show abnormal blood test results for alpha-fetoprotein (AFP). (Patients who are known to have chronic hepatitis or cirrhosis usually have an AFP test and an ultrasonogram once or twice a year, as a way of detecting HCC in the early stages.)

Clinicians suspect HCC when they see an opaque mass on an image created by ultrasound or computed tomography. A follow-up biopsy disproves or provides proof of the existence of HCC.

Evaluation of Diagnosed HCC and Surrounding Tissues

In evaluating HCC, computed tomography (CT) scans are important tools. Additional evaluations—such as blood tests and biopsies—help physicians understand the general health status of a patient, the patient's liver function, and his or her quality of life. If a patient will be treated by chemotherapy, evaluation often includes an audiogram, or hearing test, and a MUGA heart scan.

CT Scans

After HCC is diagnosed, CT scans help determine:

- The size and location of HCC in the liver
- Whether the cancer has spread beyond the liver to form satellite tumors
- The proximity of the tumor to major hepatic blood vessels and if the tumor has invaded the portal vein, the main vein that leads to the liver
- If there are blood clots (thromboses) in any of the major branches of the portal and hepatic veins
- If the lymph nodes are enlarged

A high-speed helical (spiral) triphasic CT scan of the liver allows specialists to evaluate the extent and location of the tumor. A CT scan of the chest and pelvis allow them to determine if the cancer has spread. A bone scan may be performed to exclude or confirm the presence of cancer in bone.

In evaluating CT scans of the tumor, physicians also look for evidence of cirrhosis and its complications, such as ascites, portal hypertension, and splenomegaly (an enlarged spleen).

Blood Tests

Blood tests also help doctors determine the general health status of a patient, including whether he or she has been exposed in the past to hepatitis B or C and if the hepatitis is currently active. In addition, blood test results are a measure of how well the patient's liver works.

A platelet count is a test that a doctor may order to detect cancer in its early stages. A white cell count that is below the normal range can be a sign of splenomegaly and/or portal hypertension.

Blood tests known as blood chemistries evaluate:

- Albumin level
- Prothrombin time
- Transaminase level (SGOT, SGPT, GGTP)
- Blood creatinine level

Blood tests for specific tumor "markers" include tests that detect the presence of:

- Alpha-fetoprotein (AFP)
- Desgamma carboxy prothrombin (P, or PIVKA-2)
- Neurotensin

DCP and neurotensin are markers (in the presence of a normal AFP) for the fibrolamellar variant of HCC, which often occurs in children.

Biopsies

In addition to a biopsy of the tumor, radiologists perform a biopsy on a specimen taken from the non-tumorous part of the liver. The liver biopsy helps determine the presence or degree of cirrhosis. A core-needle biopsy, rather than a fine-needle aspiration biopsy, is usually necessary to evaluate the make-up of the tumor.

If the CT scan suggests thrombosis (clotting), then a needle-aspiration biopsy of the portal vein may be necessary. This type of biopsy helps doctors determine if the tumor is actually invading the portal vein. Invasion of the portal vein by a tumor has profound consequences for the long-term outcome of liver transplantation for HCC.

Treatment Options

- Chemotherapy
- Resection
- Bile duct reconstruction
- Transplantation

These treatments are often used in combination. If a tumor is large, patients will receive chemotherapy to shrink the tumor before undergoing resection or transplantation. Also, chemotherapy can sensitize a tumor, making it more responsive to destruction by therapeutic radiation.

Liver tumors generally show little response to chemotherapeutic drugs that are given through the veins (intravenously). These drugs do tend to be effective, however, when they are delivered to the tumor directly, through the hepatic artery. (Hepatocellular carcinomas, or HCC, receive most of their oxygenated blood from the hepatic artery; the normal liver receives more than 80 percent of its oxygenated blood from the hepatic vein.) When chemotherapeutic drugs are delivered through an artery, the delivery is called intra-arterial.

Intra-arterial therapy allows specialists to give chemotherapy selectively to administer it at high concentrations to the tumor while sparing the non-cancerous liver.

Chemotherapeutic Options

Embolization

If a patient's liver is normal, specialists usually treat a vascular tumor, such as an HCC, with chemotherapy and embolization. An embolization agent, such as Gelfoam, slows down the blood supply to the tumor, cutting off its oxygen and nutrient supply. Use of an embolization agent also allows the chemotherapy to be concentrated in the tumor.

Specific Drug Regimens

For patients with less healthy livers, radiologists often administer the chemotherapeutic drugs cisplatin and adriamycin, alone or in combination. Patients with bile duct or gallbladder tumors commonly receive gencitabine or cisplatin and gencitabine. The appropriate chemotherapeutic regimen for each patient is determined by the oncologist's clinical experience.

Side Effects of Chemotherapy

Chemotherapeutic agents are strong drugs that have side effects. The most common side effects of chemotherapy include:

- Abdominal pain
- Fever from embolization
- Thrombocytopenia (a decrease in the number of platelets, fragments of red blood cells that aid in blood clotting)
- Hypomagnesemia (low magnesium levels)
- Neutropenia (a decrease in neutrophils, a specific type of white blood cell).

Liver resection is surgical removal of a section of the liver. Of all the treatment options for hepatocellular carcinoma (HCC), resection has the best long-term outcome. Resection is also the preferred treatment option for cancers of the biliary tree, or cholangiocarcinomas, that involve underlying liver tissue. To be selected for resection, removal of the tumor from the liver must be technically feasible and the amount of liver that would remain after the surgery must be sufficient to support life. Resection is usually possible for patients who do not have underlying cirrhosis or who have mild cirrhosis.

Types of Liver Resection

The removal of a section of a patient's diseased liver is called a partial hepatectomy or, if an entire lobe is removed, a lobectomy. The liver segments are filled with many sinuses and a complex network of blood vessels. Because of the anatomic complexity of the liver and the need for meticulous operative technique, hepatectomy or lobectomy is best performed by a transplantation surgeon.

Potential Complications of Liver Resection

The potential complications of liver resection include:

- *Blood loss or hemorrhage:* Improved techniques and surgical experience make this complication rare at the Thomas E. Starzl Transplantation Institute.
- *Jaundice:* Jaundice, a yellowish coloring to the skin, can result from surgical problems with the ducts leading from the liver or from reduced liver function in remaining liver tissue.
- *Sepsis:* This condition, toxicity caused by systemic infection, has been reported in 10 to 15 percent of patients nationwide after surgery. The occurrence of sepsis at the Thomas E. Starzl Transplantation Institute ranks well below the national average.
- *Wound infection:* This complication can be minimized by careful surgical techniques and strict environmental control in the operating room.
- *Leakage of bile from the cut surface of the resected liver:* To address this problem, fluid is drained from the abdomen.

After resection, patients may have two to four temporary drains in the abdomen. The drains are attached to bulblike collecting units that can be emptied. The drains are called J.P., or Jackson-Pratt, drains.

Some patients may also have another drainage tube, called a T-tube, coming from their bile duct. At first the T-tube drains bile into an attached bag. The color and consistency of the bile collected in the bag allows the surgical team to monitor liver function; the tube also allows technicians to take x-rays of the bile ducts.

Some patients may have the T-tube removed before leaving the hospital. For others, the tied off T-tube remains in place for a longer period. Before the tube is removed, a T-tube cholangiogram–a radiographic image of the bile ducts—is usually made to check the bile ducts.

After the T-tube is removed, patients may have a small amount of drainage at the tube site for a day or two; this is normal. Patients who experience abdominal pain, fever, nausea or vomiting, or upper back pain on the right side should call their coordinators immediately.

If drainage develops around a T-tube site, a patient or his or her caretaker may clean the site with hydrogen peroxide. Patients are cautioned not to use peroxide if the skin around the T-tube becomes red and irritated. T-tube dressings should be changed every day.

Bile duct reconstruction surgery may be needed as the result of a malignancy in the duct or surrounding tissue or as a result of injury to the duct.

Reconstruction as a Result of Malignancy

In bile duct reconstruction surgery, the anesthetized patient is placed on his or her back with both arms drawn away from the body. The surgeon makes an incision across the upper abdomen, below the ribcage. If necessary, the incision may be extended up to the right chest.

The approach depends upon the location of the tumor—whether it is inside or outside the liver—as well as the size and extent of metastasis, or tumor spread (if any).

Reconstruction can be quite complicated: Surgeons carefully tie off and remove tumorous ducts and involved underlying tissue. Removal of a section or lobe of the liver is often required.

Depending on the extent of duct removal, surgeons may reconstruct ducts and reconnect them directly to the intestine in a procedure known as Roux-en-Y.

Owing to the complexity of the procedure, bile duct reconstruction surgery generally takes from eight to 10 hours. The surgery may be supplemented by chemotherapy and radiation treatments.

Liver Transplant

Transplantation may be considered for treatment of primary liver tumors, also called hepatocellular carcinomas, and for hepatoblastoma limited to the liver.

Reasons for Liver Transplantation in Adults and Children

Liver failure occurs when the liver can no longer perform its many functions. Many diseases and conditions can cause liver failure.

The most common diseases that cause liver failure and require liver transplantation are chronic viral hepatitis, primary biliary cirrhosis, and primary sclerosing cholangitis. Other common reasons for liver transplantation are chronic liver diseases, fulminant (acute) hepatic failure, liver tumors, and metabolic disorders.

Chronic Liver Disease

Chronic liver diseases cause liver failure by damaging the liver over a period of time. This type of liver failure is usually irreversible. Chronic liver diseases often cause cirrhosis, which develops when normal liver cells are damaged and die and then are replaced by scar tissue. Because there are less healthy liver cells, the liver cannot work properly. Types of chronic liver diseases include:

- *Cholestatic liver diseases:* Cholestatic liver diseases usually involve problems with the excretion of bile from the liver.
  - o primary biliary cirrhosis
  - o primary sclerosing cholangitis
  - o secondary biliary cirrhosis
  - o carolis disease
  - o Alagille's syndrome
- *Hepatocellular liver diseases:* Hepatocellular liver diseases involve damage to liver cells (also called hepatocytes or parenchymal cells).
  - o chronic viral hepatitis (hepatitis B, C, D)
  - o autoimmune hepatitis
  - o alcoholic liver disease
  - o cryptogenic cirrhosis
  - o drug-induced liver disease
  - o congenital hepatic fibrosis
- *Vascular diseases:* Vascular diseases of the liver involve the veins and restricted blood flow, which may keep the liver from working properly. Restricted blood flow can result in:
  - o portal hypertension (high blood pressure)
  - o Budd-Chiari syndrome
  - o veno-occlusive disease

Fulminant (Acute) Hepatic Failure

This type of liver failure occurs suddenly and is severe. Liver failure progresses rapidly, and without transplantation the death rate is high. Fulminant hepatic failure may be caused by:

- Viruses
- Wilson's disease
- Exposure to drugs or environmental toxins

Liver tumors

Transplantation may be considered for treatment of primary liver tumors, also called hepatocellular carcinomas, and for hepatoblastoma limited to the liver.

Metabolic Disorders

Liver transplantation can usually cure metabolic or genetic diseases that cause liver failure. Such diseases include:

- Alpha-1-antitrypsin deficiency
- Wilson's disease
- Hemochromatosis
- Tyrosinemia
- Glycogen storage disease

Cancers of the Biliary Tree

Gallbladder Cancer

Half of all liver and biliary passage tumors are tumors of the gallbladder. Tumors that begin in the gallbladder often spread into the liver.

Detection

Many people who have gallbladder cancers have nonspecific symptoms. Some have symptoms that are similar to those of advanced primary liver cancer. Other symptoms sometimes associated with gallbladder tumors include abdominal cramping, intolerance of fatty foods, and pain in the right upper abdomen. New-onset jaundice often appears as a result of a gallbladder tumor. Jaundice is a yellowish coloring of the skin that results from excess bile.

Oftentimes, gallbladder cancers are discovered only as a consequence of surgery for removal of gallstones or removal of a dysfunctional gallbladder. Surgeons may see the cancer during gallbladder surgery or the cancer may be detected by a pathologist's review of the removed tissue after surgery.

Evaluation

Evaluations of gallbladder cancer may involve blood tests that measure liver function as well as tests to evaluate the extent and location of the tumor. These may include computed tomography (CT) scans of the liver, chest, and pelvis to exclude or confirm the presence of tumors that have spread from another area. A bone scan is also performed to exclude or confirm the presence of cancer in the bone. Based on these tests, physicians note the size of the tumor, its location within the liver, its proximity to major hepatic blood vessels of the liver, and whether there are metastatic tumors or nodules.

For patients who will be treated by chemotherapy, an audiogram (hearing test) and a MUGA heart scan may be required.

Duct Tumors

One third of all liver and biliary passage tumors are tumors of the intrahepatic and extrahepatic ducts. Tumors can originate in large collecting ducts, such as the bile ducts and hepatic ducts, or smaller ducts throughout the liver.

Associated Conditions

Diseases associated with bile duct tumors include liver fluke infections, gallstones (which may cause persistent irritation of the ducts), ulcerative colitis, and primary sclerosing cholangitis. Less commonly associated diseases include cystic liver disease and Carolis disease.

Detection

People with a malignant tumor in a hepatic duct often have symptoms that are similar to those of advanced primary liver cancer. Because blockage of the ducts is common, a characteristic symptom of hepatic duct cancer is new-onset jaundice. Jaundice is a yellowish coloring of the skin that results from excess bile.

Blood tests may not by themselves may not detect liver duct cancer. Additional tests may be necessary.

Duct tumors may be detected during evaluations prompted by complaints of gastrointestinal pain or discomfort. A computed tomography (CT) scan may discover a dilated bile duct. During an endoscopic examination of the gastrointestinal tract, a gastroenterologist may detect a tumor or note a narrowing of a duct—such a narrowing could indicate the presence of a tumor. Such an examination is called endoscopic retrograde cholangiopancreatography (ERCP).

Evaluation

If an ERCP yields evidence of a tumor, the gastroenterologist may use a brush to take a tissue sample during the ERCP. The sample will undergo a biopsy.

Blood tests may not by themselves detect liver duct cancer. Additional tests may be necessary.

Additional evaluations include cholangiography, enhanced CT scans, an angiogram (to determine blood vessel involvement and blood flow to the tumor), and an MRI cholangiogram. These tests provide information about the extent and location of the tumor, its proximity to major hepatic blood vessels, whether the tumor is spreading, and the quality of liver function. Knowing the location of the tumor is important because tumor location helps determine the course of treatment.

Blood tests to measure bilirubin levels may be needed to determine whether a tumor is blocking the duct.

If tests indicate increased bilirubin and duct obstruction, specialists may place a stent, or tube, in the duct to relieve the blockage. As a result of this procedure, bilirubin levels should return to normal.

Patients who will be treated by chemotherapy, an audiogram (hearing test) and a MUGA heart scan may be required.

Oesophageal Carcinoma

Oesophageal carcinoma is becoming more common, unlike the trend observed in gastric carcinoma. It is most strongly linked to alcohol, especially spirits, and smoking.

Physical signs are rare apart from wasting and perhaps a palpable supraclavicular node. The principal symptom is dysphagia.

Patients are often able to locate the level of the obstruction in their oesophagus quite accurately. For example, a carcinoma of the oesophagus in its lower third will be a described as a feeling of a blockage behind the lower part of the sternum.

Tumours tend to arise in areas of partial narrowing, i.e. at the pharyngo-oesophageal junction (40%); the junction of the upper and middle third (40%); and where the oesophagus passes through the diaphragm (20%).

Aetiology

The principle aetiological factor appears to be chronic local tissue irritation.

Possible risk factors for oesophageal cancer include:

- Alcohol
- Smoking
- Achalasia
- Caustic stricture of the oesophagus
- Geographical location e.g. China and Northern Iran
- Barrett's oesophagus
- Plummer-Vinson syndrome

- Coeliac disease
- Tylosis—hyperkeratosis of the palms and soles.

Squamous carcinomas form the majority of cancers in the proximal and middle third of the oesophagus.

Adenocarcinomas are more likely to occur in the lower third of the oesophagus and are associated with chronic gastro-oesophageal reflux and the change to columnar epithelium associated with this.

Pathology

An oesophageal carcinoma commences as a nodule which then develops into either a papilliferous mass (60%), an ulcer (25%), or an annular constriction, usually of the cardia.

Historically, the large majority of oesophageal carcinomata were squamous. Today the incidence of adenocarcinoma is rising rapidly and now accounts for 50% of all oesophageal carcinomata in the USA.

Squamous carcinoma typically arises in the upper two thirds of the oesophagus. Adenocarcinoma usually arises in a region of specialised columnar epithelium (SCE) metaplasia in the lower third of the oesophagus—Barrett's oesophagus.

DISTRIBUTION FREQUENCY % CELL TYPE

Cervical 10 squamous upper third 20 squamous middle third 20 squamous lower third 50 90% adenocarcinoma

Staging

The staging of oesophageal carcinoma is important in order to try to prevent unnecessary surgical intervention.

There are several complimentary means of determining the stage:

- Chest radiography
- Barium swallow
- Ultrasound examination
- CT and MRI scanning
- Bronchoscopy

Given the data from these techniques, the tumour can be sited on the following standard scale:

- *Stage I:* limited to oesophagus and less than 5 cm in length
- *Stage II:* limited to oesophagus, greater than 5 cm in length and with resectable nodes
- *Stage III:* lesion greater than 10 cm in length, extension through oesophagus into adjacent structures, inoperable nodes or inoperable lesion.
- *Stage IV:* lesion as in stage III with evidence of perforation, fistula or distant metastasis.

Clinical Features

Dysphagia is the most frequently presented feature of oesophageal carcinoma:

- The patient may recount a short history of progressive dysphagia, initially affecting solids only, but gradually affecting the swallowing of fluids.
- The interruption of the passage of food may cause the individual to slowly alter the diet from solid to liquid nutrition; success with this approach may be at the expense of early medical self-referral.
- The level at which difficulty in swallowing is encountered may be identifiable by the patient.
- A short history of dysphagia in an elderly male is almost certainly carcinoma of the oesophagus or the cardia of the stomach.
- An infrequent presentation is of the obstruction of a large bolus of food with no prior history of dysphagia.

Other local features may include:

- Regurgitation of food or blood-stained vomit
- Aspiration pneumonia
- Pain:
  - classically, retrosternally and in the interscapular region
  - it may radiate to the jaws and arms.

General manifestations of malignant disease may include:

- Loss of weight, due to the metabolic effects of the tumour and a reduced intake of food
- Anorexia
- Anaemia
- Coughing, due to regurgitation or a fistula
- Oedema, due to a severe reduction in protein intake in the late stages.

Secondary deposits occur in:

- Lymph nodes
- In the liver causing jaundice.

Diagnosis

The diagnosis of oesophageal carcinoma is made on:

- History and examination
- Barium swallow:
  - the first-line investigation after the history of dysphagia
  - characteristic image of an irregular stricture with shouldered margins, 4-10 cm long and often tortuous
  - a tracheo-oesophageal fistula may also be demonstrated.
- Endoscopy and biopsy:
  - establishes histology and limits of lesion
  - can be used therapeutically to dilate, so improving nutrition before a definitive operative intervention.
- Cytology by washing/abrasion technique—used for screening in China.
- CT scanning helps to determine mediastinal involvement and whether metastasis has occurred to the liver.
- Bronchoscopy may be needed to exclude bronchial involvement in upper and middle-third lesions.
- Ultrasound may be used to identify secondary liver deposits.

Management

Management of oesophageal carcinoma is dependent on the level of the lesion and the stage of the disease.

Upper third lesion—high dose radiotherapy is indicated for lesions up to 5 cm long. Vital structures in the mediastinum closely related to the upper third make surgical clearance and resection very difficult.

Middle third lesion—early tumours are resectable. Again, radical radiotherapy may be indicated if the lesion is up to 5 cm long.

Lower third lesion—most accessible surgically; adenocarcinomas are radioresistant.

Extensive disease requires palliation of dysphagia:

- Endoscopic laser surgery for lesions less than 8 cm long.
- Oesophageal stenting—e.g. with a Celestin tube—if longer than 8 cm.
- Alternatives include:
  - oesophago-gastrostomy or oesophago-jejunostomy
  - short course radiotherapy.

Prognosis

The prognosis for oesophageal carcinoma is dependent on the site of the tumour. Approximate 5-year survival figures are:

- Upper third tumours have a 20% 5-year survival.
- Middle third tumours have a 6% 5-year survival.
- Lower third tumours have a 15% 5-year survival.

The prognosis also depends on:

- Tumour size and site
- Depth of invasion
- Node metastases
- Widespread metastases

- Tumour grade
- Lymphocytic response
- General health of the patient.

Small Intestine Tumours

Tumours of the small intestine are very rare. Although this region comprises 80% of the luminal surface area of the gut, fewer than 2% of all primary gastrointestinal malignancies arise here.

Classification is as follows:

- Benign
- Hamartomatous
- Intermediate
- Malignant.

Hamartomatous Lesions

Hamartomata of the small intestine include the following conditions:

- ectopic pancreas—usually seen along the anti-mesenteric border of the bowel or in a Meckel's diverticulum.
- Hereditary haemorrhagic telangiectasia:
  - Osler-Weber-Rendu disease
  - associated with Turner's syndrome.
- Neurofibromas and arteriovenous malformation—likely to cause symptoms such as obstruction, bleeding and intussception.
- Peutz-Jeghers syndrome:
  - polypoid lesions mainly reside in the jejunum, but can occur at any point in the gastrointestinal tract
  - intussusception of the polyps can give rise to small bowel obstruction.

Hereditary Haemorrhagic Telangiectasia

Hereditary haemorrhagic telangiectasia is a rare autosomal dominant condition where multiple small telangiectases occur on the skin and mucous membranes, most commonly on the lips and the tongue. Lesions are also often scattered over the pulps of fingers. The size and number of lesions increases with age.

Epistaxis is the most common complaint.

When telangiectases are present in the gastrointestinal tract they may cause chronic blood loss with iron deficiency anaemia. Occasionally there may be torrential bleeding.

Arteriovenous malformations may occur in the:

- Liver
- Lungs, causing:
  - clubbing
  - murmurs
  - paradoxical emboli.

Oestrogen may be used to reduce the severity and frequency of epistaxes (via induction of metaplasia of nasal mucosa).

Embolization may be used if there are pulmonary arteriovenous malformations.

Benign Tumours

Every type of cell type within the wall of the small intestine has the potential for neoplasia. The most common are:

- Adenoma, especially in the duodenum:
  - tubular: low premalignant potential
  - villous: strong potential for malignancy
  - Brunner's gland adenoma: no potential for malignancy.
- Lipoma
- Angioma
- Leiomyoma
- Fibromyoma.

They are seldom discovered during the patient's lifetime because they are generally asymptomatic. When symptomatic, problems include ulceration and haemorrhage. Treatment is by local resection.

Intermediate

There are four types of benign small bowel tumours that have a strong tendency for malignant change. Each shows a spectrum of activity from truly benign to frank cancer. They include:

- Villous adenoma:
  - closely associated with carcinoma
  - small bowel polyps may accompany up to half of all cases of Gardner's syndrome.
- Smooth muscle tumours:
  - may present with haemorrhage, obstructive symptoms or a palpable mass
  - treated by wide resection and occasionally respond to chemotherapy.
- Duodenal apudomas:
  - 10% of all gastrinomas arise at this site
  - treated by local excision or pancreatoduodenectomy.
- Carcinoid tumours:
  - the ileum is the second most frequent site of occurrence
  - approximately one third have metastasized by the time of diagnosis.

Malignant

The key three malignant neoplasms of the small intestine are:

- Adenocarcinoma
- Lymphoma
- Secondaries from other sites.

Adenocarcinoma of the Small Intestine

The adenocarcinoma is the commonest type of malignant tumour of the small intestine. They are clustered within 25 centimetres either side of the duodenojejunal flexure; ileal carcinoma is rare except for that which is secondary to Crohn's disease.

The peak frequency of carcinoma is within the seventh decade with an equal sex distribution. The clinical presentation is one of occult bleeding and partial obstruction, or, if more proximally in the duodenum, epigastric pain, vomiting and jaundice.

Investigative measures include endoscopy with biopsy and barium studies. Treatment is by surgical resection: more proximally, a pancreaticoduodenectomy may suffice; more distally, bowel and mesenteric resection is required.

Prognosis is poor—15-25% at 5 years—mainly due to the insidious progression of the tumour.

COLONIC DISEASES AND CONDITIONS

Angiodysplasia of the Colon

Colonic angiodysplasia is a common cause of acute or chronic rectal bleeding and iron deficiency anaemia.

Angiodysplasias are tiny—1-5 mm in diameter—hamartomatous capillary lesions in the colonic wall which produce bleeding out of proportion to their size. They are believed to be acquired, possibly as a result of tension on the veins where they pass through the muscularis.

Diagnosis:

- Subtraction mesenteric arteriography may demonstrate bleeding if rapid
- Colonscopy: may visualise lesion.

Treatment:

- Electrical coagulation via the colonoscope.
- Resection of segment of colon if the above is unsuccessful.

Colonic Polyps

Colonic polyps may be single or multiple. Familial polyposis coli is a condition that is inherited in autosomal dominant manner in which there is extensive polyposis of the large bowel.

Polyps are a common finding in the colon. All polyps have malignant potential although the majority are adenomas, i.e. benign neoplasms. A polyp may have undergone malignant change but still be at an early stage, and hence is potentially curable. All polyps should be assumed to be malignant until proved otherwise.

Types of Colonic Polyp

Colonic polyps may be:

- Neoplastic:
  - adenomas—single or associated with familial polyposis syndrome
- Hamartomatous:
  - juvenile—singly and as a juvenile polyposis syndrome
  - Peutz-Jegher's—singly and as part of Peutz-Jegher's syndrome.
- Hyperplastic
- Reactive:
  - inflammatory polyps—associated with inflammatory bowel disease and ulcerative colitis more than Crohn's disease
  - lymphoid.

Diagnosis and Management

The diagnosis and management of colonic polyps consist of:

- History and examination
- Sigmoidoscopy: about half of colonic polyps are within reach of the rigid 25cm instrument. Use of a fibreoptic sigmoidoscope allow the colon to be examined as far as the splenic flexure and any polyps can be removed at the same time with a diathermy snare.
- Barium enema: will show polyps of significant size. This is the investigation of choice for polyps of the transverse and ascending colon. Note that it may not be possible to see the whole colon well—this is particularly true of the transverse colon.
- Colonoscopy; indicated if:
  - barium enema technically unsatisfactory
  - barium enema demonstrates polyps.
- Histology; vital because:
  - reveals whether the whole polyp was removed
  - reveals whether the polyp was malignant.

Colonic Tumours

Colonic tumours may be:

- Benign:
  - adenomatous polyp
  - papilloma
  - lipoma
  - neurofibroma
  - haemangioma.
- Malignant:
  - primary:
    - § carcinoma
    - § lymphosarcoma
    - § carcinoid tumour.
- Secondary:
  - invasion from adjacent tumours, e.g. stomach, bladder, uterus and ovary.

Colon Carcinoma

The symptoms of cancer of the colon differ according to the part of the colon affected and the type of tumour, but pain is common to all types. Unexplained weakness and anaemia are characteristic of right colonic carcinoma whilst a change in bowel habit feature in left colonic carcinoma.

The majority of colon cancers are found in the sigmoid colon and at the rectosigmoid junction. These cancers are usually small, annular and ulcerated. The next common site is the caecum, where the tumours tend to be bulky and papilloform.

Types of Colon Carcinoma

The types of colonic carcinoma are divided into left-sided, right-sided and transverse types.

Colon Carcinoma (on left side of colon)

Left-sided colonic carcinoma is characterised by a change in bowel habit due to obstruction. Pain is felt in the left side of the abdomen because there is commonly involvement of the sigmoid colon and the rectosigmoid junction, and there is gross blood in the stool. The carcinoma tend to be small, annular and ulcerated. It appears as a fixed filling defect with an annular "apple core" configuration on barium enema. Usually, the patient is over 40 and commonly, over 70 years of age. Men are affected slightly more than women.

The patient with left-sided colonic carcinoma may be pale due to chronic blood loss and anaemia, and may show weight loss. The left supraclavicular lymph nodes may be enlarged.

The abdomen may be distended and the caecum palpable. The liver may be enlarged due to metastases.

Masses may be felt in the left iliac fossa which may be hard and indentable because of faeces above the tumour. They will be tender if there is surrounding inflammation, and will be dull to percussion, but the abdomen will feel normal on palpation if the mass is small and lying in the paravertebral gutter. A mass may be noted anteriorly on rectal examination if the tumour is down into the pelvis.

Hyperactive bowel sounds indicate chronic intestinal obstruction. During an attack of colic, loud high-pitched continuous gurgl.

Symptoms

The symptoms of left-sided colonic carcinoma include:

- Change in bowel habit due to obstruction.
- Cycle of alternating constipation and diarrhoea: constipation from the hold-up of faeces at the site of the tumour, which then liquefies and the patient develops spurious, offensive diarrhoea.
- Lower left abdominal pain: initially, a mild abdominal colic or ache, which after some weeks or months, becomes persistent with severe colicky exacerbations.
- A lump in the left iliac fossa or localized tenderness
- Painful micturition and change in frequency indicating involvement of the bladder.
- Darkly-coloured faeces streaked with blood, often containing mucus.

Less commonly:

- Loss of weight then anorexia
- Rectal bleeding and iron deficient anaemia
- Tenesmus.

Aetiology

The cause of colorectal carcinoma is unknown except for a small proportion of cases where there is malignant change in previous polyposis coli or ulcerative colitis. However, this disease is almost unknown in third world rural communities.

Some risk factors for the development of colorectal carcinoma are:

- Pre-existing colonic polyps
- Familial polyposis coli
- Ulcerative colitis
- Crohn's disease
- Schistosomal colitis
- Family history—first-degree relatives of patients with colorectal cancer have 2-3 fold increased risk, especially if relative was diagnosed under the age of 50.
- Environment—exposure to radiation; asbestos.
- Presence of ureterocolostomy.
- Diet—high fat, high calories, low dietary calcium, low fermentable fibre.
- Genetic markers, e.g. the chromosome 2 locus of de la Chapelle and Volgelstein may define a subset of colorectal cancer patients—hereditary non-polyposis colon cancer—that constitute about 5% of all colorectal carcinomas.

Other possible factors:

- Previous cholecystectomy—by increased presentation of bile acids to colonic bacteria for conversion into potential carcinogens.
- Previous gastric surgery for benign peptic ulcer.

Treatment

The treatment of left-sided colonic cancer is by surgery, when feasible. The aim is to resect the colon. The patient must be warned of the possibility of a permanent colostomy if the growth is unresectable or resectable and on the left-hand side. A temporary colostomy is sometimes necessary in order to protect an anastomosis made under difficult conditions.

The patient is admitted 2-3 days before the operation in order to prepare the bowel. The colon is cleared of exogenous material using laxatives and/or enemas, and cleansed of infective organisms using broad spectrum, poorly-absorbed antibiotics such as neomycin.

Usually, a left hemicolectomy or a Paul-Mickulicz procedure is performed. If the growth cannot be resected, a Hartmann's procedure is performed and a permanent colostomy created.

Colon Carcinoma (on right side of colon)

Right-sided colonic cancer implies carcinoma in the caecum, and the ascending and proximal transverse colon.

The patient usually presents with unexplained pain in the right iliac fossa plus or minus general symptoms such as anaemia, malaise and weakness. Abdominal pain often develops late in the disease because the tumour may remain silent until it has grown a considerable size.

In general, patients are over 40 years of age, and commonly the condition is seen in 70-80 year olds. Women are more affected than men.

Aetiology

The cause of colorectal carcinoma is unknown except for a small proportion of cases where there is malignant change in previous polyposis coli or ulcerative colitis. However, this disease is almost unknown in third world rural communities.

Some risk factors for the development of colorectal carcinoma are:

- Pre-existing colonic polyps.
- Familial polyposis coli.
- Ulcerative colitis.
- Crohn's disease.
- Schistosomal colitis.
- Family history—first-degree relatives of patients with colorectal cancer have 2-3 fold increased risk, especially if relative was diagnosed under the age of 50.
- Environment—exposure to radiation; asbestos
- Presence of ureterocolostomy.
- Diet—high fat, high calories, low dietary calcium, low fermentable fibre.
- Genetic markers, e.g. the chromosome 2 locus of de la Chapelle and Volgelstein may define a subset of colorectal cancer patients—hereditary non-polyposis colon cancer—that constitute about 5% of all colorectal carcinomas.

Other possible factors:

- Previous cholecystectomy—by increased presentation of bile acids to colonic bacteria for conversion into potential carcinogens.
- Previous gastric surgery for benign peptic ulcer.

Symptoms

Possible symptoms of right-sided colonic carcinoma include:

- Pallor, debility, breathlessness—due to iron deficiency anaemia caused by prolonged bleeding.

- Loss of weight and anorexia.
- Occult blood in faeces.
- Persistent, dull ache in right iliac fossa, often postprandial and mistakenly attributed to gallbladder or gastroduodenal disease. This is a late symptom.

Less commonly:

- Intestinal colic and intestinal obstruction if the growth occludes the ileocaecal valve.
- Acute appendicitis if the tumour blocks the mouth of the appendix, causing it to dilate.
- Change in bowel habit, either constipation or diarrhoea but not both alternately.

Signs

The patient with a right-sided colonic carcinoma may be pale and thin, possibly jaundiced.

The supraclavicular nodes may be palpable.

The abdomen may be generally distended or 'full' in the right iliac fossa. The right iliac fossa is often tender with some guarding of the covering muscles. A firm irregular mass may be felt which may be fixed or freely mobile. When it is mobile it tends to slip upwards into the paravertebral gutter or medially and downwards into the pelvis. It is dull to percussion.

The liver may be palpable and irregular.

The bowel sounds should be normal. Hyperactivity indicates obstruction of the ileo-caecal valve.

The faeces may contain blood.

Spread

The spread of colonic cancer is variably:

- Lymphatic:
  - most common
  - through mesenteric and para-aortic nodes, and eventually, the thoracic duct
  - may involve supraclavicular nodes in late stages.
- Direct extension:
  - through the bowel wall into adjacent structures, e.g. small intestine, stomach, duodenum, ureter, bladder, uterus, abdominal wall.
- Haematogenous spread:
  - 10-15% of cases
  - to liver in 75%, lung, or bone.
- Transcoelomic spread:
  - through the serosa and tumour cells into the peritoneal cavity forming local deposits of malignant nodules
  - the recto-vesical or recto-uterine pouches are often involved and on digital rectal examination can be felt as a hard shelf—Plummer's shelf
  - other common sites include omentum, and ovaries—Krukenberg tumour.
- Intraluminal metastasis:
  - exfoliated cells may become trapped in an anastomotic suture or staple line during operation "anastomotic recurrence.

Investigations

The preferred investigations for rectal carcinoma are:

- Full blood count.
- Blood film: test for iron-deficiency anaemia.
- Rectal examination: palpable mass in less than 50% of cases.
- Rigid sigmoidoscopy and proctoscopy: performed at the initial consultation—reveals tumours in sigmoid region and enables positive evidence by biopsy to be obtained.
- Flexible sigmoidoscopy.
- Stool sample: test for occult blood.
- *Colonoscopy:* enables inspection and biopsy of the higher reaches of the colon. Gives high sensitivity if used by an experienced operator.
- Requires a full bowel preparation.
- Barium enema: usually reveals the tumour as a stricture or filling defect. But negative results are not uncommon, so if this occurs when the condition is suspected, repeat the investigations after a few weeks.

- *IVU:* a useful preoperative investigation if there is a risk of ureteric involvement.

A barium enema and other invasive tests can be particularly distressing and should not be undertaken lightly.

Differential Diagnosis

An initial erroneous diagnosis of colonic carcinoma is made in as many as 25% of patients once gastrointestinal symptoms appear.

Diseases producing similar local symptoms:
- Diverticular disease
- Ulcerative colitis
- Crohn's disease
- Ischaemic colitis
- Amoebiasis.

Diseases producing similar general manifestations:
- Carcinoma of stomach
- Carcinoma of pancreas
- Uraemia
- Pernicious anaemia.

Treatment

Right-sided colonic carcinoma is treated surgically, if at all feasible. The aim is to resect the affected segment of bowel.

The patient is admitted 2-3 days before the operation in order to prepare the bowel. The colon is cleared of exogenous material using laxatives and/or enemas, and cleansed of infective organisms using broad spectrum, poorly absorbed antibiotics such as neomycin.

Care is taken to look for metastases. Liver function tests, a liver scan, chest X-ray, and barium enema are valuable pre-operative investigations. Evidence of metastasis may not prevent planned surgery. Blood transfusion may be necessary if the anaemia is severe.

The terminal ileum, ascending colon and hepatic flexure are removed by right hemicolectomy. The patient can usually resume normal activities after 6 weeks.

Prognosis

The staging of colonic carcinoma is the most important determinant of survival rate and is normally expressed via Dukes classification. The overall 5 year survival rate is 35%:
- Operation for cure can be performed on about 70% of patients:
  - 10% of lesions not resectable at operation
  - 20% have liver or other distant metastases.
- Operative mortality rate is 2-6%
- 5 year survival rate for curative resection is 55%.

Complications such as obstruction or perforation adversely affect survival. Patients should be followed for recurrent, metastatic, or metachronous lesions. Faecal occult blood should be tested every 6-12 months and colonoscopy performed 1 year after operation. Surgical resection for recurrent lesions should be considered.

Once colorectal cancer has metastasised, the average survival duration without chemotherapy is 3-9 months (1). Systemic chemotherapy is rarely curative in patients with metastatic colorectal cancer except, sometimes, where metastatic disease is confined to the liver and potentially resectable after chemotherapy.

Colon Carcinoma (Transverse)

The patient with carcinoma of the transverse colon presents with a picture intermediate between that of left-sided and right-sided lesions.

A palpable mass may be noticed in the abdomen which is freely mobile in the early stages. A distended caecum indicates obstruction.

The tumour may be treated surgically by transverse colectomy.

Screening for Colon Carcinoma

Screening could potentially have a beneficial effect on outcome as only half the patients presenting with large bowel cancer have the potential for cure; earlier detection and treatment secures an improved prognosis.

Flexible sigmoidoscopy and colonoscopy are too labour-intensive, but faecal occult blood testing is a more promising technique. The 'Haemoccult' method, for example, uses guaiac resin that has been stabilised on filter paper to detect as little as 2-5 ml of blood passed per 24 hours. However, false positives can result if meat has been eaten in the last three days, and compliance with testing is often poor.

Research is targeting more sensitive and specific means of indicating occult bleeding, e.g. enzyme immunoassays, and of increasing compliance, e.g. a pad that is used to wipe the anus and is then developed. However, the debate on whether screening is cost-effective continues. Using methods that detect occult blood loss assume that all tumours bleed but this is not the case.

Treatment of Colon Cancer

Treatment of colonic carcinoma consists of wide surgical resection of the lesion.

Colorectal carcinomas are relatively unresponsive to chemotherapy but palliative chemotherapy in patients with locally advanced or metastatic disease has been shown to reduce death and progression at 12 months (1). The findings translate into a 16% absolute difference in survival and a 25% increase in progression free survival (increases in 3.7 months in median survival and 6 months in median progression free survival) in patients treated with palliative chemotherapy e.g. 5-fluorouracil alone or in combination with other chemotherapeutic agents.

The response to radiotherapy is limited by the difficulty of directing the radiation beam at the tumour without damaging surrounding structures, e.g. the bladder.

Surgical Treatment of Colon Cancer

Treatment of colonic carcinoma consists of wide surgical resection of the lesion and its regional lymphatic drainage after preparation of the bowel. The primary tumour is resected, even if distant metastases have occurred, since prevention of obstruction or bleeding may offer palliation for long periods.

The abdomen is explored to determine resectability of the tumour and to search for multiple primary carcinomas of the colon, distant metastases, and associated abdominal disease. Care is taken not to contribute to the spread of the tumour by unnecessary palpation. Some authors have even advocated occlusion of the bowel with encircling tape on either side of the lesion in order to contain exfoliated cancer cells within the segment to be resected.

The cancer-bearing portion is mobilised and removed.

Non-surgical Ttreatment of Colorectal Cancer

Colorectal carcinomas are relatively unresponsive to chemotherapy but liver metastases may occasionally be controlled by 5-fluorouracil (5 FU). At the time of the operation and for a week postoperatively, the portal vein is infused with heparin and 5 FU. This approach seems to be particularly beneficial for Dukes' C tumours.

5 FU is usually given in combination with Leucovirin. Recently other agents e.g. irinotecan, oxaliplatin have been found to also have a beneficial effect.

The response to radiotherapy is limited by the difficulty of directing the radiation beam at the tumour without damaging surrounding bowel. Also, if radiotherapy is to be useful, there must be only local invasion—sterilization of local lymph nodes will have no effect on prognosis, for example, if there is already hepatic involvement.

Raltitrexed is an inhibitor of thymidylate synthase. It is licensed for use as monotherapy when fluorouracil-based palliative therapy for colorectal cancer is inappropriate or not tolerated.

Irinotecan

Irinotecan inhibits topoisomerase-1 which catalyses the breaking and rejoining of DNA strands.

Irinotecan is licensed for first-line use in patients with advanced colorectal cancer, in combination with fluorouracil and folinic acid, and as second-line monotherapy when fluorouracil-based therapy has failed (1).

A regime of 5-fluorouracil and leucovirin and Irinotecan has been shown to be beneficial compared to a regime without Irinotecan. There was an objective response in 39% vs 21%, a longer time before tumour progression 7 months vs 4 months and a longer median survival 15 months vs 13 months (2).

Oxaliplatin

This is a diaminocyclohexane platinum compound which forms crosslinks in DNA, so inhibiting DNA replication.

Treatment with Oxaliplatin is associated with a 10% probability of an objective response when given alone or in combination with 5-fluorouracil and leucovirin in patients who have already received 5-fluoruracil.

Occult Hepatic Metastases (colorectal cancer)

Accurate preoperative staging is very important in predicting the prognosis of colorectal cancer. Significant occult hepatic metastases carry a poor prognosis. If the hepatic metastases group are subtracted from the group of apparently better-classified tumours, the prognosis of these tumours is much improved.

Intraoperative ultrasound is useful in finding occult hepatic metastases.

Prognosis

The staging of colonic carcinoma is the most important determinant of survival rate and is normally expressed via Dukes classification. The overall 5 year survival rate is 35%:

- Operation for cure can be performed on about 70% of patients:
  - 10% of lesions not resectable at operation
  - 20% have liver or other distant metastases
- Operative mortality rate is 2-6%
- 5 year survival rate for curative resection is 55%

Complications such as obstruction or perforation adversely affect survival. Patients should be followed for recurrent, metastatic, or metachronous lesions. Faecal occult blood should be tested every 6-12 months and colonoscopy performed 1 year after operation. Surgical resection for recurrent lesions should be considered.

Once colorectal cancer has metastasised, the average survival duration without chemotherapy is 3-9 months (1). Systemic chemotherapy is rarely curative in patients with metastatic colorectal cancer except, sometimes, where metastatic disease is confined to the liver and potentially resectable after chemotherapy.

Pancreatic Carcinoma

A disease of later life, pancreatic carcinoma is the third most common cancer of the gastrointestinal tract and the sixth most common cause of cancer deaths.

Seventy percent of tumours occur in the head of the pancreas in proportion to the amount of tissue in different parts of the pancreas.

Progress is insidious. There is early regional lymph node involvement and spread to the liver. The tumour may metastasize to bone and lung.

Less common endocrine tumours of the pancreas such as glucagonomas and insulinomas may occur.

Aetiology

The cause of pancreatic carcinoma is unknown.

Factors which have been associated with the development of pancreatic carcinoma include:

- Smoking
- Chronic pancreatitis, possibly secondary to alcohol consumption
- High fat diet, which may explain the rising incidence in affluent countries
- Diabetes mellitus

Certain industries seem to impart a high risk to their workers; occupational exposure to coal gas and aluminium increase the risk.

Coffee consumption is no longer considered to be a risk factor.

Clinical Features

Presenting features of pancreatic carcinoma include:

- Weight loss in 80%.
- Deep epigastric pain, which in 60% of cases, radiates to the back. It is a very hard pain to treat.
- Jaundice with pruritis if tumour affects head of the pancreas and obstructs the biliary system; occurs in 50%.
- Ascites with a knobbly liver in 30%.
- Anorexia, nausea, vomiting.
- Palpable gallbladder—Courvoisier's law.

Less common presentations:

- Steatorrhoea.
- Thrombophlebitis migrans: may also occur in glucagonomas.
- Acute pancreatitis.
- Gastric outlet obstruction, causing pyloric stenosis.
- Gastrointestinal haemorrhage due to duodenal erosion.
- Symptoms of hypoglycaemia may occur if the tumour is an insulinoma—very rare.

Investigations

- Biochemistry:
  - raised serum bilirubin and alkaline phosphatase in obstructive jaundice
  - may be impaired glucose tolerance or diabetes.
- Ultrasound—to look for dilated ducts and stones .
- ERCP or transhepatic percutaneous cholangiography.
  - allows a pancreatogram to be taken
  - pancreatic juice can be collected for cytology.
- CT scan—the most reliable method of diagnosis—may show metastatic disease.
- CT or US guided biopsy—may be used to confirm the diagnosis.
- carcinoembryonic antigen—may be raised if hepatic metastases.

Management of Pancreatic Carcinoma

The management of pancreatic carcinoma can be divided into steps able to cure or palliate:

- *Curative:* surgery offers the only possibility of cure. A radical pancreaticoduodenectomy—Whipple's operation—may be used in this condition. Surgery should be performed in specialist centres. There is evidence that surgery plus adjuvant therapy with 5-fluorouracil, alone or in combination, may prolong survival (from around 11-14 months to 20-23 months) but this requires confirmation (1).
- Palliative:
  - jaundice and associated itching can be relieved by procedures such as endoscopic or percutaneous stenting. Surgical intervention requires the creation of a biliary diversion via a cholecystojejunostomy.
  - vomiting may be due to duodenal involvement and thus a gastroenterostomy may be necessary

- pain relief is achieved using opiates and/or coeliac plexus block.
- chemotherapy (1)—for patients with advanced disease, gemcitabine is easily administered in the outpatient setting, is relatively well tolerated, and is a useful first-line treatment in patients able to manage most, or all, self-care. However, the overall treatment benefits are limited.

Prognosis

The prognosis of pancreatic carcinoma is very poor. Without surgical treatment, less than 3% of all patients survive for 5 years.

The benefit of surgical intervention is dependent on the site of the tumour. A Whipple's resection for carcinoma of the head of the pancreas can give, at best, a 5-year survival of 19%. An absence of lymph node involvement was associated with an improved prognosis. Tumours of the body and tail of the pancreas are associated with a worse prognosis, whatever the mode of intervention, 1-year survival was 8-9%.

Glucagonoma

This is a result of a tumour of the alpha 2 cells of the islets of Langerhans. The majority of these tumours are malignant.

This tumour may present with attacks of hyperglycaemia, stomatitis, vulvitis, anaemia, a rash and diarrhoea. Necrolytic migratory erythema is specifically associated with this condition.

This tumour forms of part of a multiple endocrine neoplasia syndrome (MEN I).

Insulinoma

This is a result of a tumour of the APUD cells of the islets of Langerhans. The majority of these APUD tumours are benign.

The most common of these rare tumours is an insulinoma which are derived from beta cells. This tumour may present with attacks of hypoglycaemia, especially when fasting and exercising. Attacks are treated with oral or intravenous glucose. The vast majority (90%) are benign.

Diagnosis is based on:

- Inappropriate hyperinsulinaemia
- High ratio of proinsulin to insulin in a fasting blood sample (due to defective post-translational processing of proinsulin which allows proinsulin to be secreted in addition to insulin and C-peptide).
- CT scanning and/or pancreatic arteriography to identify the site of the lesion—usually in distal 2/3 of pancreas (occasionally in head of pancreas or ectopic site such as duodenal wall).

This tumour forms of part of a multiple endocrine neoplasia syndrome (MEN I).

Management: surgery or medical treatment with diazoxide.

Sixteen

Tumors of Genitourinary Trac

OVARIAN CANCER

Ovarian cancer is cancer that begins in the ovaries. In women, the ovaries produce eggs *(ova)*. The ovaries are also the main source of the female hormones, estrogen and progesterone. One ovary is located on each side of the uterus in the pelvis.

Types of Ovarian Tumors

There are many types of tumors that can start growing in the ovaries. Some are *benign* (noncancerous) and never spread beyond the ovary. These patients can be treated successfully by surgically removing one ovary or the part of an ovary containing the tumor. Other types of ovarian tumors are *malignant* (cancerous) and may spread to other parts of the body. Their treatment is more complex, and is discussed later in this document.

In general, ovarian tumors are named according to the kind of cells the tumor started from and whether the tumor is benign or cancerous. There are three main types of ovarian tumors:

Epithelial tumors start from the cells that cover the outer surface of the ovary.

Germ cell tumors start from the cells that produce the *ova* (eggs).

Stromal tumors start from connective tissue cells that hold the ovary together and produce the female hormones estrogen and progesterone.

Epithelial Ovarian Tumors

Benign epithelial ovarian tumors: Most epithelial ovarian tumors are benign and therefore, do not spread and usually do not lead to serious illness. There are several types of benign epithelial tumors, including *serous adenomas, mucinous adenomas,* and *Brenner tumors.*

Tumors of low malignant potential: When viewed under the microscope, some ovarian epithelial tumors do not clearly appear to be cancerous—these are called *tumors of low malignant potential (LMP tumors).* They are also known as *borderline tumors.*

Epithelial ovarian cancers: Cancerous epithelial tumors are called *carcinomas*. About 85 percent of ovarian cancers are *epithelial ovarian carcinomas.* Epithelial ovarian carcinoma cells have several features that can be recognized under the microscope. These features are used to classify epithelial ovarian carcinomas into *serous, mucinous, endometriod,* and *clear cell* types. *Undifferentiated* epithelial ovarian carcinomas don't look like any of these four subtypes and they also tend to grow and spread more quickly. In addition to their classification by cell type, epithelial ovarian carcinomas are also given a grade and a stage. The grade is on a scale of 1, 2, or 3. Grade 1 epithelial ovarian carcinomas more closely resemble normal tissue and tend to have a better *prognosis* (outlook). Grade 3 epithelial ovarian carcinomas less closely resemble normal tissue and usually have a worse outlook. The tumor stage describes how far the tumor has spread from where it started in the ovary. Staging is explained in detail in a later section.

Primary Peritoneal Carcinoma

Primary peritoneal carcinoma, also called *extra-ovarian primary peritoneal carcinoma (EOPPC)* and *serous surface papillary carcinoma,* is a cancer closely related to epithelial ovarian cancer. It develops from cells that line the pelvis or abdomen, which are very similar to epithelial cells on the surface of the ovaries. Because EOPPC tends to spread along the surfaces of the pelvis and abdomen, it is often difficult to tell exactly where the cancer first started. Under a microscope, EOPPC looks just like epithelial ovarian cancer. Women who have had their ovaries removed can still develop this type of cancer.

Symptoms of EOPPC are similar to those of ovarian cancer, including abdominal pain or bloating, nausea, vomiting, indigestion, and a change in bowel habits. Also like ovarian cancer, EOPPC may cause an elevation in the tumor marker CA-125.

Treatment for people with EOPPC usually includes surgery to remove as much of the cancer as possible, followed by chemotherapy like that given for ovarian cancer. Information on prognosis is limited since it is a newly recognized type of cancer, but early studies suggest that prognosis is similar to ovarian cancer.

Germ Cell Tumors

Germ cells are the cells that usually form the *ova* or eggs. There are several subtypes of germ cell tumors. Most germ cell tumors are benign, although some are cancerous and may be life threatening. The most common germ cell tumors are teratoma, dysgerminoma, endodermal sinus tumor, and choriocarcinoma. Malignant germ cell tumors account for about 15 percent of ovarian cancers.

Teratoma: This germ cell tumor has a benign form called *mature teratoma* and a cancerous form called *immature teratoma.* The mature teratoma is by far the most common ovarian germ cell tumor, usually affecting women of reproductive age (teens through forties). It is often called a *dermoid cyst* because its lining resembles skin. These tumors or cysts also contain a variety of other benign tissues that may resemble adult respiratory passages, bone, nervous tissue, teeth, and other tissues. Surgical removal of the cyst is curative.

Immature teratomas occur in girls and young women, usually younger than 18. These are rare cancers that resemble embryonic or fetal tissues such as connective tissue, respiratory passages, and brain. Tumors that are not very immature *(grade 1 immature teratoma)* and have not spread beyond the ovary are cured by surgical removal of the ovary. When they have spread beyond the ovary and/or much of the tumor has a very immature appearance (*grade 2 or 3 immature teratomas*), chemotherapy is recommended in addition to surgical removal of the ovary.

Dysgerminoma: Although this is the most common ovarian cancer of germ cells, it represents only 2% of all ovarian cancers. It usually affects women in their teens and twenties. Although dysgerminomas are considered malignant (cancerous), most do not grow or spread very rapidly. When they are limited to the ovary, over 95% are cured by surgical removal of the ovary, without any further treatment. Even when the tumor has spread further, the combination of surgery and chemotherapy is effective in about 90% of patients.

Endodermal sinus tumor (yolk sac tumor) and choriocarcinoma: These very rare tumors typically affect girls and young women. They tend to grow and spread rapidly but are usually very sensitive to chemotherapy. Choriocarcinomas more commonly start in the placenta (during pregnancy) rather than in the ovary. Placental choriocarcinomas are usually even more responsive to chemotherapy than ovarian choriocarcinomas.

Stromal Tumors

These tumors account for about 5 percent of ovarian cancers. More than half are found in women over age 50, but some occur in young girls. Some, but not all, of these tumors produce female hormones or, less often, male hormones. They can cause vaginal bleeding to resume after menopause, or can cause menstrual periods and breast development in young girls. If male hormones are produced, the tumors can disrupt normal periods and cause facial and body hair to grow. Types of malignant (cancerous) stromal tumors include *granulosa cell tumors, granulosa-theca tumors,* and *Sertoli-Leydig cell tumors,* which are usually considered low-grade cancers. Thecomas and fibromas are benign stromal tumors.

Ovarian Cysts

An ovarian cyst is a collection of fluid inside an ovary. Many cysts are completely normal. These are called functional cysts and occur as a normal part of ovulation. The fluid will usually be absorbed and the cyst will disappear without any treatment over a few months. If a woman develops a cyst, the doctor may want to check it again in a few months to see if the size has gotten smaller. If however, the mass is large, or occurs in childhood or after menopause, or does not go away, further testing is usually advised since a small number of these may be cancer. Treatment of benign cysts may consist of observation (follow-up with physical exams and imaging tests), medications, or surgical removal.

THE KEY STATISTICS ABOUT OVARIAN CANCER

Ovarian cancer is the sixth most common cancer among women, excluding non-melanoma skin cancers. The American Cancer Society estimates that about 23,400 new cases of ovarian cancer will be diagnosed in the United States during 2001. Ovarian cancer accounts for 4% of all cancers in women.

The good news is that the ovarian cancer *incidence rate* has been slowly decreasing since 1991. The incidence rate is a precise way for scientists to describe how common or rare a disease is. The ovarian cancer incidence rate is defined as the number of new cases diagnosed each year per 100,000 women.

Ovarian cancer ranks fifth in cancer deaths among women, accounting for more deaths than any other cancer of the female reproductive system. It is estimated that there will be about 13,900 deaths from ovarian cancer in the United States during 2001.

The five—year survival rate is used to provide a standard way of discussing prognosis. It refers to the percentage of patients who live at least 5 years after their cancer is diagnosed, although many of these patients live much longer than 5 years after diagnosis. Five-year *relative* survival rates exclude from the calculations patients dying of other diseases, and are considered to be a more accurate way to describe the prognosis for patients with a particular type and stage of cancer. Of course, 5-year survival rates are based on patients diagnosed and initially treated more than 5 years ago. Improvements in treatment often result in a more favorable outlook for recently diagnosed patients.

About 78% of ovarian cancer patients survive one year after diagnosis and over 50% survive longer than five years after diagnosis. If diagnosed and treated while the cancer has not spread outside the ovary, the five-year survival rate is 95%. However, only 25% of all ovarian cancers are found at this early stage. Older women with ovarian cancer tend to have a poorer prognosis than younger ones. For example, the five-year survival rate is 64% in women under 65 years of age and 30% in women over 65.

RISK FACTORS FOR OVARIAN CANCER

Researchers have discovered several specific factors that increase a woman's likelihood of developing epithelial ovarian cancer. These risk factors do not apply to other less common types of ovarian cancer such as germ cell tumors and stromal tumors.

Most women with ovarian cancer do not have any known risk factors. It is important to remember that risk factors increase the odds of getting a disease but do not guarantee it will occur. Only a small number of women who have risk factors will develop ovarian cancer.

Age: Most ovarian cancers develop after menopause. A woman is considered to be menopausal when she has gone a year without a menstrual period. Half of all ovarian cancers are found in women over the age of 65.

Reproductive history: Women who started menstruating at an early age (before age 12), had no children or had their first child after age 30, and/or experienced menopause after age 50, may have an increased risk of ovarian cancer. There seems to be a relationship between the number of menstrual cycles in a woman's lifetime and her risk of developing ovarian cancer.

Fertility drugs: In some studies, researchers have found that prolonged use of the fertility drug *clomiphene citrate,* especially without achieving pregnancy, may increase a woman's risk for developing ovarian tumors, particularly a type known as tumors of *low malignant potential* (LMP tumors). A woman taking this drug should discuss its potential risks with her doctor. However, infertility also increases the risk of ovarian cancer, even without use of fertility drugs. More research to clarify these relationships is now underway.

Family history of ovarian cancer: Ovarian cancer risk is increased among women whose mother, sister, or daughter have, or have had, ovarian cancer, especially if they developed ovarian cancer at a young age. A woman can inherit an increased risk for ovarian cancer from relatives on her mother's side or father's side of the family. About 10% of ovarian cancers result from an inherited tendency to develop the disease. Many cases of familial epithelial ovarian cancer are due to inherited gene mutations that can be identified by genetic testing. Women with ovarian cancers due to these inherited gene mutations tend to have a better prognosis than patients who do not have any family history of ovarian cancer. Refer to the section on causes of ovarian cancer for information on these gene mutations. Genetic counseling, genetic testing, and strategies for preventing familial ovarian cancer are discussed in the prevention section of this document.

Breast cancer: Women who have had breast cancer also have an increased risk of developing ovarian cancer. There are several reasons for this observation. Some of the reproductive risk factors for ovarian cancer may also increase breast cancer risk. Also, inherited mutations of the BRCA1 and BRCA2 genes greatly increase a woman's risk for both cancers.

Talcum powder: It has been suggested that talcum powder applied directly to the genital area or on sanitary napkins may be *carcinogenic* (cancer-causing) to the ovaries. Most, but not all studies suggest a slight increase in risk of ovarian cancer in women who used talc on the genital area. In the past, talcum powder was sometimes contaminated with asbestos, a known cancer-causing mineral. This may explain the association with ovarian cancer in some studies. Body and face powder products have been required by law for over 20 years to be asbestos-free. However, proof of the safety of these newer products will require follow-up studies of women who have used them over a period of many years. There is no evidence at present linking cornstarch powders with any female cancers.

Hormone replacement therapy (HRT): Some studies suggest the use of estrogens by women after menopause may slightly increase their risk of developing ovarian cancer, while other studies have not found any effect on ovarian cancer risk. A recent review that recalculated results of other studies that have been previously published suggested that use of hormone replacement for over ten years increases ovarian cancer risk by about 30 percent, and that use for shorter periods of time increase ovarian cancer risk by about 15 percent. On the other hand, HRT reduces the risk of heart attacks and bone fractures. The decision to use hormone replacement therapy after menopause should be made by a woman and her doctor after weighing the possible risks and benefits. Factors to consider include her other risk factors for heart disease, ovarian cancer, breast cancer, osteoporosis (thinning and weakening of bones), and the severity of menopausal symptoms.

WHAT CAUSES OVARIAN CANCER?

Researchers have made great progress in understanding how certain mutations (changes) in DNA can cause normal cells to become cancerous. DNA is the chemical that carries the instructions for nearly everything our cells do. We usually resemble our parents because they are the source of our DNA. However, DNA affects more than our outward appearance. Some *genes* (parts of our DNA) contain instructions for controlling when our cells grow and divide. Certain genes that promote cell division are called *oncogenes*. Others that slow down cell division, cause cells to die at the appropriate time, or help repair DNA damage are called *tumor suppressor genes.* It is known that cancers can be caused by DNA *mutations* (defects) that turn on oncogenes or turn off tumor suppressor genes.

Inherited Genetic Factors

During the past few years, scientists have learned much about how certain genes inherited from a woman's parents can greatly increase her ovarian cancer risk. These include the BRCA1 and BRCA2 genes, and several genes related to hereditary nonpolyposis colon cancer (HNPCC).

BRCA1 and BRCA2 genes: Although these inherited gene mutations were originally found in women with breast cancer, they are also responsible for about 9% of ovarian cancers. Normally, these genes help to prevent cancer by making proteins that keep cells from growing abnormally. However, if a person has inherited a mutated gene from either parent, this cancer-preventing protein is less effective, and chances of developing breast and/or ovarian cancer increase. Between 56 and 87 percent of women with inherited BRCA1 or BRCA2 mutations will develop breast cancer by the age of 70. The lifetime ovarian cancer risk for women with BRCA1 or BRCA2 mutations has been estimated to be between 17 percent and 44 percent. These estimates vary considerably because they are based on studies of women of various racial and ethnic groups living in different countries. The impact of BRCA mutations on ovarian cancer risk is modified by the other risk factors discussed earlier in this document, as well as by other genes that have not yet been discovered. Differences in these other factors among the groups of women participating in each of these studies account for much of the variation in estimates of cancer risk. In comparison, the ovarian cancer lifetime risk for the general population of women is about two percent.

Hereditary nonpolyposis colon cancer (HNPCC): This syndrome is also caused by inherited gene mutations that reduce the body's ability to repair damage to its DNA. This results in very high risks for colorectal cancer and *endometrial* (lining of the uterus) cancer, and a somewhat increased risk for developing ovarian cancer. The risk for ovarian cancer with HNPCC syndrome is much less than with BRCA1 or BRCA2 defects. This gene mutation causes about 1% of all ovarian epithelial cancers.

Acquired Genetic Changes

Most DNA mutations related to ovarian cancer occur during a woman's life rather than having been inherited. *Acquired mutations* of oncogenes and/or tumor suppressor genes may result from radiation or cancer-causing chemicals. So far, studies have not been able to identify any single chemical in the environment, or in our diets, that is specifically linked to cause mutations that cause ovarian cancer. The cause of most acquired mutations remains unknown.

Most ovarian cancers have several acquired gene mutations. Research has suggested that tests to identify acquired changes of certain genes, such as the p53 tumor suppressor gene or the HER2 oncogene, in ovarian cancers may help in predicting a woman's prognosis. The role of these tests is still not certain, and some cancer specialists feel that more research is needed. Recently, a monoclonal antibody therapy called trastuzumab (Herceptin) has been developed that specifically interrupts the growth-promoting action of the HER2 oncogene. This new treatment has been approved as a treatment for breast cancer, and is currently being tested in clinical trials to determine whether it is useful in treating ovarian cancer.

CAN OVARIAN CANCER BE PREVENTED?

Most women have one or more risk factors for ovarian cancer. However, most of the common factors only slightly increase a woman's risk, so they only partly explain the frequency of the disease. So far, knowledge about risk factors has not been translated into practical ways to prevent most cases of ovarian cancer.

Researchers have found several ways a woman can reduce her risk of developing epithelial ovarian cancer. Much less is known about ways to lower the risk of developing germ cell and stromal tumors of the ovaries. The remainder of this section refers to epithelial ovarian cancer only. It is important to realize that some of these strategies reduce the risk only slightly while others decrease it much more. Some strategies are easily followed and others require surgery. If you are concerned about your risk of ovarian cancer, you may want to discuss this information with your health care providers. They can help you consider these ideas in the context of your own situation.

Oral contraceptives: The use of oral contraceptives (birth control pills) decreases the risk of developing ovarian cancer, especially among women who used them for several years. Compared to women who never used oral contraceptives, those who used oral contraceptives for more than five years have about a 60 percent lower risk of developing ovarian cancer.

Tubal ligation or hysterectomy: Tubal ligation is a surgical procedure to "tie" the fallopian tubes to prevent pregnancy. When performed after childbearing, tubal ligation may reduce the chance of developing ovarian cancer. A hysterectomy may also reduce your risk.

One theory to explain why tubal ligation and hysterectomy reduce ovarian cancer risk is that some cancer-causing substances may enter the body through the vagina and pass through the uterus and fallopian tubes to reach the ovaries. This may explain the effect of removing the uterus or blocking the fallopian tubes on ovarian cancer risk. However, the impact of these operations on ovarian cancer risk is relatively small and they cannot prevent all or even most cases. We emphasize that these operations should be done only when there are valid medical reasons, and not exclusively for their effect on ovarian cancer risk.

If you are having a *hysterectomy* (removal of the uterus) for a valid medical reason and you have a strong family history of ovarian or breast cancer, you may wish to consider having a *bilateral oophorectomy* (removal of both ovaries) as part of that procedure. If you are *postmenopausal* (after menopause) or *perimenopausal* (near menopause), the ovaries should be removed at the same time as the hysterectomy even if you do not have an increased risk of ovarian cancer. If you are having a hysterectomy and are older than 40, you should discuss the issue of ovarian removal with your doctor.

Pregnancy and breast-feeding: Having one or more children, particularly if your first is born before you are age 30, plus prolonged (one year or more) breast-feeding, also may decrease your risk. Although these measures slightly reduce risk, they do not guarantee protection against ovarian cancer. Doctors do not recommend making choices about when to have a child specifically for the purpose of reducing ovarian cancer risk, especially since using oral contraceptives will have a greater impact on this risk.

Diet: results of some studies suggest that a high fat diet may increase ovarian cancer risk. Other studies disagree, however. The American Cancer Society recommends choosing most foods from plant sources (fruits, vegetables, whole grain products) and limiting intake of high fat foods, especially those from animal sources. Even though the impact of these dietary recommendations on ovarian cancer risk remains uncertain, following these recommendations can help prevent several other diseases, including some types of cancer.

Prevention strategies for women with a family history of ovarian cancer: Genetic counseling can predict whether a woman is likely to have one of the gene mutations associated with an increased ovarian cancer risk. If a woman's family history suggests that she might have one of these gene mutations, genetic testing can be done. Before undergoing genetic testing, a woman should discuss its benefits and potential drawbacks. Genetic testing can determine if you or members of your family carry certain gene mutations that cause a high risk of ovarian cancer. For some women with a strong family history of ovarian cancer, knowing that they do not have a mutation that increases their ovarian cancer risk can be a great relief for them and their children. Knowing that you do have such a mutation can be very stressful, but many women find this information very helpful in making important decisions about certain prevention strategies for them and their children.

Use of oral contraceptives is one way to decrease ovarian cancer in women at high risk for this disease. However, some studies have indicated that oral contraceptives might increase breast cancer risk in women with a strong family history of breast cancer. Other studies, on the other hand, have not found any increase in breast cancer risk among women with BRCA mutations who take oral contraceptives. Other studies, on the other hand, have not found any increase in breast cancer risk among women with BRCA mutations who take oral contraceptives. Additional research is needed to learn more about the risks and benefits of oral contraceptives to women at high ovarian and breast cancer risk.

Surgery to remove one or both ovaries is called an *oophorectomy*. A *prophylactic oophorectomy* is surgery to remove both of the ovaries before an ovarian cancer occurs. This is a controversial operation because it causes premature menopause in premenopausal women, and may be unnecessary. It generally is recommended only for certain very high-risk patients over age 40. This operation lowers ovarian cancer risk a great deal but does not entirely eliminate it. In some women with a very high risk of ovarian cancer (due to a strong family history) who have had both ovaries removed, cancers can still form from the lining cells of the pelvic cavity where the ovaries were previously located. This type of cancer, known as *primary peritoneal carcinoma* occurs more often in women with BRCA gene mutations. Recent studies suggest that having both ovaries removed can also lower the risk of developing breast cancer among women with BRCA gene mutations.

About 25% of ovarian cancers are found at an early stage. Early detection improves the chances that ovarian cancer can be treated successfully. When ovarian cancer is found early at a localized stage, about 90% of patients live longer than 5 years after diagnosis.

Routine pelvic examination: Annual pelvic examinations and Pap smears to check the pelvic area both internally and externally should begin at age 18 or when a women becomes sexually active, whichever is earlier. During this exam, the health care professional feels the ovaries and uterus for size, shape, and consistency. Although the Pap test is effective in early detection of cervical cancer, it cannot detect most ovarian cancers. Most of the ovarian cancers that are detected through Pap smears are already advanced. Although a pelvic examination is routinely recommended because it can find some reproductive system cancers at an early stage, most early ovarian tumors are difficult or impossible for even the most skilled examiner to feel.

Seek medical attention if symptoms appear: The ovaries are deep inside the pelvis and cannot be seen directly without surgery. Small ovarian tumors are difficult for even the most skilled examiner to feel. Early cancers of the ovaries tend to cause symptoms that are relatively nonspecific. These symptoms include swelling of the abdomen (due to a mass or accumulation of fluid), unusual vaginal bleeding, pelvic pressure, back pain, leg pain, and digestive problems such as gas, bloating, indigestion, or long-term stomach pain. Most of these symptoms can also be caused by other less serious conditions. By the time ovarian cancer is considered as a possible cause of these symptoms, it may have already spread beyond the ovaries. Also, some types of ovarian cancer can rapidly spread to the surface of nearby organs. Nonetheless, prompt attention to symptoms can improve the odds of early diagnosis and successful treatment. If you have symptoms of ovarian cancer, report them to your health care provider right away.

Screening tests for ovarian cancer: *Screening* refers to tests and examinations used to detect a disease, such as cancer, in people who do not have any symptoms. Women with a high risk of developing epithelial ovarian cancer, such as those with a very strong family history of this disease, may be screened with *transvaginal sonography* (an ultrasound test performed with a small instrument placed in the vagina) and blood tests. Transvaginal sonography is helpful in finding a mass in the ovary, but it does not accurately predict which masses are cancers and which are due to benign diseases of the ovary. Blood tests for ovarian cancer may include measuring the amount of CA-125 (also known as OC-125). The amount of this protein is increased in the blood of many women with ovarian cancer. However, some noncancerous diseases of the ovaries can also increase the blood levels of CA-125 and some ovarian cancers may not produce enough CA-125 to cause a positive test. When these tests are positive, it may be necessary to do more X-ray studies or to take samples of fluid from the abdomen or tissue from the ovaries to find out if a cancer is really present.

In preliminary studies of women at average risk of ovarian cancer, these tests did not make any difference in the number of deaths caused by ovarian cancer. For this reason, transvaginal sonography and the CA-125 blood test are not recommended for ovarian cancer screening of women without known strong risk factors. However, some recent studies found that cancers detected by these tests tend to be somewhat less advanced than cancers of women who did not have any screening tests. Additional research is in progress to improve ovarian cancer screening tests. It is hoped that further improvements will make these tests effective enough to lower the ovarian cancer death rate.

There are no tests recommended for screening women for germ cell tumors or stromal tumors. Some germ cell cancers release certain markers (proteins) such as human chorionic gonadotropin (HCG) and alpha-fetoprotein (AFP) into the blood. After these tumors have been treated by surgery and chemotherapy, blood tests for these markers can be used as a sign that the cancer may be coming back.

Signs and Symptoms of Ovarian Cancer

There are several signs and symptoms that may be caused by ovarian cancer. However, most of these may also be caused by benign (noncancerous) diseases and by cancers of other organs.

- Prolonged swelling of the abdomen (due to a mass or accumulation of fluid)
- Digestive problems including gas, loss of appetite, bloating, long-term abdominal pain, or indigestion
- Unusual vaginal bleeding is a rare sign of ovarian cancer. It is a strong warning of some type of abnormality, although not necessarily ovarian cancer. Bleeding that occurs between periods, is heavier, or lasts longer than usual, is considered abnormal. Any postmenopausal bleeding, staining, or persistent vaginal discharge is abnormal. A woman of any age who has unusual vaginal bleeding should alert her doctor immediately.
- Pelvic pressure (feeling as though you have to urinate or defecate all the time)
- Pelvic pain is a nonspecific symptom. It may be caused by ovarian cancer, other cancers, or by several benign conditions.
- Leg pain
- Back pain

If there is reason to suspect you may have ovarian cancer, your doctor will use one or more methods to be absolutely certain that the disease is present and to determine the stage of the cancer.

Consultation with a Specialist

If your pelvic examination or other tests suggest that you may have ovarian cancer, you will need a doctor or surgeon who specializes in treating women with this type of cancer. A *gynecologic oncologist* is an obstetrician/gynecologist who is specially trained in treating cancers of the female reproductive system.

Imaging Studies

Imaging methods such as computed tomography (CT) scans, magnetic resonance imaging (MRI) scans, and ultrasound studies can confirm whether a pelvic mass is present. Although these studies cannot confirm if the mass is a cancer, they are useful in looking for spread of ovarian cancer to other tissues and organs.

Ultrasound: *Ultrasound* or *ultrasonography* uses sound waves to create an image on a video screen. Sound waves are released from a small probe placed in the woman's vagina or on the surface of her abdomen. The sound waves create echoes as they enter the ovaries and other organs. The same probe detects the echoes that bounce back and a computer translates the pattern of echoes into a picture. Because ovarian tumors and normal ovarian tissue often reflect sound waves differently, this test may be useful in detecting tumors and in determining whether a mass is solid or a fluid-filled cyst.

Color-flow Doppler: This procedure uses a special type of ultrasound instrument to assess blood flow to the ovaries. In ovarian cancer there is usually an increase in blood flow. However, several benign conditions can also increase blood flow to the ovaries.

Computed tomography: Commonly referred to as a CT or CAT scan, this test uses a rotating X-ray beam to create a series of pictures of the body from many angles. A computer combines the information from these pictures, producing a detailed cross-sectional image. *Contrast material* is usually injected into a vein before CT scanning to help produce clearer pictures.

Chest X-ray: This test may be done to determine whether ovarian cancer has spread to the lungs. This spread may cause one or more tumors in the lungs and often causes fluid to collect around the lungs. This fluid, called a *pleural effusion*, can be seen with chest X-rays.

Magnetic resonance imaging (MRI): Like computed tomography, MRI displays a cross-section of the body. However, MRI uses powerful magnetic fields instead of radiation. The procedure can present cross-sectional views from several angles.

Tissue Sampling

The only way to determine for certain if a growth in the pelvic region is cancer is to *biopsy* (removing a sample of tissue) the suspicious area and examine the tissue sample under a microscope. In patients with *ascites* (collection of fluid inside the abdomen), samples of fluid can also be used to diagnose the cancer. A biopsy is usually done at the time of surgery. Depending on the extent of disease, the surgical procedure may be a *laparotomy* (surgery through an abdominal incision) or *laparoscopy* (surgery done through a lighted tube inserted into a very small incision in the pelvis). The goal of surgery for ovarian cancer is to obtain tissue samples for diagnosis and staging, and to remove all deposits of cancer larger than 1 cm (about one-half inch). Another diagnostic method is to obtain small samples of the cancer using CT scanning or ultrasound to guide a thin biopsy needle. This method might be used if the patient cannot have surgery because of advanced cancer or some other serious medical condition.

STAGING

Most ovarian cancers that are not obviously widespread are staged at the time of surgery. This is done by sampling tissues from different parts of the pelvis and abdomen to be examined under the microscope. Staging is very important because ovarian cancers of different stages have a different prognosis and are treated differently. The accuracy of the staging may determine whether or not a patient will be cured. If the cancer is not properly staged, then cancer that has spread outside the ovary may be missed and not treated. Once a stage has been assigned, it does not change, even when the cancer recurs or spreads to new locations in the body.

Ask your cancer care team to explain the staging procedure. Also ask them if they will perform a thorough staging procedure. After surgery, ask what your cancer's stage is. In this way, you will be able to take part in making informed decisions about your treatment.

Staging of ovarian cancer is described using the *FIGO system.* FIGO stands for International Federation of Gynecologists and Obstetricians.

Stage I: The cancer is still contained within the ovary (or ovaries).

Stage IA: Cancer has developed in one ovary and the tumor is confined to the inside of the ovary. There is no cancer on the outer surface of the ovary. Laboratory examination of washings from the abdomen and pelvis did not find any cancer cells.

Stage IB: Cancer has developed within both ovaries without any tumor on their outer surfaces. Laboratory examination of washings from the abdomen and pelvis did not find any cancer cells.

Stage IC: The tumor is present in one or both ovaries and one or more of the following are present: (1) cancer on the outer surface of at least one of the ovaries, (2) in the case of cystic tumors (fluid-filled tumors), the capsule (outer wall of the tumor) has ruptured (burst), (3) laboratory examination found cancer cells in fluid or washings from the abdomen.

Stage II: The cancer involves one or both ovaries and has involved other organs (such as the uterus, fallopian tubes, bladder, the sigmoid colon, or the rectum) within the pelvis.

Stage IIA: The cancer has extended to, or has actually invaded the uterus or the fallopian tubes, or both. Laboratory examination of washings from the abdomen did not find any cancer cells.

Stage IIB: The cancer has extended to other nearby pelvic organs such as the bladder, the sigmoid colon, or the rectum. Laboratory examination of fluid from the abdomen did not find any cancer cells.

Stage IIC: The cancer involves pelvic organs as in stages IIA or IIB and one or more of the following are present: (1) cancer on the outer surface of at least one of the ovaries, (2) in the case of cystic tumors (fluid-filled tumors), the capsule (outer wall of the tumor) has ruptured (burst), (3) laboratory examination found cancer cells in fluid or washings from the abdomen.

Stage III: The cancer involves one or both ovaries, and one or both of the following are present: (1) cancer has spread beyond the pelvis to the lining of the abdomen, (2) cancer has spread to lymph nodes (glands that fight infection and produce some types of blood cells.)

Stage IIIA: During the staging operation, the surgeon can see cancer involving the ovary or ovaries, but no cancer is grossly visible (can be seen without using a microscope) in the abdomen and the cancer has not spread to lymph nodes. However, when biopsies are checked under a microscope, tiny deposits of cancer are found in the lining of the upper abdomen.

Stage IIIB: There is cancer in one or both ovaries, and deposits of cancer are present in the abdomen which are large enough for the surgeon to see but smaller than 2 cm (about 3/4 inch) across. Cancer has not spread to the lymph nodes.

Stage IIIC: The tumor is in one or both ovaries, and one or both of the following is present: (1) cancer has spread to lymph nodes, (2) deposits of cancer larger than 2 cm (about 3/4 inch) across are seen in the abdomen.

Stage IV: This is the most advanced stage of ovarian cancer. The tumor is in one or both ovaries. Distant *metastasis* (spread of the cancer to the inside of the liver, the lungs, or to other organs located outside of the peritoneal cavity) has occurred. Finding ovarian cancer cells in *pleural fluid* (from the cavity that surrounds the lungs) is also evidence of stage IV disease.

CANCER OF CERVIX

Cervical cancer is a disease caused by the abnormal growth and division of cells that make up the *cervix*, which is the narrow, lower end of the *uterus* (womb). he cervix is composed of three layers of tissue:

- An *outer lining* known as the serous membrane (slippery covering)
- A *middle, muscular layer*
- An *inner lining* known as the mucous membrane, which is composed of thin, flat, scaly cells called squamous cells. This inner lining has many tiny glands that secrete a clear, lubricating mucous.

Nearly all cervical cancers arise from the cells of the inner lining of the cervix.

Normally, cervical cells grow in an orderly fashion. However, when control of that growth is lost, cells divide too frequently and too fast.

Certain well-defined cellular changes may progress to cervical cancer:

- *Mild cervical dysplasia* results when irregular cells are limited to the deepest one-third of the surface cell layer (known as the *epithelium*) that lines the cervix.
- *Moderate cervical dysplasia* occurs when uncontrolled cell growth continues, and up to two-thirds of the surface cell layer is abnormal.
- If abnormal cell growth progresses to include the full thickness of the surface cell layer, the condition is known as *severe cervical dysplasia,* or *carcinoma in situ, or CIS.* Carcinoma in situ does not penetrate surrounding tissues, stays within the confines of the epithelium, and is considered *benign.*

A tumor is considered *malignant* (cancerous) if abnormal cells:

- Penetrate the membrane that separates the surface cell layer and the underlying supportive tissue (called the stroma) of the cervix.
- Spread to the surrounding tissues or organs.

There are several types of cervical cancer:

- *Squamous cell carcinoma (SCC)* is the most common type of cervical cancer, accounting for 85% to 90% of all cases. It develops from the cells that line the inner part of the cervix, called the squamous cells. It usually begins where the part of the cervix that connects with the *vagina* (called the ectocervix) meets the part of the cervix that opens into the uterus (called the endocervix).
- *Adenocarcinoma* develops from the column-shaped cells that line the mucous- producing glands of the cervix. In rare instances, adenocarcinoma originates in the supportive tissue around the cervix. Adenocarcinoma accounts for about 10% of all cervical cancers.
- *Mixed carcinomas* (for example, adenosquamous carcinomas) combine features of both squamous cell carcinoma and adenocarcinoma.

Cervical cancer is most often diagnosed in women who are between the ages of 50 and 55.

- Girls under age 15 rarely develop the disease, but the risk of cervical cancer does rise between the late teen years and the early 30's.
- In both white and black women, cervical *carcinoma in situ* (a *benign* tumor) is most common between the ages of 25 and 30.

Some individuals are more likely to develop cervical cancer:

- City-dwellers and women who are members of racial or cultural minorities develop cervical cancer more often than other women do.
- Vietnamese women have the highest cervical cancer rate in the United States.
- Hispanics, Native Americans, and African Americans develop cervical cancer more often than white women do.

These statistics may reflect that:

- Many recent immigrants and other minority groups wrongly believe that a woman who isn't sexually promiscuous doesn't need to have a *Pap test*.
- African American women tend to have Pap tests less often than white women.

The most significant risk factors are:

- Human papillomavirus (HPV)
- Sexual history

Various other risk factors have also been identified.

Human Papilloma Virus (HPV)

Human papillomavirus (HPV) is a virus that can infect:

- The genital tract
- The external genitals
- The area around the anus

HPV has nothing to do with HIV, the virus that causes AIDS. There are 46 genetic types of HPV, but not all are dangerous. Only certain types of HPV, which can be transmitted from one person to another during sexual contact, increase the risk of cell *dysplasia* (abnormal cell growth) and/or progression to cervical cancer.

The HPV types that produce *genital warts* (lesions that are raised and bumpy, or flat and almost impossible to see) are different from those that cause cervical cancer. However, women who have a history of genital warts have almost twice the risk of an abnormal Pap smear as other women.

Other Risk Factors

It is probable that other factors contribute to cervical cancer, such as:

- *Poverty* Women who are poor may not have access to medical services that detect and treat *precancerous* cervical conditions. When such women develop cervical cancer, the disease usually remains undiagnosed and untreated until it has spread to other parts of the body.

  Women who are poor are often undernourished, and poor nutrition can also increase cervical cancer risk.
- *Pap test history* Not having regular *Pap tests* increases the chance of unrecognized cervical cancer. Between 60% and 80% of women with newly diagnosed cervical cancer have not had a Pap test in at least five years.
- *Tobacco use* Women who smoke are about twice as likely to develop cervical cancer as women who do not. The more a woman smokes - and the longer she has been smoking - the greater the risk.
- *Eating habits:* A diet that doesn't include ample amounts of fruits and vegetables can increase a woman's risk of developing cervical cancer.
- *Weakened immune system:* A woman whose immune system is weakened has a higher-than-average risk of developing cervical lesions that can become cancerous. This includes women who are HIV-positive (infected with the virus that causes AIDS). It also includes women who have received organ transplants and must take drugs to suppress the immune system so that the body won't reject the new organ.
- *Hormonal medications:* Some experts suggest that hormones in oral contraceptives (birth control pills) can make women more susceptible to *Human papillomavirus (HPV)*. At least one study has indicated that taking birth control pills significantly increases a woman's risk of developing HPV-related *genital warts*. Other research suggests that using oral contraceptives for five years or longer slightly elevates a woman's risk of developing cervical cancer, especially if she began taking the Pill before the age of 25.
- *Diethylstilberstrol (DES):* A rare type of cervical cancer has been diagnosed in a small number of women whose mothers took

diethylstilbestrol (DES), a medicine that was once used to prevent miscarriage.

- *Douching:* Because douching may destroy natural antiviral agents normally present in the *vagina,* women who douche every week are more apt to develop cervical cancer than women who do not.
- *Chemical exposure:* Women who work on farms or in the manufacturing industry may be exposed to chemicals that can increase their risk of cervical cancer.

Women with a weakened immune system due to the virus that causes AIDS are more likely to develop cervical cancer:

- Cervical cancer is very common in women who are positive for human immunodeficiency virus *(HIV).*
- Cervical cancer is sometimes the disease that first suggests a diagnosis of acquired immunodeficiency syndrome (AIDS)
- HIV can compound the effects of *Human papillomavirus (HPV),* causing cervical changes to progress more rapidly into cervical cancer than they otherwise might.

Early-stage cervical cancer and *precancerous* cervical conditions are almost 100% curable.

The most common forms of cervical cancer begin with changes in cervical cells.

If these changes are detected early enough, treatment can be started immediately to prevent cervical cancer from developing.

The best way to detect early cervical cancer and precancerous conditions of the cervix is to have a gynecologic examination and Pap test.

Because cervical cancer usually progresses slowly, some physicians feel that a woman doesn't need to have a Pap test every year if she:

- Is 65 years of age or older
- Has had normal Pap tests for three years in a row

Many experts recommend a Pap test every three years for women who have had a *hysterectomy* (removal of the *uterus*) for reasons unrelated to cervical disease.

Symptoms of cervical cancer don't usually appear until the abnormal cells invade nearby tissue.

Symptoms can include:

- Abnormal bleeding
- Heavier, long-lasting periods
- Unusual vaginal discharge
- Pelvic pain

Abnormal bleeding may occur:

- Between menstrual periods
- After menopause
- After intercourse
- After a pelvic examination

These symptoms are not always a sign of cervical cancer. They can be caused by sexually transmitted diseases (STDs) or other conditions. Your doctor can determine the cause of these symptoms.

Routine screening for cervical abnormalities can detect early-stage cancer and *precancerous* conditions that could progress to invasive disease. The process begins with a *Pap test,* also known as a Pap smear.

This painless office procedure detects about 95% of all cervical cancers and precancerous cervical conditions.

To perform a Pap test, a health professional uses a spatula, brush, or cotton swab to collect cells from the cervix and cervical canal. The cells are then "smeared" on a slide, preserved with a fixative, stained, and sent to a laboratory for microscopic analysis by a cytopathologist (a specialist who studies cells in order to diagnose disease).

If The Pap Test Suggests A Problem

If the Pap test results suggest a problem, the physician will then conduct additional tests. These may include:

- *ThinPrep Pap test*
- *Speculoscopy*

- *Schiller test and colposcopy*
- *Colposcopy-directed biopsy*
- *Endocervical curettage*
- *Cone biopsy*
- *Dilation and curettage (D&C)*
- *Cervicography*

Thinprep Pap Test

This test is performed only after an initial Pap test has indicated the presence of abnormal cervical cells. Cells are collected the same way as in a traditional Pap test, but this newer procedure improves slide-preparation techniques and provides more accurate results.

Speculoscopy

Recently approved by the US Food and Drug Administration (FDA), this procedure involves the use of a magnifier and a special wavelength of light. Speculoscopy allows the physician to see cervical abnormalities that would otherwise be undetectable when performing a Pap test.

Schiller Test and Colposcopy

A physician performing the Schiller test applies a vinegar-like solution to the cervix and then coats it with iodine. Next, the physician performs a colposcopy, which is an examination of the cervix with a magnifying instrument called a colposcope.

Healthy cervical cells look brown, whereas abnormal cells appear white or yellow. The Schiller test and colposcopy are painless office procedures that have no side effects.

If colposcopy reveals abnormal areas on the cervix, the physician will order a biopsy-the removal of tissue for examination under a microscope by a cytopathologist (a specialist who studies cells in order to diagnose disease).

Coloposcopic-Directed Biopsy

The physician uses forceps to remove small pieces of cervical tissue from areas of the cervix where abnormal-looking tissue has been detected. Local anesthetic is sometimes used to numb the cervix, and a woman who undergoes this office procedure may briefly experience pain, mild cramping, or light bleeding.

Endocervical Curretage

This procedure-which generally is performed at the same time as colposcopic biopsy - removes cells from the endocervix (part of the cervix that opens into the *uterus*).

- Local anesthetic may be used to numb the cervix before the physician proceeds.
- Next, a narrow instrument called a curette is inserted into the endocervix.
- Cells are then removed from this region, which cannot be seen during colposcopy.

A woman who has endocervical curettage may experience menstrual-type cramping or light bleeding for a short time afterward.

Cone Biopsy

This procedure consists of removing a cone-shaped piece of tissue from the cervix. Tissue is removed from the area between the ectocervix (the part of the cervix that connects with the *vagina*) and the endocervix (the part of the cervix that opens into the *uterus*). This "transformation zone" is the area where cancerous and precancerous conditions most often develop.

The two methods commonly used to perform cone biopsy are:

- Loop electrosurgical excision procedure (LEEP): This procedure is conducted in a physician's office under local anesthesia (the woman will be awake but pain will be blocked). A wire heated by electrical current is used to remove cervical tissue for laboratory analysis. The procedure takes about 10 minutes. Mild cramping may occur during the procedure and afterward. Mild or moderate bleeding may persist for several weeks.

- *Cold knife cone biopsy:* The physician uses a surgical scalpel or laser (intense, focused light beam) to remove abnormal cervical tissue. Cold knife cone biopsy is performed in a hospital under general anesthesia. A woman who undergoes the procedure can go home the same day but may experience cramping and bleeding for a few weeks afterward.

Dilation And Curettage (D&C)

If a Pap test doesn't clearly indicate whether abnormalities are caused by problems in the cervix or in the endometrium (lining of the uterus), the physician may conduct a dilation and curettage (D&C). During a "D&C," the physician enlarges the cervix (dilation) and scrapes the inside of the uterus and cervical canal (curettage) to remove tissue for microscopic analysis.

This procedure may be performed in a doctor's office without anesthesia or in an outpatient facility or hospital with epidural, spinal, or general anesthesia. When a D&C is performed without anesthesia, most women report cramps as the cervix is opened. After a D&C, some women experience complications such as bleeding, infection, or-in rare cases-perforation (piercing) of the uterus. D&C's have been performed for many years and, in general, are very safe.

Cervicography

This diagnostic procedure enables a physician to obtain and examine a photographic image of the cervix. Cervicography may clarify abnormal Pap test results in women at above-average risk of developing cervical cancer. It could eventually reduce the need for colposcopy.

If the Cancer has Spread

If the physician suspects that *tumor* cells have spread to regions outside of the cervix, he or she may decide that additional tests are needed. In particular, the physician may want to examine the lymph nodes, pelvic area, bladder, and rectum using the following methods:

- Cystoscopy
- Proctoscopy
- Computed tomography (CT scan)
- Magnetic resonance imaging (MRI)
- IVP
- Barium enema
- Chest X-ray

Cystoscopy

This procedure (also known as cystourethroscopy) lets the physician see the inside of the bladder, bladder neck, and urethra.

During cystoscopy, a cystoscope (thin, telescope-like tube with a tiny attached camera) is inserted into the bladder through the urethra (the passage through which urine passes from the bladder out of the body). This allows the physician to see whether cancer has spread from the cervix to the bladder or urethra.

Conducted under local or general anesthesia, cystoscopy can also be used to remove small tissue samples for microscopic examination.

Proctoscopy

During this procedure, the physician uses a proctoscope (a lighted tube), which is inserted into the *rectum* to examine the rectum or pelvis. In this way, the doctor can determine whether cancerous cells have spread to these organs from the cervix.

Computed Tomography (CT Scan)

Computed tomography is an imaging technique in which an X-ray rotates around the body and takes pictures ("scans") at many angles. A computer puts the scans together and creates detailed images of the body's organs in cross-section.

Sometimes a special dye known as contrast medium is injected or drunk to highlight body parts during CT scanning. For example, contrast medium may be used to highlight the intestines and emphasize any spread of cervical cancer within the pelvic cavity and/or to the lymph nodes.

Magnetic Resonance Imaging (MRI)

An MRI is another computer-assisted imaging method. It uses a powerful electromagnet to activate the water molecules within the body and create finely detailed images of tissue. This technique is sometimes used to determine whether cancer has spread from the cervix to the lymph nodes or other nearby organs.

IVP

An intravenous pyelogram (IVP), also called intravenous urography, is a urinary system X-ray conducted to detect abnormalities in the urinary tract. Contrast dye is injected into a vein. Then the physician traces the route of the dye as it is removed from the kidneys and passed through the ureters (tubes that carry urine from the kidneys to the bladder) to the bladder.

This procedure may be used to identify urinary tract abnormalities caused by cancer that may have spread from the cervix.

Baruim Enema

This is a radiographic procedure in which contrast medium is introduced into the bowels through the anus so that the lower intestinal tract is visible on an X-ray.

Chest X-Ray

This imaging procedure shows whether cancer has spread from the cervix to the lungs.

"Staging" is a method that has been developed to describe the extent of cancer growth. The stage of cervical cancer describes the tumor's:

- Size
- Depth of penetration within the cervix
- Spread within and beyond the cervix

Staging allows the physician to customize cancer treatment and to predict how a patient will fare over time. *In general, the lower the stage, the better the person's prognosis (expected outcome).*

The physician uses all available findings to choose a stage that best describes the woman's condition.

Cervical cancer is staged by information that is obtained through:

- Biopsy (removal of tissue for examination)
- Information gathered from the pathology report that accompanies a biopsy
- Cystoscopy (visual examination of the urinary tract with a camera-like instrument called an endoscope)
- Abdominal ultrasound (which uses high-frequency sound waves to produce an image of the inner body)
- Computed tomography (CT) scan (a computer-assisted technique that produces cross-sectional images of the body)
- Magnetic resonance imaging (or MRI, which uses powerful magnets to create finely detailed images of body tissue)

Staging With the FIGO System

Cervical cancer staging is usually described in terms of the FIGO system, a staging scheme developed by the International Federation of Gynecology and Obstetrics. The FIGO classifications are grouped within basic stages labeled stage 0 through stage IV (0-4):

- Stage 0–Carcinoma in situ. *Tumor* is present only in the epithelium (cells lining the cervix) and has not invaded deeper tissues.
- Stage I–Invasive cancer with tumor strictly confined to the cervix.
  - o Stage IA–In this earliest form of stage I, a very small amount of tumor can be seen under a microscope.
  - o Stage IA1–Tumor has penetrated an area less than 3 millimeters deep and less than 7 millimeters wide.

  - Stage IA2–Tumor has penetrated an area 3 to 5 millimeters deep and less than 7 millimeters wide.
  - Stage IB–This stage includes tumors that can be seen without a microscope. It also includes tumors that cannot be seen without a microscope but that are more than 7 millimeters wide and have penetrated more than 5 millimeters of connective cervical tissue.
  - Stage IB1–Tumor that is no bigger than 4 centimeters.
  - Stage IB2–Tumor that is bigger than 4 centimeters. Tumor has spread to organs and tissues outside the cervix but is still limited to the pelvic area.
- Stage II–Invasive cancer with tumor extending beyond the cervix and/or the upper two-thirds of the *vagina*, but not onto the pelvic wall.
  - Stage IIA–Tumor has spread beyond the cervix to the upper part of the vagina.
  - Stage IIB–Tumor has spread to the tissue next to the cervix.
- Stage III–Invasive cancer with tumor spreading to the lower third of the vagina or onto the pelvic wall; tumor may be blocking the flow of urine from the kidneys to the bladder.
  - Stage IIIA–Tumor has spread to the lower third of the vagina.
  - Stage IIIB–Tumor has spread to the pelvic wall and/or blocks the flow of urine from the kidneys to the bladder.
- Stage IV–Invasive cancer with tumor spreading to other parts of the body. This is the most advanced stage of cervical cancer.
  - Stage IVA–Tumor has spread to organs located near the cervix, such as the bladder or *rectum*.
  - Stage IVB–Tumor has spread to parts of the body far from the cervix.

The lower the stage number, the less the cancer has grown and spread. For example, a "stage I" cervical cancer is relatively small and has not yet spread beyond the pelvic area. By contrast, a "stage IV" cancer is much more serious, as it has already spread to the lymph nodes (the body's drainage system) as well as to other locations.

The main types of cervical cancer treatment are:

- *Surgery,* which may include a hysterectomy
- *Radiation therapy*
- *Chemotherapy*

Also used in cervical cancer treatment are *biological therapy* and other *therapies* such as clinical trials.

The type of treatment that is most appropriate for each case depends primarily on how early the cervical cancer is diagnosed. Other factors that affect treatment options are:

- Location of the *tumor* within the cervix
- Tumor type
- The woman's age
- Her general health
- Her childbearing plans
- Whether or not the woman is pregnant

All treatments for invasive cervical cancer are associated with potentially serious side effects. In addition, women of childbearing age who have invasive cervical cancer must cope with the emotional consequences of premature menopause and infertility. Many people find strength in the support of counselors, clergy, medical personnel, and other women who share their fight and their fears.

In addition to standard treatments, women with cancer that has spread to distant organs/sites may decide to participate in clinical trials (experimental studies) that offer new medications or other therapies.

Surgery

Both surgery and radiation therapy are equally effective strategies for women who have early cervical cancer. Each form of treatment has a survival rate of 85 to 90%. The factors that influence the choice between radiation therapy and surgery include the woman's age, health, and the extent of the disease.

The surgical procedures used to treat early cervical cancer include:

- *Laser surgery:* This outpatient treatment for cancer that has not spread uses a laser (a focused, high-energy light beam) to vaporize abnormal cells. Laser surgery can also be used to remove small pieces of tissue for laboratory analysis. It is not used to treat invasive cervical cancer.
- *Cryosurgery:* Cryosurgery kills abnormal cervical cells by freezing them with a metal probe cooled with liquid nitrogen. This procedure, which can be performed in a physician's office, is used to treat cancer that has not penetrated deep layers of cervical tissue or spread beyond the cervix.
- *Conization (cone biopsy):* This procedure, which can be used for diagnosis as well as treatment, uses a surgical scalpel, laser knife (cold cone knife), or LEEP (LEETZ) procedure to remove a small amount of cone-shaped tissue from the cervix. Physicians usually use this procedure to establish a diagnosis of cervical cancer before performing surgery or initiating radiation therapy.

  Conization rarely is used as the sole treatment for this disease unless a woman wants to preserve her ability to have children and the microscopic amount of cancer present hasn't spread beyond her cervix.
- *LEEP (LEETZ).* This procedure removes abnormal tissue with a thin wire heated by electricity. It is used to treat cancer that has not spread beyond the area where it originated.

Laser surgery, cryosurgery, LEEP, and conization almost always remove or destroy all *precancerous* tissue and prevent abnormal cells from becoming malignant (cancerous). These procedures may cause cramping and a watery brown discharge that lasts for several weeks. Regular post-operative examinations are necessary to make sure the condition does not recur and require additional treatment.

Some individuals who undergo surgery may require additional radiation therapy or chemotherapy afterward. Women with very advanced cancers often require combinations of surgery, radiation, and chemotherapy.

Hysterectomy

Although women with later-stage cervical cancers usually receive radiation therapy, some individuals select *hysterectomy* (surgical removal of the *uterus*) as a primary treatment. Hysterectomy may:

- Preserve the ovaries and vagina
- Reduce treatment time
- Allow for a more thorough examination of cancerous lesions

Women who have had a hysterectomy cannot become pregnant.

There are several types of hysterectomy:

- Simple (total) hysterectomy
- Radical hysterectomy
- Pelvic exenteration

1. *Simple (total) hysterectomy* is used to treat microscopic cancer that hasn't spread beyond the *uterus*, and also some cases of *carcinoma in situ*. In simple hysterectomy:
   - The uterus (including the cervix) is removed.
   - The vagina remains intact.
   - The ovaries (the two reproductive glands in which the eggs and the female sex hormones are made) and the fallopian tubes (which carry the eggs into the uterus) are also left intact. They are removed only if they are affected by some other disease.
   - Pelvic lymph nodes, the parametrium (tissue surrounding the uterus), and the ligaments in the pelvis are not removed.

   A simple hysterectomy can be performed in two ways:

- A vaginal hysterectomy involves removing the organs through the vagina.
- An abdominal hysterectomy involves removing the organs through an incision in the abdomen.

  Although this operation usually doesn't affect sexual desire or the ability to have intercourse, a woman who has had a total hysterectomy no longer menstruates (has periods) and can't become pregnant. Yet, because the ovaries remain, she will not experience early menopause, which is the end of menstruation.

2. *Radical hysterectomy* is performed once cancer has spread beyond the cervix. It involves the removal of the:
   - Uterus
   - Cervix
   - Parametrium (tissue surrounding the uterus)
   - Ovaries
   - Fallopian tubes
   - Upper vagina
   - Some or all of the local lymph nodes
3. *Pelvic exenteration* This rare and extreme procedure is used to treat recurrent cervical cancer that has spread to surrounding organs. Pelvic exenteration removes the same organs and tissues as radical hysterectomy. In addition, though, pelvic exenteration may remove the bladder, rectum, part of the colon, and/or vagina.

   If the bladder needs to be removed:

- Surgeons who must remove the bladder may connect a short segment of the intestine to the abdominal wall. This allows urine to periodically drain into a catheter (small tube) that is placed within a small opening in the abdomen. Or,
- The surgeon may attach a small plastic bag to the front of the abdomen to collect a continuous flow of urine.

If the rectum (end of the large intestine) needs to be removed, surgeons must create a new way for the woman to eliminate solid waste. This can be done by:

- Attaching the remaining intestine to the abdominal wall. This procedure, known as a colostomy, allows solid waste to pass through the opening in the abdomen into a small plastic bag at the front of the abdomen.
- Reconnecting the healthy sections of the colon. A woman who undergoes this procedure doesn't have to wear a bag or other external appliance to collect waste.

If the vagina has to be removed, plastic surgery must be performed to create an artificial vagina. Surgeons will use skin, muscle and/or intestinal tissue grafts to accomplish this. Such vaginal reconstruction is a very rare procedure.

Radiation Therapy (Radiotherapy)

Radiation therapy uses high-energy X-rays to destroy cancer cells. Cancers that extend beyond the cervix into the pelvis, lower vagina, and urinary tract typically receive radiation.

- Radiation therapy can be combined with surgery or chemotherapy to treat early cervical cancers and more invasive stages of the disease.
- Radiation also can be used to relieve symptoms caused by advanced cancer.

Physicians treat cervical cancer with external beam radiation, radioactive implants, or a combination of these therapies.

External beam radiation is administered the same way as a diagnostic X-ray. External beam radiation is usually given five times a week for five or six weeks, with an extra boost of radiation at the end of that time.

Women are encouraged to remain as active as possible during the course of this therapy, but they may experience side effects in the target area such as hair loss, dry or irritated skin, or permanent darkening of the skin. Therefore, women who undergo radiation therapy should: practice good personal hygiene, use lotions or creams only with a physician's approval, wear loose clothing, and expose the target area to air whenever possible.

Implant radiation (brachytherapy) puts cancer-killing radiation as close to the tumor as possible, but spares the healthy tissue nearby. The radioactive material is either placed in a capsule and inserted into the cervix, or placed in thin needles that are inserted directly into the tumor.

The woman stays in the hospital for one to three days while the implants remain in place. Repeated several times over a period of one to two weeks, brachytherapy can cause the treated area to look and feel sunburned. Treated tissues regain their normal appearance within 6 to 12 months.

A woman should not have sex until a few weeks after completing radiation therapy. These treatments can cause numerous side effects that can be severe but usually disappear after treatment is completed. Side effects include:

- Fatigue
- Diarrhea
- Frequent or uncomfortable urination
- Vaginal dryness
- Itching
- Burning

Other complications of external beam radiation and brachytherapy include:

- Proctitis (inflammation of the rectum)
- Cystitis (inflammation of the bladder)
- Vaginal scarring
- Anemia and/or bruising
- Increased risk of infection
- Sexual difficulties
- Premature menopause
- Vesicovaginal fistula (development of an abnormal tunnel between the vagina and the bladder or rectum)

Medications and special techniques can help a woman successfully manage the side effects and complications of radiation therapy. Regular medical monitoring can help to prevent cancer recurrence.

Chemotherapy

Chemotherapy is the treatment of choice for cervical cancer that has:

- Spread too far from its origin to be treated by surgery or radiation
- Recurred (come back) after surgery or radiation therapy

Chemotherapy also may be used to:

- Relieve pain associated with advanced cervical cancer
- Shrink cancer to an operable size before surgery is performed. This is called neo-adjuvant chemotherapy. It can help prevent cervical cancer from spreading.

The Drugs Most Often Used

The cytotoxic (cancer-killing) drugs most often used to treat advanced or recurrent cervical cancer are *cisplatin (Cisplatinum®, Platinol®), ifosfamide (Ifex®)*, and *5-fluorouracil (5-FU)*. Taken by mouth or injected into a vein, these drugs enter the bloodstream and destroy cancer cells that have spread from the cervix to distant parts of the body.

Other drugs that have been used to treat cervical cancer include *carboplatin (Paraplatin®), methotrexate, bleomycin, mitomycin C (Mutamycin®),* and *vincristine (Oncovin®).*

Paclitaxel (Taxol®), a drug used in breast cancer, is also being tested in clinical studies of cervical cancer.

Chemotherapy usually is administered at an outpatient facility, physician's office, or in the patient's home; but a woman who is in poor health may be hospitalized for treatment. Chemotherapy treatments alternate with recovery periods that allow a woman to rest and regain her strength before the next round of therapy begins.

Combination chemotherapy (a combination of two or more chemotherapy drugs) may be more effective than any single drug. When used in association with surgery or radiation, chemotherapy can help to prevent the spread or recurrence of cervical cancer. Recent clinical trials have shown that *cisplatin* combined with radiation therapy improves survival rates for women with advanced cervical cancer.

A woman undergoing chemotherapy may experience side effects such as:

- Nausea and vomiting
- Appetite changes
- Mouth sores
- Vaginal sores
- Hair loss (temporary)
- Fatigue
- Bruising and bleeding
- Susceptibility to infection
- Anemia
- Menstrual cycle changes
- Early menopause
- Infertility

Side effects generally subside after treatment is completed Most women who undergo chemotherapy for cervical cancer are already infertile as a result of surgery or radiation therapy. Physicians may prescribe hormones to help with symptoms of premature menopause.

Biological Therapy

Biological therapy can be used to treat cancer that has spread from the cervix to other parts of the body. Interferon-a cell protein that provides immunity to viral infections-is the type of biological therapy most often used. Biological therapy is usually administered on an outpatient basis and is sometimes combined with chemotherapy.

"Flu-like" side effects, among other complaints, have been reported by women who undergo biological therapy. These include:

- Fever and/or chills
- Muscle aches
- Weakness
- Diarrhea
- Rash
- Appetite loss
- Nausea or vomiting
- Easy bleeding or bruising

Side effects can be severe, but they generally subside after treatment is completed.

Other Therapies

A woman whose cancer is advanced and whose chance of survival is poor may choose to:

- Combine standard therapies with experimental treatment
- Enroll in a clinical trial designed to measure the effectiveness of new treatments for cervical cancer

The recurrence (return) of cervical cancer can be:

- Localized-confined to the pelvic organs near the cervix, or
- Metastatic-widespread throughout the bloodstream or lymphatic system to distant organs like the lungs, or bone.

Pelvic exenteration is a treatment option for recurrent cervical cancer that is limited to the pelvic area. This rare procedure involves the removal of the *uterus*, related lymph nodes and tissues, and, possibly, the bladder, rectum, part of the colon, and/or vagina. Recurrent cancer cannot be eliminated in about 60% of affected women. In such cases, palliative (pain-relieving) radiation therapy or chemotherapy may reduce symptoms.

Chemotherapy and radiation are also used to relieve symptoms associated with cervical cancer that has spread to distant organs. These treatments can provide temporary relief in 15 to 25% of women with this disease.

Some women with cervical cancer that has spread may choose to enroll in clinical trials designed to evaluate *systemic* (whole-body) chemotherapy and other new treatments for this form of the disease.

Fibroids

A fibroid is the most common tumor (abnormal mass of tissue) found in the pelvis. Such a tumor develops most often between the ages of 35 and 45 years, seldom before age 20. Fibroids do not occur at all before puberty. After a woman completes menopause, they generally stop growing and may even disappear.

Usually a fibroid is found in the uterus where it is the most common form of uterine mass. A fibroid can also develop on another structure that contains smooth muscle cells. In very rare cases, it can even "invade" another organ when it grows too large to confine itself to its original location.

A fibroid is a solid tumor that contains mostly smooth muscle held together by fibrous tissue. (That's how it came by its popular name.) Other names for fibroids are *leiomyomas, myomas, fibromas,* and *fibromyomas.*

Fibroids usually occur as multiple tumors that tend to grow very slowly. Sometimes, however, a woman may have a single fibroid the size of a grapefruit or even one so large that it fills the entire abdomen. On the other hand, a fibroid tumor may be so small that it can be seen only under a microscope. It can weigh as much as 25 or 50 pounds, with the largest fibroid tumor ever reported weighing more than 140 pounds.

It is difficult to know just how many women have fibroids, since unless they cause a problem, a woman may never realize she has them. It is, however, estimated that fibroids occur in about 30 percent of women aged 25 to 45. They are more common in women who are overweight. Your risk is lower if you have had a baby or if you smoke.

For some reason, black women seem more likely to develop fibroids than women in other racial groups. Almost half of all black women more than 30 years of age have fibroids compared with 20 percent of white women of the same age group. Interestingly, studies have found a low incidence of fibroids among women in Africa. Overall, however, fibroids tend to be larger and more numerous in black women at diagnosis.

TYPES

The type of problems that fibroids cause depends on their location. Therefore, your doctor's first concern will be to pinpoint the exact location of the tumors. It is this information that determines the best course of treatment.

Fibroids are categorized by their location. The various types include:

- Submucous fibroid
- Intramural fibroid
- Subserous fibroid
- Pedunculated fibroid
- Interligamentous fibroid
- Parasitic fibroid

Submucous fibroid: This type occurs just beneath the lining of the uterus and can displace the lining as it grows. This displacement can lead to menstrual irregularities and discomfort. After a while, this fibroid may develop a thin stalk called a pedicle. The stalk remains attached to the uterine wall, but the fibroid is able to "travel." When this happens, the tumor may protrude into the uterus, which will then contract in an attempt to rid itself of this foreign body. The fibroid may also enter the vagina. As the fibroid moves around, the stalk may become twisted and lose blood, causing bleeding between periods. Infection may also occur.

Intramural fibroid: This round tumor is most commonly found within the uterine wall. The uterus can become enlarged as the intramural fibroid grows.

Subserous fibroid: This type grows on the outer wall of the uterus, sometimes jutting out from the lining. A subserous fibroid can grow overly large without causing any recognizable symptoms—until it interferes with other organs, creating problems there.

Pedunculated fibroid: Such a tumor develops when a subserous fibroid grows a stalk called a peduncle. As these tumors get bigger and bigger, the original blood supply may not be sufficient to feed the fibroid. If the tumor becomes twisted or begins to degenerate as the blood supply diminishes, it can cause severe pain.

Interligamentous fibroid: This tumor, which grows sideways between the layers of the broad ligament (band of fibrous connective tissue) supporting the uterus, is extremely difficult to remove without interfering with important organs or the blood supply to the uterus.

Parasitic fibroid: When a fibroid attaches itself to another organ, it transforms itself into the rarest of all types, the parasitic fibroid. As the tumor establishes a new source of blood, its uterine stalk gradually degenerates until the fibroid is no longer attached to the uterus at all.

Fibroids: The Five Major Types (Fig. 16.1)

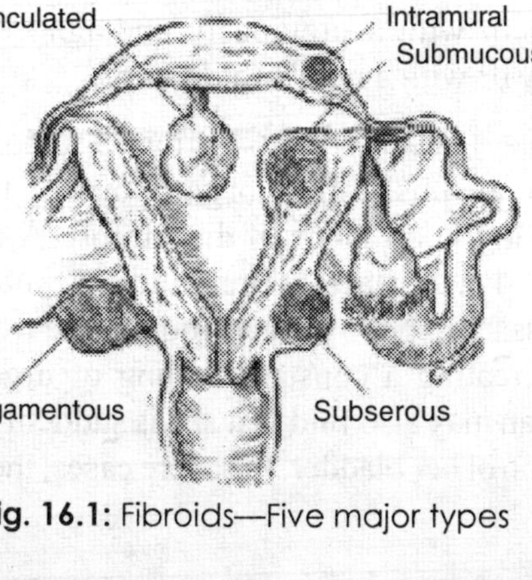

Fig. 16.1: Fibroids—Five major types

Classified by their location within and around the uterus, the noncancerous growths known as fibroids can grow for years without causing a problem—and may vanish after menopause. *Submucous* fibroids lie just below the inner lining of the uterus, *subserous* below the outer lining, and *intramural* deep within the uterine wall. If one of these growths develops a stalk, it's called a *pedunculated* fibroid. When found in the ligaments that support the uterus, it's an *interligamentous* fibroid. If a fibroid causes any symptoms at all, the first one is likely to be excessive menstrual bleeding.

SYMPTOMS AND DIAGNOSIS

A fibroid tumor, one of the masses a physician most frequently feels during a pelvic examination, is easily recognized during exploratory surgery. Many, many fibroid tumors, however, are discovered while a physician is looking for something else—or simply are not discovered at all. If a woman experiences no unpleasant symptoms, there may be no reason to look for them.

On the other hand, the mere presence of fibroid tumors can interfere with the doctor's general assessment of your health. Fibroid tumors that grow near the ovaries can make it impossible for the doctor to feel the ovaries and determine whether they are healthy—a big concern for women older than 40 years of age.

Ultrasound scanning enables physicians to distinguish these tumors. This diagnostic procedure can confirm the presence of fibroids when a woman has symptoms that raise suspicion of the tumors. However, because certain types of fibroids look similar to ovarian tumors, and the fibrous tissue can interfere with the sound waves, it's possible for the ultrasound reading to be in accurate.

A basic pelvic exam—during which the physician determines whether the uterus has become unusually large—provides a diagnosis most of the time. However, after reviewing the results of the examination and considering your specific symptoms, the physician may conduct additional procedures. For example, *hysteroscopy* allows the physician to "see" inside the uterus by using a small, lighted tube. *Sonohysterography,* a sort of "internal ultrasound," is performed through the vagina after filling the uterus with sterile water.

In rare cases the only way a physician can be sure is to look inside via an operation. The decision to operate depends on the particular symptoms, on what the doctor suspects is the cause, and on considerations such as a woman's likelihood of developing ovarian cancer or other disorders that might be overlooked because of the fibroids. The Classic Symptoms

Though most fibroids do not produce any symptoms, when they do cause problems—as happens in about 25 percent of those with fibroids—women are most likely to complain of (1) excessive bleeding, (2) pain, and (3) a swollen abdomen. (Actually the stomach isn't any bigger—the problem is the uterus, which stretches as the fibroids grow, pushing the intestines upward.) If symptoms develop, physicians typically find six or seven tumors in the uterus.

- Excessive bleeding
- Pain
- Swollen Abdomen
- Infertility

Excessive bleeding occurs in about 30 percent of the women with fibroids. Most often the bleeding is caused by a type of fibroid tumor that grows underneath the endometrium, or lining of the uterus. As the tumors grow, the lining stretches, thins, and becomes distorted, all of which produce bleeding.

When a woman develops abnormal bleeding, she notices that her menstural flow is heavier, but that it lasts—at least at first—for the same number of days. She frequently will find, however, that after a while her periods are lasting longer. Some women, in fact, bleed almost constantly. Excessive blood loss drains iron from a woman's body causing anemia.

To determine whether the bleeding is related to fibroid tumors or to some other problem, the doctor may prescribe a certain type of birth control pills. It may also be necessary for the doctor to scrape the inside of the uterus and examine the tissue in a procedure called dilation and curettage or a D&C. One of the physician's major concerns is to make sure that a cancerous growth is not present alongside fibroids.

Pain, if it accompanies fibroids, will generally occur during the menstrual cycle but, more commonly, will not occur at all. With fibroid-related pain, women who have had relatively pain-free menstrual cycles for years may suddenly become very uncomfortable. They experience painful spasms or cramps similar to those felt during labor. Indeed, the fibroid may act like a foreign body, and the uterus responds by contracting, trying to get rid of it.

If a fibroid presses on the pelvic nerves, the woman may feel hip or back pain. If the tumor becomes twisted or begins to deteriorate, the pain may be felt as a sudden severe stabbing in the lower abdomen. Sexual intercourse may also become uncomfortable.

Pain that occurs between menstrual periods is seldom caused by uncomplicated fibroid tumors. When this kind of pain is the problem, the doctor needs to seek another cause. There could be a problem with a previously undiagnosed pregnancy or with a nonfibroid tumor.

Swollen Abdomen: As fibroid tumors grow, they can push other organs out of the way resulting in all kinds of discomfort. A growing fibroid can flatten the bladder, making it necessary to go to the bathroom more frequently and creating a constant feeling of urgency. A woman may also find that she is suddenly unable to control her bladder. In severe cases, the fibroid may push on the urethra or urinary canal so hard that she cannot urinate at all and has to be catheterized. If the tumor extends towards the back and leans on the lower bowel, a woman is likely to develop a backache, become constipated, and find it difficult to have a bowel movement.

Infertility: Fibroids can make it difficult for a woman to become pregnant or, if she does become pregnant, to carry the baby for the full nine months. Many things can happen to interfere with conception, with the fertilized egg's implantation in the uterus, and with the baby's growth. Tumors can block the sperm's pathway to the egg by distorting the uterus or pushing the cervix, or opening of the birth canal, out of alignment with the uterus. Large tumors can pinch the fallopian tubes, interfering with the egg's journey to the uterus.

Most fibroids are found underneath the lining of the uterus. As they grow, the lining above them stretches and may not receive enough nourishment. A fertilized egg may not be able to implant itself properly on the fibroid-distorted lining; and even if the egg does manage to attach itself to the thinned out lining, it may not hold on for the full nine months. The pregnancy will then end in a miscarriage. It is also difficult for the egg to attach itself to the lining if the woman constantly suffers bleeding.

As the pregnancy progresses, fibroids may occupy space meant for the baby. The tumors may also keep the uterus from expanding to accommodate a growing baby. Either of these situations could result in miscarriage or premature labor.

Fibroids may also interfere with the baby's birth, making it necessary for delivery by cesarean section. For example, the uterus may not be able to contract sufficiently, resulting in ineffective labor. Or the baby may not have enough room to assume the proper position for a normal birth. Tumors in or near the birth canal can block the baby's progress. After the baby is born, fibroids may also increase the amount of maternal bleeding.

Fibroids do not prevent most women from conceiving and delivering healthy babies. But when fibroids do cause problems, they are likely to be serious. Indeed, when a woman has a history of miscarriages, a physician will think "fibroids" and try to establish or rule out the presence of these tumors. However, there are many causes of infertility, so only a thorough evaluation can determine whether fibroids are the culprit. If they do prove to be the reason, surgery to remove them will take care of the problem for many women.

TREATMENT

The decision to actively treat fibroids can only be made on an individual basis. Most women require no treatment at all. If the tumors are small and cause no problems, most physicians will simply schedule an examination every six months to make sure the fibroids aren't growing. Reasons for Treatment

Your doctor may decide to treat fibroids if they start growing rapidly, cause serious pain or discomfort, or may interfere with your ability to become pregnant. In the following situations, physicians are likely to proceed more aggressively:

- Bleeding
- Sudden enlargement of fibroids
- Pain, pressure and other discomfort
- Location of the tumors
- Myomectomy
- Hysterectomy

Bleeding: This is often the primary indication for surgery particularly if the woman is experiencing an extremely heavy flow during her menstrual period and notices blood clots. Persistent bleeding greatly reduces the amount of iron in the body, producing anemia that does not respond well to treatment.

Sudden enlargement of fibroids: Rapid growth of fibroids at any age is cause for concern, but this is particularly so after menopause, when the tumors should be shrinking due to decreased estrogen production. The doctor must make sure that not a single one of the tumors is malignant. Although almost all fibroids are benign, a malignant tumor could be hidden among them. It is important to note that malignancy is not the only explanation for sudden enlargement of fibroids. This often happens during pregnancy. In women who are not pregnant, bleeding and deterioration inside the tumor are commonly at fault.

Pain, pressure and other discomfort: If the symptoms caused by fibroids become intolerable, the fibroids must be treated. Each woman must decide for herself whether she has reached this stage.

If the fibroids interfere with other organ systems, surgery may clearly be necessary. For example, fibroid tumors that encroach on the urinary system may cause so much pressure and crowding that a woman is almost unable to urinate.

Location of the tumors: Sometimes fibroids must be removed because their location is likely to cause serious problems sooner or later, as with tumors that obscure the ovaries. In addition, certain types of fibroids resemble ovarian tumors—a fact of particular concern for women over the age of 40, when the danger of ovarian tumors increases. Surgery

When the problems caused by fibroids are severe enough to require treatment, it may be necessary to remove not only the tumors, but also the uterus. The type of surgery performed depends on the woman's age; the type of symptoms she is experiencing; the size, number, and location of the fibroids; and whether she plans to have children in the future. Following are descriptions of two forms of surgery—myomectomy and hysterectomy.

Myomectomy: Understandably, the prospect of any type of gynecologic surgery is upsetting to a woman who hopes to become pregnant. Yet continued presence of fibroids may in itself make pregnancy impossible. For women faced with this dilemma, a myomectomy is the procedure of choice.

A myomectomy is the surgical removal of each tumor separately without damaging or disturbing the uterus. The procedure is successful in almost all women who choose to have it performed. Generally, it doesn't matter how numerous or how big the fibroids are or where they are located.

When performing a myomectomy, the surgeon tries to remove as many tumors as possible while making as few surgical cuts as possible. It is sometimes feasible to remove certain tumors through the vagina, or belly button, but in most cases the surgeon has to make an abdominal incision. During the operation, the surgeon closes up the spaces in the uterine lining where the fibroids used to be so that blood will not collect there afterward.

The possibility of blood loss is a major concern during surgery, but there are procedures and drugs that allow surgeons to limit bleeding during and after the operation. Because the fibroids are removed one at a time, surgery can take several hours—much longer than removal of the entire uterus.

It is important to remember that women who have had fibroids once are likely to have them again. The likelihood of a recurrence depends on a woman's age, race, and whether most of her tumors were removed during the procedure. Estimates vary, but one quarter to half of the women who have a myomectomy can expect to eventually develop additional tumors.

While a second—or even a third—myomectomy is an option if the tumors return, multiple myomectomies can lead to problems. The walls of the uterus, for example, can stick together due to scarring which can make it harder to become pregnant. Or the bowel may become blocked. Or there could be so much bleeding that a transfusion is necessary. Unfortunately, many, if not most, of the women who develop additional fibroids eventually have to undergo a hysterectomy.

Despite these possible drawbacks, the improved outlook for preserving a woman's fertility makes myomectomy an increasingly popular choice for younger patients. And, the fact is that most women who have fibroids will *not* have to have a hysterectomy.

Hysterectomy: When fibroids cause severe complications, a hysterectomy, or removal of the uterus, will probably be necessary. Removing the uterus effectively removes the fibroids, because most of these tumors are attached to the uterus. Hysterectomy is generally considered the procedure of choice when:

- A woman who has completed her family and whose uterus has grown to the size that would accommodate a 12-week old fetus suffers from severe symptoms
- There are extensive or especially large tumors
- The bleeding caused by fibroids is debilitating
- The fibroids are creating problems with other organs in the body

Because a hysterectomy leaves the ovaries intact, a woman does not automatically face menopause after the operation. The decision to preserve or remove a woman's ovaries generally depends on her age at the time of surgery. The current practice is to perform the procedure as a last resort.

There has been much criticism of unnecessary hysterectomies; and fibroids are the justification in an estimated 30 percent of cases. Limiting this surgery—which remains the only true cure for fibroids—to older women who do not plan to become pregnant and who have serious symptoms should naturally reduce the number of hysterectomies performed. Other Options

Physicians have been evaluating less invasive surgical procedures, as well as ways to treat fibroid tumors without any surgery at all. Some doctors have begun using lasers to either shrink or remove these tumors. Others have been experimenting with techniques such as myolysis. In this procedure, a small needle is snaked to the tumor through a tube inserted in the abdominal wall. The needle delivers electrical current to cauterize the blood supply that feeds the tumor, prompting the fibroid to gradually shrink and possibly even disappear. Cryomyolysis is essentially the same procedure, except that a probe is used to freeze the tumor. These techniques, which could be performed at an outpatient facility, seem to be promising. However, research is still needed to make sure they can be used in women who may want to become pregnant afterward.

Another new technique, uterine artery embolization, also aims to starve the tumor by blocking its blood supply. This procedure, which is considered to be low-risk, is performed by a radiologist. A catheter is inserted into the femoral artery in the thigh through a small incision in the groin. With the help of an X-ray picture, the catheter is then guided up into the uterine artery. Small, plastic sand-like particles are then released through the catheter to block the tiny arteries supplying the tumor. Currently recommended only for women who have severe fibroid-related bleeding, the procedure doesn't require anesthesia, enjoys a high success rate, and does not appear to interfere with fertility. However, we don't know whether this approach will actually improve a woman's chances of becoming pregnant if failure to conceive has been a problem.

Endometrial ablation also has proved effective in women who experience excessive bleeding. One method involves inserting a balloon catheter into the uterus. Once in place, the catheter is filled with sterilized liquid, which is then heated. The heat destroys the endometrial tissue, and the bleeding stops. The good news is that destroying the lining of the uterus eliminates the fibroid problem. The bad news, of course, is that the procedure also eliminates the option of subsequent pregnancies. Although ablation is generally safer than using lasers or cauterization, this approach is still under investigation. It is possible that the bleeding could return.

In several scientific studies, fibroids have responded quite dramatically to treatment with synthetic forms of the naturally occurring substance known as gonadotropin-releasing hormone (also called GnRH). These agents, which include the drugs Lupron, Synarel, and Zoladex, work by decreasing blood flow to the uterus, thereby starving the tumors. Most women who have used Lupron, for instance, have had their fibroids shrink to half their starting size.

The treatments do have drawbacks. The drugs have to be taken regularly, either by self-injection or as a nasal spray. Once treatments stop, the tumors grow back within 4 to 6 months; and while some women have no problems during treatment, potential side effects can be severe. The drugs suppress the amount of estrogen in the body, so patients often suffer the complaints commonly associated with menopause, including hot flashes, vaginal dryness, mood swings, and trouble concentrating.

Sustained suppression of estrogen can also lead to weakening of the bones (osteoporosis), so the drug is typically used for only 3 to 6 months. Preliminary studies, however, have shown that it may be possible to counteract bone loss (and other menopausal-like side effects) by adding back small amounts of estrogen and progesterone. By doing this, physicians should be able to maintain uterine and fibroid shrinkage and control fibroid-related bleeding for longer periods of time. The best results in these studies occur when the "add-back" hormones are given in the lower menopausal replacement dosages (compared to the higher hormone doses commonly used in birth control pills) *and* when the hormones are added *after* the uterus and fibroids have had a chance to shrink.

Drug therapy is regarded as especially helpful for women who are trying to become pregnant or plan to have surgery. The treatments can also be used as a "holding action" for women who are nearing menopause—when the fibroids will shrink on their own. It will effectively delay surgery until it becomes unnecessary.

CANCERS OF THE PENIS

Each of the tissues in the penis contains several types of cells. Different types of penile cancer (cancer of the penis) can develop in each kind of cell. The differences are important, because they determine the seriousness of the cancer and the type of treatment needed. About 95% of penile cancers develop from flat, scale-like skin cells called *squamous* cells.

Like most other forms of nonmelanoma skin cancer, these tumors tend to grow slowly. When detected in the early stages, these tumors can usually be cured. Squamous cell penile cancers can develop anywhere on the organ, but most develop on the foreskin (in men who have not been circumcised) or on the glans.

Verrucous carcinoma is an uncommon form of squamous cell cancer that can occur on the male or female genitals, skin, mouth, larynx, and anus. Verrucous carcinoma of the genitals is sometimes also called a *Bushke-Lowenstein tumor*. Due to its appearance, it is often difficult to distinguish from a benign genital wart (see the section "Benign and Precancerous Conditions" for more information). These low-grade cancers can spread deeply into surrounding tissue but very rarely do they metastasize.

A very rare type of penile cancer called *adenocarcinoma* can develop from sweat glands in the skin of the penis. *Paget's disease* of the penis is a condition in which adenocarcinoma cells are found in the penile skin. The cancer cells at first spread within the skin, but may eventually invade underneath the skin and spread to lymph nodes. Paget's disease can affect skin anywhere in the body but most often affects skin of the perianal area, vulva, and the breasts. This condition should not be confused with Paget's disease of the bone, an entirely different disease also named after Dr. James Paget.

The earliest stage of squamous cell cancer of the penis (or any other organ) is called squamous cell *carcinoma in situ* (abbreviated as *CIS*). Penile CIS is contained entirely within the skin of the penis and has not yet spread to deeper tissues of the penis. Depending on the exact location of a CIS of the penis, doctors may give additional names to the disease. CIS of the glans is sometimes called *erythroplasia of Queyrat*. The same condition, when found on the shaft of the penis (or skin of other parts of the body), is called *Bowen's disease*.

About 2% of penile cancers develop from pigment-producing skin cells called *melanocytes*. Cancers of these cells are called *melanoma*. These cancers are more dangerous because they grow and spread more rapidly. Melanomas usually develop from sun-exposed areas of skin. Although sun exposure is an important risk factor for melanoma, a few of these cancers can develop on the penis, or other areas not likely to become sunburned.

Basal cell cancers are most common cancers of sun exposed areas of skin, such as the face, neck and arms. Basal cell cancers represent less than 2% of penile cancers. They are slowly growing tumors that very rarely spread to other parts of the body.

The remaining 1% of penile cancer consists mostly of sarcomas, cancers that develop from the blood vessels, smooth muscle, and other connective tissue cells of the penis.

Benign and Precancerous Conditions

Sometimes abnormal growths develop on the penis which are benign (not cancerous). Some of these benign growths may eventually evolve into invasive cancer if they are not treated. These premalignant conditions can resemble warts or irritated patches of skin. Like penile cancer, they usually develop on the glans or on the foreskin, but they can also occur along the shaft of the penis.

Condylomas are wart-like growths that resemble tiny cauliflowers. Some are so small that they are apparent only when the skin is viewed under a magnifying lens. Others may reach an inch or more in diameter.

Squamous cell cancer of the penis usually forms slowly over many years, and is usually preceded by precancerous changes that may last for several years. The medical terms for this precancerous condition are *penile intraepithelial neoplasia*, or dysplasia. "Intraepithelial" means that the precancerous cells are confined to the epithelium (surface layer of the penile skin).

WHAT ARE THE KEY STATISTICS ABOUT PENILE CANCER?

The American Cancer Society estimates that in 2001 about 1,200 new cases of penile cancer will be diagnosed in the United States. An estimated 300 men will die of penile cancer during 2001 in the United States. The incidence rate of penile cancer in the United States is about 0.001%, which means it occurs in about 1 man out of 100,000.

Penile cancer is very rare in North America and Europe. It accounts for about 0.2% of cancers in men and 0.1% of cancer deaths in men in the United States. However, penile cancer is much more common in some parts of Africa and South America, where it accounts for up to 10% of cancers in men.

The overall 5-year survival rate for all stages of penile cancer together is about 50%. When penile cancer is detected early, treatment is simplest, most effective and less likely to result in significant side effects or complications.

The 5-year survival rate refers to the percent of patients who live at least 5 years after their cancer is diagnosed. Many of these patients live much longer than 5 years after diagnosis, and 5-year rates are used to produce a standard way of discussing prognosis. Five-year *relative* survival rates exclude from the calculations patients dying of other diseases, and are considered to be a more accurate way to describe the prognosis for patients with a particular type and stage of cancer. Of course, 5-year survival rates are based on patients diagnosed and initially treated more than 5 years ago. Improvements in treatment often result in a more favorable outlook for recently diagnosed patients.

TESTICULAR CANCER

Testicular cancer (also called cancer of the testicle, or cancer of the testis) is a *malignant*, or cancerous, growth of the testicle, one of the male sex organs.

Cancer of the testicle is rare, occurring most commonly in young to middle-aged men. It is very rare before puberty or in old age.

There are two basic types of testicular cancer:

- *Seminoma:* Made of a single type of cell-most likely from the same type of cell that produces sperm. Makes up about 40% of testicular cancers
- *Nonseminoma:* A group of cancers that consist of several different cell types. Makes up about 60% of testicular cancers

Other cancers affecting the testicle are extremely rare and develop from:

- Testicular tissue
- Lymphatic tissue (tissue associated with the lymph nodes of the immune system).

Testicular cancer is one of the most common cancers in young men between the ages of 15 and 34. However, other age groups are also susceptible, so all men should be aware of its symptoms.

In the fairly recent past, testicular cancer was considered a dangerous and difficult cancer to treat. Advances in treatment have drastically altered the picture.

Today, most men diagnosed with testicular cancer-especially when diagnosed at an early stage-can expect to survive the disease. *In fact, when detected early, the overall cure rate for testicular cancer is greater than 90 percent.*

Even for those men with advanced testicular cancer, the cure rate is about 70 percent.

Facts About Testicular Cancer

- Testicular cancer usually strikes men between the ages of 15 and 35, and is one of the most common cancers in men in this age group.

- Testicular cancer is rare; it accounts for only about 1% of all cancers in men.
- Testicular cancer is more common in Caucasian men than in men of other ethnic groups.
- When found and diagnosed early, testicular cancer has a cure rate of 90%.
- It has been suggested that the risk of testicular cancer may be higher in men affected with the HIV virus (the virus that causes AIDS), but the evidence is weak and unsubstantiated so far.
- About 7500 cases are reported annually in the USA

The cause of testicular cancer is largely unknown. As yet, there is no identifiable link between testicular cancer and genetics, habits, lifestyles, or activities.

There is some evidence that the risk of testicular cancer is higher in men whose testicles failed to descend normally through the *inguinal canal* to the scrotum before birth or by the age of three.

Because of this slightly higher risk for testicular cancer, if a testicle has not descended by birth, or an undescended testicle is detected in a child, surgery is performed to place the testicle into its normal position soon after it is detected.

SYMPOMATOLOGY OF TESTICULAR CANCER

The earliest symptoms of testicular cancer are:

- Pain, swelling, or hardness in the testicle, or some combination of these symptoms
- A small, painless lump on the testicle
- A "heaviness" in the scrotum
- An ache in the lower abdomen or groin
- An accumulation of blood or fluid in the scrotum
- Any change in the way a testicle feels.

In rare cases, a man will feel tenderness in his breast area. When this happens, it is usually caused by one variety of testicular cancer, in which high levels of a particular hormone called human chorionic gonadotropin, or HCG, are secreted by the growth in the testicle

None of these symptoms are positive signs of cancer. But if any of these symptoms last longer than two weeks, a doctor should be consulted.

All cancers should be diagnosed and treated as soon as possible, but it is especially important in testicular cancer. The sooner cancer is found and treated, the better the chances of complete recovery.

One of the most effective ways of finding a tumor is by testicular self-examination on a monthly basis.

Most lumps in the testicle are cancerous, but noncancerous masses and cysts can arise from other causes, such as infection.

If a suspicious lump is found, the initial steps toward diagnosis include:

- Physical examination
- Specialized tests.

Physical Examination

When symptoms suggest a cancer in a testicle, the doctor:

- Will ask about personal and family history
- Will perform a complete physical examination
- May order a blood test, urine test, and/or chest X-ray.

Specialized Tests

These may include:

- *Ultrasound of testicles:* The doctor also may order an ultrasound of the testicles. Ultrasound is a painless test that uses sound waves to produce images of the inner body, and can usually distinguish between normal and abnormal structures. It cannot tell whether any abnormal tissue is actually cancer.

- *CT scan or MRI,* high tech tests in which computers are used to produce precise images of the inside of the testis.

If these tests are inconclusive, or if cancer is strongly suspected, an operation called an inguinal orchiectomy is performed.

The outlook for testicular cancer is excellent.

- Researchers have found more and better ways to diagnose and treat this disease, and recovery has dramatically improved.
- The majority of men treated for testicular cancer today are cured by their initial treatment.
- Many of those who experience a recurrence can be cured as well.
- Doctors emphasize that, while the cure rate is very high for all types and stages of testicular cancer, many of the drastic measures undertaken to cure later-stage disease can be avoided if the cancer is diagnosed early.

The best way to find testicular cancer is through regular self-examination.

Testicular Self-Examination (TSE)

A simple procedure called testicular self-examination (TSE), undertaken just once a month, can improve the chance of finding a testicular tumor.

TSE should be performed after a warm bath or shower, because heat relaxes the scrotum and makes it easier to find anything unusual.

The National Cancer Institute recommends following these simple steps every month:

1. Stand (without clothing) in front of a mirror. Visually check for any swelling on the skin of the scrotum.
2. Examine each testicle with both hands. Place the index and middle fingers under the testicle with the thumbs placed on top. Roll the testicle gently between the thumbs and fingers. It's normal for one testicle to be slightly larger than the other.
3. Locate the epididymis-a soft, tube-like structure behind the testicle. If a man is familiar with the epididymis, he won't mistake it for a suspicious lump. Cancerous lumps are usually found on the sides of the testicle, but some appear on the front.
4. If you find a lump-or anything suspicious-see the doctor immediately. The abnormality may not be cancer, but if it is, the chances are great it can spread if not stopped by treatment. Remember that testicular cancer is highly curable when diagnosed and treated promptly.

One of the first things the doctor does when testicular cancer is diagnosed is to determine the stage of the disease. This investigation is called "staging" and was developed to describe the extent of the cancer growth. It allows the physician to customize the treatment.

Testicular cancer is "staged' by information obtained from the surgical findings as well as from one or more of the following tests:

- Tumor marker tests
- Computed tomography (CT) scan
- Magnetic Resonance Imaging (MRI)
- Ultrasound
- Surgery

There are three stages of testicular cancer:

- *Stage 1:* The cancer is confined to the testicle only.
- *Stage 2:* The cancer has spread to the retroperitoneal lymph nodes, which are the lymph nodes located in the rear of the body, below the diaphragm (the muscular wall that separated the abdomen from the chest cavity).
- *Stage 3:* Cancer has spread beyond the lymph nodes to other areas of the body.

Tumor Marker Tests

Tumor markers are substances found in abnormal amounts in the blood in people with certain types of cancer. Specialized laboratory tests have been designed to identify tumor markers.

Tumor marker tests may help to determine the type of testicular cancer by identifying blood levels of the tumor markers present.

The tumor marker sought is *HCG* (human chorionic gonadotrophin), a hormone secreted by certain types of testicle tumors.

Computed Tomography (CT) Scan

CT scans are diagnostic techniques that use X-rays passed through the body at different angles to produce images.

A computer analyzes the images of the testis and shows them as cross-sections, or "slices," of the tissue being studied.

Magnetic Resonance Imaging (MRI)

Magnetic Resonance Imaging is a diagnostic technique that produces high-quality cross-sectional images of organs and structures within the body, in this case the testis, without X-rays or other radiation.

During the imaging, the patient lies within a large, hollow, cylindrical magnet and is exposed to short, harmless bursts of a powerful magnetic field.

Ultrasound

Ultrasound is a technique that uses very high frequency sound waves inaudible to the human ear. After the sound waves are passed into the body, the reflected echoes are detected and analyzed by computer to produce a picture of the tissue or organ being studied.

Surgery

When testicular cancer is suspected, the recommended procedure is to examine the suspicious tissue under a microscope. The tissue is obtained through an operation called an inguinal *orchiectomy* (surgical removal of the testicle), during which the affected testicle is removed for examination.

A biopsy by itself is usually rarely done. The proper procedure is removal of the entire testicle to confirm that cancer is present and to determine the exact type. Studies show that cutting through just the outer layer of a testicle to obtain a tissue sample can cause the spread of cancer, if it is present.

The doctor also may recommend additional surgery to remove abdominal lymph nodes. After surgery, the nodes are sent to a pathologist to determine if the testicular cancer has spread.

No one treatment works for all testicular cancer. This is because the two basic types of testicular cancer-seminomas and nonseminomas-differ in:

- Their tendency to spread
- The way they spread
- How they respond to radiation therapy

Because of these different characteristics, seminomas and nonseminomas require different treatments. The treatment combinations are chosen depending on the tumor type and the stage of the disease.

Once the stage of testicular cancer has been determined, the cancer can be treated in several different ways:

- Surgery to remove the testicle
- Radiation therapy
- Chemotherapy
- A combination of the above

Surgery

When testicular cancer is suspected, the affected testicle is removed and examined under a microscope. This procedure is called an inguinal *orchiectomy* (surgical removal of the testicle), and it involves removing the testicle from the scrotum.

Presurgical preparations include:

- The patient is instructed to have nothing to eat or drink after midnight the night before the procedure.
- Sometimes (depending on the doctor and/or the insurance) the patient is admitted to the hospital the day or night before the procedure; on other occasions, the patient is admitted the day of the surgery.

The operation is performed either with general anesthesia (in which the patient is asleep) or local anesthesia (in which the area of surgery is numbed, and the patient is sedated but awake).

- An incision is made in the groin and the testicle is "delivered" from the scrotal sac up into the groin incision. This is to avoid an incision through the scrotum to the cancerous testicle, which may lead to spreading of the cancer.
- The testicle is "delivered" after the spermatic cord (which connects the testicle to structures within the abdomen) has been clamped. Once delivered, the testicle with its cord clamped can be more safely handled without spreading the cancer.
- The entire suspected testicle is removed because if the problem is cancer, cutting through the outer layer of the testicle to obtain a tissue sample might cause spreading of the disease.
- After removal of the testicle, the incision is closed with stitches.

After Surgery

- Complete healing can be expected without complications.
- The patient is advised to wear an athletic supporter and to avoid vigorous exercise for a month or so after the operation.

Radiation Therapy

Radiation therapy (also called radiotherapy, cobalt treatment, or irradiation) uses high-energy X-rays to treat cancer. Like surgery, radiation therapy is a local treatment, only affecting cells in the treated area.

Chemotherapy

Chemotherapy is the use of specialized drugs to treat cancer. Chemotherapy is used when:

- There are signs that the cancer has spread
- The doctor suspects that cancer remains after surgery or radiation

The drugs used for treatment are usually a combination of *cisplatin* and *etoposide*, two drugs that control the disease with minimal side effects.

Other drugs approved for use with testicular cancer include:

- Ifosamide (*Ifex*)
- Vinblastine sulfate (*Velban*)
- Bleomycin sulfate (*Blenoxane*)

Treatment For Seminomas

Seminomas are generally slow growing, with a tendency to stay localized-that is, in the testicle-so it is not usually necessary to remove lymph nodes.

Seminomas are especially susceptible to radiation, which effectively destroys any cancer cells that might be in the retroperitoneal lymph nodes.

When seminomas are diagnosed in Stage 1 or 2, treatment is usually a combination of:

- Testicle removal
- Radiation
- Chemotherapy

When seminomas are diagnosed in Stage 3, treatment is usually chemotherapy.

Treatment For Nonseminomas

Most nonseminomas are diagnosed in the later stages. Even so, when confined to the testicle, this type of cancer is usually treated with:

- Testicle removal
- Careful follow-up for at least two years

About 10% of Stage 1 nonseminomas recur (come back again). If this happens, treatment includes chemotherapy.

When nonseminoma cancer is diagnosed in Stage 2, and patients have had testicle and lymph node removal, they may need no further therapy. However, some specialists recommend a short course of chemotherapy to reduce the risk of recurrence.

Stage 3 nonseminomas is usually treated with chemotherapy.

Kidney Tumors

Renal cell cancer, also called renal adenocarcinoma, or hypernephroma, can often be cured if it is diagnosed and treated when still localized to the kidney and to immediately surrounding tissue. The probability of cure is directly related to the stage or degree of tumor dissemination. Even when regional lymphatics or blood vessels are involved with tumor, a significant number of patients can achieve prolonged survival and probable cure. When distant metastases are present, disease-free survival is poor, although occasional selected patients will survive after surgical resection of all known tumor. Because a majority of patients are diagnosed when the tumor is still relatively localized and amenable to surgical removal, approximately 40% of all patients with renal cancer survive 5 years. Occasional patients with locally advanced or metastatic disease may exhibit indolent courses lasting several years. Late tumor recurrence many years after initial treatment occasionally occurs.

Renal cell cancer is one of the few tumors in which well-documented cases of spontaneous tumor regression in the absence of therapy exist, but this occurs very rarely and may not lead to long-term survival. Surgical resection is the mainstay of treatment of this disease. Even in patients with disseminated tumor, locoregional forms of therapy may play an important role in palliating symptoms of the primary tumor or of ectopic hormone production. Systemic therapy has demonstrated only limited effectiveness.

CELLULAR CLASSIFICATION

Approximately 85% of renal cell cancers are adenocarcinomas, for the most part of proximal tubular origin. Most of the remainder are transitional cell carcinomas of the renal pelvis. Adenocarcinomas may be separated into clear cell and granular cell carcinomas, although the 2 cell types may occur together in some tumors. Some investigators have found that granular cell tumors have a worse prognosis, but this finding is not universal. The distinction between well-differentiated renal adenocarcinomas and renal adenomas can be difficult. The diagnosis is usually made arbitrarily on the basis of size of the mass, but size alone should not influence the treatment approach, since metastases can occur with lesions as small as 0.5 centimeters.

STAGE INFORMATION

The staging system for renal cell cancer is based on the degree of tumor spread beyond the kidney. Involvement of blood vessels may not be a poor prognostic sign if the tumor is otherwise confined to the substance of the kidney. Abnormal liver function test results may be due to a paraneoplastic syndrome that is reversible with tumor removal and do not necessarily represent metastatic disease. Except when computed tomography (CT) examination is equivocal or when iodinated contrast material is contraindicated, CT scanning is as good as or better than magnetic resonance imaging (MRI) for detecting renal masses.

TNM definitions

Primary Tumor (T)

- TX: Primary tumor cannot be assessed
- T0: No evidence of primary tumor
- T1: Tumor 7 cm or less in greatest dimension limited to the kidney

- T2: Tumor more than 7 cm in greatest dimension limited to the kidney
- T3: Tumor extends into major veins or invades adrenal gland or perinephric tissues but not beyond Gerota's fascia
  - § T3a: Tumor invades adrenal gland or perinephric tissues but not beyond Gerota's fascia
  - § T3b: Tumor grossly extends into the renal vein(s) or vena cava below the diaphragm
  - § T3c: Tumor grossly extends into the renal vein(s) or vena cava above the diaphragm
- T4: Tumor invades beyond Gerota's fascia

Regional Lymph Nodes (N)

- NX: Regional lymph nodes cannot be assessed
- N0: No regional lymph node metastasis
- N1: Metastasis in a single regional lymph node
- N2: Metastasis in more than 1 regional lymph node
- [*Note: Laterality does not affect the N classification.*]

Distant Metastasis (M)

- MX: Distant metastasis cannot be assessed
- M0: No distant metastasis
- M1: Distant metastasis

AJCC stage groupings

Stage I:

- T1, N0, M0

Stage II:

- T2, N0, M0

Stage III:

- T1, N1, M0
- T2, N1, M0
- T3a, N0, M0
- T3a, N1, M0
- T3b, N0, M0
- T3b, N1, M0
- T3c, N0, M0
- T3c, N1, M0

Stage IV:

- T4, N0, M0
- T4, N1, M0
- Any T, N2, M0
- Any T, any N, M1

Stage I Renal Cell Cancer

AJCC T1 or T2, N0, M0

Surgical resection is the accepted, often curative therapy for stage I renal cell cancer. Resection may be simple or radical. The latter operation includes removal of the kidney, adrenal gland, perirenal fat, and Gerota's fascia, with or without a regional lymph node dissection. Some, but not all, surgeons believe the radical operation yields superior results. In patients who are not candidates for surgery, external radiation therapy or arterial embolization can provide palliation. In patients with bilateral stage I neoplasms (concurrent or subsequent), bilateral partial nephrectomy or unilateral partial nephrectomy with contralateral radical nephrectomy when technically feasible may be a preferred alternative to bilateral nephrectomy with dialysis or transplantation.[1] There is increasing evidence that a partial nephrectomy is curative in selected cases. It is important to have a pathologist examine the gross specimen as well as the frozen section from the parenchymal margin of excision.

Stage II Renal Cell Cancer

AJCC TNM T3a, N0, M0

A surgical resection is the accepted, often curative therapy for stage II renal cell cancer. Resection should be radical. The operation includes removal of the kidney, adrenal gland, perirenal fat, and Gerota's fascia, with or without a regional lymph node dissection. Lymphadenectomy is commonly employed, but its effectiveness has not been definitively proven. External-beam irradiation has been given before or after nephrectomy without conclusive evidence that this improves survival compared with results of surgery alone, but may be of benefit in selected patients with more extensive tumors. In patients who are not candidates for surgery, arterial embolization can provide palliation. In patients with bilateral stage T3a neoplasms (concurrent or subsequent), bilateral partial nephrectomy or unilateral partial nephrectomy with contralateral radical nephrectomy when technically feasible may be a preferred alternative to bilateral nephrectomy with dialysis or transplantation.

Stage III Renal Cell Cancer

AJCC TNM T3b, N0, M0

A surgical resection is the accepted, often curative therapy for this stage of renal cell cancer. Resection should be radical. The operation includes removal of the kidney, adrenal gland, perirenal fat, and Gerota's fascia, with or without a regional lymph node dissection. Lymphadenectomy is commonly employed, but its effectiveness has not been definitively proven. Surgery is extended to remove the entire renal vein and caval thrombus and a portion of the vena cava as necessary. External-beam irradiation has been given before or after nephrectomy without conclusive evidence that this improves survival compared with results of surgery alone, but may be of benefit in selected patients with more extensive tumors. In patients who are not candidates for surgery, arterial embolization can provide palliation. In patients with stage T3b neoplasms who manifest concurrent or subsequent renal cell carcinoma in the contralateral kidney, a partial nephrectomy when technically feasible may be a preferred alternative to bilateral nephrectomy with dialysis or transplantation.

For patients with any T, N1-3, M0 disease: This stage of renal cell cancer is curable with surgery in a small minority of cases. A radical nephrectomy and lymph node dissection is necessary. The value of preoperative and postoperative external irradiation has not been demonstrated, but external-beam radiation therapy may be used for palliation in patients who are not candidates for surgery. Arterial embolization of the tumor with gelfoam or other materials may be employed preoperatively to reduce blood loss at nephrectomy or for palliation in patients with inoperable disease.

Stage IV Renal Cell Cancer

AJCC TNM T4, N0, M0;
or any T, any N, M1

Almost all of these patients are incurable. Tumor embolization, external-beam irradiation, and nephrectomy can aid in the palliation of symptoms due to the primary tumor or related ectopic hormone production. There is minimal evidence that nephrectomy induces regression of distant metastases. Hence, nephrectomy, in the hope that it will be followed by spontaneous regression of metastases is not advised. Spontaneous regressions occasionally occur; indeed, a prospective surveillance series of 73 patients with advanced renal cell cancer demonstrated apparent temporary objective regression in 5 (7%) patients without nephrectomy or any therapy. Selected patients with solitary or a limited number of distant metastases can achieve prolonged survival with nephrectomy and surgical resection of the metastases. This has been shown to be the case even for patients with brain metastases. The likelihood of achieving therapeutic benefit with this approach appears enhanced in patients with a long disease-free interval between the initial nephrectomy and the development of metastatic disease.

Responses to cytotoxic chemotherapy generally do not exceed 10% for any regimen that has been studied in adequate numbers of patients. Because of early reports of success, progestational agents have been administered to patients with metastatic renal cell cancer, but the frequency of response is disappointingly low, and there is no rationale for their use as anticancer therapy. They may offer subjective palliation, however. Various biologic therapies have been evaluated. Interferon alfas have approximately a 15% objective response rate in appropriately selected individuals. In general, these patients have non-bulky pulmonary and/or soft tissue metastases with excellent performance status (ECOG 0,1) and no weight loss. The interferon alfa doses used in studies reporting good response rates have been in an intermediate range, 6-20 MU-TIW. These responses are rarely complete or durable. More promising are treatments using interleukin-2 (IL-2). Administration of IL-2 appears to have a similar overall response rate to interferon alfa, but with approximately 5% of the appropriately selected patients having durable complete remissions. Combinations of IL-2 and interferon have been studied but have not been shown to be better than high-dose IL-2 alone. The optimum dose of IL-2 is unknown. High-dose therapy appears to be associated with higher response rates but with more toxic effects. Low-dose inpatient regimens can retain efficacy with fewer toxic effects, especially hypotension. Outpatient, subcutaneous administration has also demonstrated responses with acceptable toxic effects. Because of the overall poor results with drug treatment, patients with metastatic renal cell cancer should be considered for clinical trials, especially phase I and II trials evaluating newer chemotherapeutic agents and biologics such as interferons or IL-2 and strategies to modulate multidrug-resistant (MDR) phenotype, which is highly expressed in renal cell cancers.

TRANSITIONAL CELL CARCINOMA

Transitional cell carcinoma of the renal pelvis, accounting for only 7% of all kidney tumors, and transitional cell cancer of the ureter, accounting for only 1 of every 25 upper tract tumors, are curable in more than 90% of patients if they are superficial and confined to the renal pelvis or ureter. Patients with deeply invasive tumors that are still confined to the renal pelvis or ureter have a 10 to 15% likelihood of cure. Patients with tumors with penetration through the urothelial wall or with distant metastases usually cannot be cured with currently available forms of treatment. The major prognostic factor at the time of diagnosis of upper tract transitional cell cancer is the depth of infiltration into or through the uroepithelial wall. However, even if ureteroscopy and pyeloscopy are successfully implemented, accurate assessment of depth of invasion is difficult. Therefore, total excision of the ureter with a bladder cuff, renal pelvis, and kidney is recommended in an attempt to provide the greatest likelihood of cure.

Most superficial tumors are likely to be well differentiated, while infiltrative tumors are likely to be poorly differentiated. The incidence of synchronous or metachronous contralateral upper tract cancers ranges from 2 to 4%; the incidence of subsequent bladder cancer after prior upper tract transitional cell cancer ranges from 30 to 50%. When involvement of the upper tract is diffuse (involving both the renal pelvis and ureter), the likelihood of subsequent development of bladder cancer increases to 75%. DNA ploidy has not added significant prognostic information beyond that provided by stage and grade.

The majority of upper tract uroepithelial tumors are of transitional cell histology. Squamous cell cancer of the urinary tract constitutes less than 15% of the tumors of the renal pelvis and a smaller percentage of ureteral tumors and is often associated with chronic calculus disease and infection.

Grade of transitional cell cancer of the upper tract has generally been found to correlate with stage. Superficial tumors are generally grade I or II, whereas the majority of infiltrative tumors are grades III and IV. Prognosis is worse for patients with high-grade (grades III and IV) tumors than for those with low-grade (grades I and II) tumors.

Though comparable in many respects to staging systems described for bladder cancer, unique structural aspects of the renal pelvis and ureter have led to several differences in the classification schema of tumors that involve the upper tracts. Clinical staging is based on a combination of radiographic procedures (e.g., intravenous pyelogram and computed tomographic scans) and, more recently, ureteroscopy and biopsy.

The advent of rigid and flexible ureteroscopic techniques has permitted endoscopic access to the ureter and renal pelvis. This may permit greater accuracy in preoperative definition of the stage and grade of an upper tract neoplasm. In addition, fulguration and endourological access permit resection or laser coagulation of highly selected low-stage, low-grade lesions of the ureters. However, this approach is still under clinical evaluation since there is the possibility of inaccurate assessment of the stage and extent of disease, and the adequacy and risks of such treatment have not yet been defined.

Localized

Patients with localized disease may be classified into 3 groups:

- *Group 1:* Low-grade tumor confined to the urothelium without lamina propria invasion ("Papilloma" Grade I transitional cell cancer).
- *Group 2:* Grade I-III carcinomas without demonstrable subepithelial invasion or focal microscopic invasion or papillary carcinomas with carcinoma *in situ* and/or carcinoma *in situ* elsewhere in the urothelium.
- *Group 3:* High-grade tumors that have infiltrated the renal pelvic wall or renal parenchyma or both, but are still confined to the kidney. Infiltration of muscle in the upper tract may not be associated with as much potential for distant dissemination as appears to be the case for bladder cancer.

Regional

- *Group 4:* Extension of tumors beyond the renal pelvis or parenchyma and invasion of peripelvic and perirenal fat, lymph nodes, hilar vessels, and adjacent tissues.

Metastatic

- Spread of the tumor to distant tissues.

Each of these classifications has been subclassified into categories of unicentricity or multicentricity, the latter indicating a more pervasive tumor diathesis and generally a less favorable prognosis.

Although the classifications listed above have prognostic significance, they can only be determined at the time of nephroureterectomy, which is the treatment of choice for patients with this disease. Because of the high incidence of tumor recurrence within the intramural ureter among patients who have had incomplete excision of this area, nephroureterectomy should include the entire ureter and a margin of periureteral orifice mucosa ("bladder cuff").

A TNM system for staging has been established and has demonstrated accurate predictions of survival. The TNM staging system may be a better predictor of prognosis than tumor grade, although both are strongly predictive of survival. Median survival for patients with tumors confined to the subepithelial connective tissue was 91.1 months compared to 12.9 months for patients with tumors invading the muscularis and beyond in 1 report. Flow cytometry analysis identifies low-stage, low-grade tumors at high risk of recurrence by virtue of their aneuploid histograms.

The rarity of synchronous bilateral renal pelvic neoplasia, the low incidence of asynchronous development of contralateral upper tract tumors, and the increased risk of tumor recurrence in the ipsilateral ureter distal to the original pelvic tumor are the rationale for total nephroureterectomy with bladder cuff for most patients with renal pelvic transitional cell cancers and ureteral cancers.

Contemplation of anything less than total excision must take into account the potential risk for tumor recurrence anywhere in the upper tract unit. In other than unifocal, low-grade, low-stage renal pelvic tumors, the probable extensive involvement of both contiguous and noncontiguous sites would appear to make segmental excision an unnecessary option with a potentially serious risk. However, an operative possibility includes segmental excision of a particular lesion. If the extent of a tumor can be determined by intraoperative assessment, and frozen section histologic diagnosis confirms low-grade, unifocal tumor of limited size, then segmental excision is possible. However, this approach should be reserved for highly selected patients. This includes those patients who have a solitary kidney or those with decreased renal function and who require maximal preservation of renal tissue. The likelihood of tumor recurrence in this setting, and of extension of disease outside the renal pelvis once the pelvis has been violated, is a serious risk that must be heavily weighed in offering a patient this therapeutic option.

Ureteral transitional cell cancer may more readily offer the possibility of segmental excision if the absence of proximal disease can be documented. In this setting, attention is focused on the ease of reconstruction of the ureter and restoration of ureterovesical continuity. This is most feasible if the cancer is in the distal ureter. If partial ureterectomy is possible and proximal disease has been excluded, then segmental excision and ureteral reimplantation can be performed.

Systematic regional lymph node dissection in conjunction with nephroureterectomy or segmental excision has not been found to enhance the effectiveness of surgery if tumors are of high grade or high stage, since in these instances the overall results are so poor. Correspondingly, lymph node involvement is uncommon in low-stage disease, and lymphadenectomy is therefore unlikely to remove additional tumor. Thus, lymph node dissection at the time of nephrectomy may offer prognostic information, but little, if any, therapeutic benefit.

LOCALIZED TRANSITIONAL CELL CANCER OF THE RENAL PELVIS AND URETER

Standard Treatment Options

1. Nephroureterectomy with cuff of bladder.
2. Segmental resection of ureter, only if the tumor is superficial and located in distal 1/3 of ureter.

Treatment Options Under Clinical Evaluation

The development of new instrumentation for endourological treatment of upper tract transitional cell cancer has provided new options for regional management of these cancers. Introduction of electrofulguration and resection instruments or laser probes either transureterally or percutaneously may permit destruction of a primary cancer. Introduction of cytotoxic agents has also been employed. Although a biopsy can be taken for staging purposes, the accuracy of this remains to be determined. The efficacy of treatment by these maneuvers has not been established.

1. Electroresection and fulguration or laser fulguration, if the tumor is superficial.
2. Any parenchymal sparing procedure (segmental resection; ureteroscopic or percutaneous resection/fulguration/laser destruction) if the renal unit is solitary or renal function is depressed.
3. Intrapelvic or intraureteral cytotoxic/immunotherapy. The dramatic successes that have been reported with intravesical cytotoxic (thiotepa, mitomycin, doxorubicin) or immunologic/inflammatory (BCG, interferon) therapy for superficial transitional cell cancers in the bladder have led to the occasional use of these agents in the treatment of upper tract cancers. Long-term follow-up of the results of such treatments has generally not been reported, and the efficacy of this approach cannot be assessed, largely because experience has been limited to those patients whose compromised clinical status (solitary kidney, renal failure, medical risks for surgery) may have influenced clinical outcome. The use of this approach will be limited by the extent of disease in the renal pelvis, the access that these agents may have to the area of disease, the sensitivity of the cancer being treated, and the adequacy and accuracy of initial tumor staging and continued monitoring.
4. Laser vaporization/coagulation. Transurethral and percutaneous access to the upper tract have permitted the use of laser therapy in the control of superficial upper tract transitional cell cancers. This approach is dependent on accurate staging and adequate visualization of the lesions that need to be coagulated. Results of this approach are at present too preliminary to assess. Therapeutic efficacy, however, will depend on staging accuracy on initial treatment and ease of monitoring such patients for disease recurrence and possible progression.

METASTATIC TRANSITIONAL CELL CANCER OF THE RENAL PELVIS AND URETER

The prognosis for any patient with metastatic or recurrent transitional cell cancer is poor. The proper management of recurrence depends on the sites of recurrence, extent of prior therapy, and individual patient considerations. Chemotherapy regimens that have been shown effective for metastatic bladder cancer have generally been applied to transitional cell cancers arising from other sites. Patients with distant metastases have a poor prognosis, and can be appropriately offered treatment on a clinical trial.

In patients with metastatic or recurrent transitional cell carcinoma of the bladder, combination chemotherapy has produced high response rates and occasional complete responses. Results from a randomized trial that compared methotrexate, vinblastine, doxorubicin, and cisplatin (M-VAC) to single-agent cisplatin in advanced bladder cancer show a significant advantage with M-VAC in both response rate and median survival. The overall response rate with M-VAC in this cooperative group trial was 39%.

Other chemotherapy agents that have shown activity in metastatic transitional cell cancer include the following:

- Paclitaxel.
- Ifosfamide.
- Gallium nitrate.
- Gemcitabine.

Cancer of Urinary Bladder

Approximately 70 to 80% of patients with newly diagnosed bladder cancer will present with superficial bladder tumors (i.e., stage Ta, Tis, or T1). Those who do present with superficial, noninvasive bladder cancer can often be cured, and those with deeply invasive disease can sometimes be cured by surgery, irradiation, or a combination of modalities that include chemotherapy. Studies have demonstrated that some patients with distant metastases have achieved long-term complete response following treatment with combination chemotherapy regimens. There are clinical trials suitable for patients with all stages of bladder cancer; whenever possible, patients should be included in clinical trials designed to improve on standard therapy.

The major prognostic factors in carcinoma of the bladder are the depth of invasion into the bladder wall and the degree of differentiation of the tumor. Most superficial tumors are well differentiated. Patients in whom superficial tumors are less differentiated, large, multiple, or associated with carcinoma in situ (Tis) in other areas of the bladder mucosa are at greatest risk for recurrence and the development of invasive cancer. Such patients may be considered to have the entire urothelial surface at risk for the development of cancer. Tis may exist for variable durations. Adverse prognostic features associated with a greater risk of disease progression include the presence of multiple aneuploid cell lines, nuclear p53 overexpression, and expression of the Lewis-x blood group antigen. Patients with Tis who have a complete response to bacillus Calmette-Guerin have approximately a 20% risk of disease progression at 5 years; patients with incomplete response have approximately a 95% risk of disease progression. Several treatment methods (i.e., transurethral surgery, intravesical medications, and cystectomy) have been used in the management of patients with superficial tumors, and each method can be associated with 5-year survival in 55% to 80% of patients treated.

Invasive tumors that are confined to the bladder muscle on pathologic staging after radical cystectomy are associated with approximately a 75% 5-year progression-free survival rate. Patients with more deeply invasive tumors (which are also usually less well differentiated) experience 5-year survival rates of 20% to 40% following radical cystectomy. When the patient presents with locally extensive tumor that invades pelvic viscera or with metastases to lymph nodes or distant sites, 5-year survival is uncommon, but considerable symptomatic palliation can still be achieved. Expression of the tumor suppressor gene p53 also has been associated with an adverse prognosis for patients with invasive bladder cancer. A retrospective study of 243 patients treated by radical cystectomy found that the presence of nuclear p53 was an independent predictor for recurrence among patients with stage T1, T2, or T3 tumors.

More than 90% of bladder carcinomas are transitional cell carcinomas derived from the uroepithelium. About 6 to 8% are squamous cell carcinomas, and 2% are adenocarcinomas. Adenocarcinomas may be either of urachal origin or of nonurachal origin; the latter type is generally thought to arise from metaplasia of chronically irritated transitional epithelium. Pathologic grade, which is based on cellular atypia, nuclear abnormalities, and the number of mitotic figures, is of great prognostic importance.

The clinical staging of carcinoma of the bladder is determined by the depth of invasion of the bladder wall by the tumor. This determination requires a cystoscopic examination that includes a biopsy, and examination under anesthesia to assess the size and mobility of palpable masses, the degree of induration of the bladder wall, and the presence of extravesical extension or invasion of adjacent organs. Clinical staging, even when computed tomographic and/or magnetic resonance imaging scans and other imaging modalities are used, often underestimates the extent of tumor, particularly in cancers that are less differentiated and more deeply invasive.

Risk Factors

Several populations with a variety of exposures appear to be at higher risk for developing bladder cancer. By far the greatest known environmental risk factor in the general population is cigarette smoking, with individuals who smoke having a 4-fold to 7-fold increased risk of developing bladder cancer than individuals who have never smoked. Risk is reduced with cessation of smoking, but a relatively small decrease in incidence is seen for the first 5 to 7 years after cessation. Even after 10 years, the risk of an individual developing bladder cancer is still almost twice that of an individual who has never smoked.

Among the chemicals implicated in smoking-induced bladder cancer are aminobiphenyl and its metabolites. It is possible that inherited and inducible enzymes are important in the activation and detoxification of aminobiphenyls and other putative bladder carcinogens. These enzymes include N-acetyltransferase 2 (NAT2), cytochrome P450 1A2 (CYT 1A2), and glutathione S-transferase M 1. Several studies have indicated that specific genotypes and phenotypes of these enzymes and their activities, particularly in the liver and urothelium, are associated with susceptibility to smoking-induced bladder cancer and bladder cancer induced by other aryl amines, particularly in industrially exposed populations. Not all of these studies, however, have been well controlled for active or former smoking histories.

A variety of industrial exposures have also been implicated as risk factors for developing bladder cancer, primarily aromatic amines present in the production of dyes, and benzidine and its derivatives, combustion gases and soot from coal, possibly chlorinated aliphatic hydrocarbons, chlorination by-products in heated water, and certain aldehydes (e.g., acrolein used in chemical dyes and in the rubber and textile industries).

Occupations reported to be associated with an increased risk of bladder cancer include those that involve organic chemicals such as dry cleaners, paper manufacturers, rope and twine makers, and workers in apparel manufacturing.

Additional risk factors that predispose an individual to more aggressive forms of bladder cancer include prolonged exposures to urinary foreign bodies and infections; *Schistosoma hematobium* (Bilharzial) bladder infections; exposure to cyclophosphamide and perhaps other alkylating agents such as ifosfamide (although the use of mesna in conjunction with these agents has reduced the incidence); and pelvic radiation therapy for other malignancies. Renal transplant recipients appear to have an increased incidence of bladder cancer. Individuals with chronic acetaminophen and phenacetin exposure have a higher incidence of urothelial cancer, more often in the upper urinary tract than in the bladder. The use of Chinese herbs has been associated with a rapidly progressive interstitial nephropathy; urothelial malignancy (transitional cell carcinoma) of the upper urinary tract develops subsequently in almost half of these patients. The prime carcinogen appears to be aristolochic acid (AA) extracted from species of *Aristolochia*. Because of the diversity of the Chinese herbal regimens used, in addition to AA, other unidentified phytotoxins may also play a role.

Clinical Presentation

Bladder cancer represents a spectrum of neoplasms that can present as superficial (75%), invasive (20%) or metastatic disease (5%). Hematuria is the most common presenting sign, occurring in about 90% of cases. Other presenting symptoms include dysuria, urinary frequency or urgency, and, less commonly, flank pain secondary to obstruction, and pain from pelvic invasion or bone metastases. Diagnosis and staging usually begin with cystoscopy.

Screening Methods

Cystoscopy and Cytology

The use of cystoscopies and bladder wash/urinary cytologic examinations has proven quite successful in the surveillance and management of patients with previously treated bladder cancers. These means are not practical in individuals without a history of bladder cancer, however, because of expense and morbidity.

Hematuria

Although hematuria is the most common presenting sign of bladder cancer, most individuals with hematuria do not have bladder cancer. In the general population, the prevalence of asymptomatic gross hematuria is about 2.5% while the prevalence of asymptomatic microhematuria is about 13%.

One-time Hematuria testing

Two groups have reported on the use of testing a single urine specimen for blood to detect urologic malignancies, serious urinary tract diseases, and bladder cancers. Both studies were performed retrospectively to ascertain information from patients who were seen at a large multispecialty clinic or who subscribed to a large health maintenance organization (HMO) and were tested in a "multiphasic screening." Because of the retrospective nature of each study, neither was designed to specifically look for bladder cancer detection or to focus on the population at highest risk (men aged 50 years and older). Both studies concluded that single hematuria testing was not effective in diagnosing bladder cancer. A longer follow-up of the HMO study indicated that individuals with microhematuria were at a higher risk for subsequent development of muscle-invading bladder cancer, with a latency of 3.5 to 14.5 years. There is insufficient evidence to indicate that single hematuria testing is effective in screening for bladder cancer, and there is no evidence that single hematuria testing results in reduced mortality from the disease.

TNM Definitions

Primary Tumor (T)

- TX: Primary tumor cannot be assessed
- T0: No evidence of primary tumor
- Ta: Noninvasive papillary carcinoma
- Tis: Carcinoma *in situ*: "flat tumor"
- T1: Tumor invades subepithelial connective tissue
- T2: Tumor invades muscle
  - § pT2a: Tumor invades superficial muscle (inner half)
  - § pT2b: Tumor invades deep muscle (outer half)
- T3: Tumor invades perivesical tissue
  - § pT3a: Microscopically
  - § pT3b: Macroscopically (extravesical mass)
- T4: Tumor invades any of the following: prostate, uterus, vagina, pelvic wall, or abdominal wall
  - § T4a: Tumor invades the prostate, uterus, vagina
  - § T4b: Tumor invades the pelvic wall, abdominal wall

Note: The suffix "m" should be added to the appropriate T category to indicate multiple lesions. The suffix "is" may be added to any T to indicate the presence of associated carcinoma in situ.

Regional Lymph Nodes (N)

- NX: Regional lymph nodes cannot be assessed
- N0: No regional lymph node metastasis
- N1: Metastasis in a single lymph node, 2 cm or less in greatest dimension
- N2: Metastasis in a single lymph node, more than 2 cm but not more than 5 cm in greatest dimension; or multiple lymph nodes, none more than 5 cm in greatest dimension
- N3: Metastasis in a lymph node, more than 5 cm in greatest dimension

Distant Metastasis (M)

- MX: Distant metastasis cannot be assessed
- M0: No distant metastasis
- M1: Distant metastasis

AJCC Stage Groupings

Stage 0a

- Ta, N0, M0

Stage 0is

- Tis, N0, M0

Stage I

- T1, N0, M0

Stage II

- T2a, N0, M0
- T2b, N0, M0

Stage III

- T3a, N0, M0
- T3b, N0, M0
- T4a, N0, M0

Stage IV

- T4b, N0, M0
- Any T, N1, M0
- Any T, N2, M0
- Any T, N3, M0
- Any T, any N, M1

Prolonged survival in most patients with superficial cancers is achieved by transurethral resection (TUR) with or without intravesical chemotherapy. However, cure is not possible for the majority of patients with deeply invasive tumors and for most patients with regional or distant metastases. In North America, the standard treatment of patients with invasive bladder cancers is radical cystectomy and urinary diversion. Other treatment approaches include TUR and segmental resection with or without radiation therapy, combined chemotherapy-radiation therapy, or either followed by salvage cystectomy, when needed, for local failure. Therefore, many newly diagnosed bladder cancer patients are candidates for participation in a clinical trial. Clinical trials include studies of chemoprevention of superficial disease, adjuvant chemotherapy for advanced local or regional disease, preservation of bladder function with chemotherapy-radiation therapy, and development of more effective systemic therapy and methods of palliation for metastatic tumors.

Reconstructive techniques that fashion low-pressure storage reservoirs from the reconfigured small and large bowel eliminate the need for external drainage devices and, in some male patients, allow voiding per urethra. These techniques are designed to improve the quality of life for patients who require cystectomy.

Stage 0 bladder cancer is defined by the following TNM classifications:

- Ta, N0, M0
- Tis, N0, M0

Patients with stage 0 bladder tumors can be cured by a variety of treatments, even though the tendency for new tumor formation is high. In a series of patients with Ta or T1 tumors who were followed for a minimum of 20 years or until death, the risk of bladder cancer recurrence following initial resection was 80%. Patients at greatest risk of recurrent disease are those whose tumors are large, poorly differentiated, multiple, or associated with nuclear p53 overexpression. In addition, patients with carcinoma *in situ* (Tis) or dysplasia of grossly uninvolved bladder epithelium are at greater risk of recurrence and progression.

Transurethral resection (TUR) and fulguration are the most common and conservative forms of management. Careful surveillance of subsequent bladder tumor progression is important. One retrospective series addressed the value of performing a second TUR within 2 to 6 weeks of the first. A second TUR performed on 38 patients with Tis or Ta disease found that 9 patients (24%) had lamina propria invasion (T1) and 3 patients (8%) had muscle invasion (T2). Such information may change the definitive management options in these individuals. Patients who require more aggressive forms of treatment are those with extensive multifocal recurrent disease and/or other unfavorable prognostic features. Segmental cystectomy is applicable to only a small minority of patients because of the tendency of bladder carcinoma to involve multiple regions of the bladder mucosa and to occur in areas that cannot be segmentally resected.

Intravesical therapy with thiotepa, mitomycin, doxorubicin, or bacillus Calmette-Guerin (BCG) is most often used in patients with multiple tumors or recurrent tumors or as a prophylactic measure in high-risk patients after TUR. Administration of intravesical BCG plus subcutaneous BCG following TUR was compared with TUR alone in patients with Ta and T1 lesions. Treatment with BCG delayed progression to muscle-invasive and/or metastatic disease, improved bladder preservation, and decreased the risk of death from bladder cancer. Another randomized study of patients with superficial bladder cancer also reports a decrease in tumor recurrence in patients given intravesical and percutaneous BCG compared with controls. Two nonconsecutive 6-week treatment courses with BCG may be necessary to obtain optimal response. Patients with a T1 tumor at the 3-month evaluation after a 6-week course of BCG and patients with Tis that persists after a second 6-week BCG course have a high likelihood of developing muscle-invasive disease and should be considered for cystectomy. A randomized study that compared intravesical and subcutaneous BCG with intravesical doxorubicin showed better response rates and freedom from recurrence with the BCG regimen for recurrent papillary tumors as well as for Tis. A randomized trial from the Swedish-Norwegian Bladder Cancer Group compared 2 years of intravesical treatment with mitomycin C versus BCG. However, no difference was observed in tumor progression or overall survival between the two arms at 5 years.[Level of evidence: 1iiD] Although BCG may not prolong overall survival for Tis disease, it appears to afford complete response rates of about 70%, thereby decreasing the need for salvage cystectomy.Studies show that intravesical BCG delays tumor recurrence and tumor progression. Preliminary results from a prospective randomized trial suggest that maintenance BCG, when given to patients who are disease-free after a 6-week induction course, improves survival. One study that compared mitomycin with interferon alfa-2b showed an improved outcome with mitomycin, although interferon was better tolerated.

Stage I bladder cancer is defined by the following TNM classification:

- T1, N0, M0

Patients with stage I bladder tumors can be cured by a variety of treatments, even though the tendency for new tumor formation is high.

Stage II bladder cancer is defined by the following TNM classifications:

- T2a, N0, M0
- T2b, N0, M0

Stage II bladder cancer may be controlled in some patients by transurethral resection (TUR), but often more aggressive forms of treatment are dictated by recurrent tumor or by the large size, multiple foci, or undifferentiated grade of the neoplasm. Segmental cystectomy is appropriate only in very selected patients.

Radical cystectomy is considered standard treatment. In some reports, bladder-sparing radiation therapy with salvage cystectomy when indicated yields similar therapeutic results to those of radical cystectomy and can be delivered to patients who are not candidates for surgery.

Stage III bladder cancer is defined by the following TNM classifications:

- T3a, N0, M0
- T3b, N0, M0
- T4a, N0, M0

A few highly selected patients with stage III bladder cancer may be suitable for segmental cystectomy or interstitial irradiation. The relatively high frequency of extensive intramural tumor spread and lymph node involvement make radical cystectomy and external-beam irradiation more logical forms of treatment in most patients.

Stage IV bladder cancer is defined by the following TNM classifications:

- T4b, N0, M0
- Any T, N1, M0
- Any T, N2, M0
- Any T, N3, M0
- Any T, any N, M1

Currently, only a small fraction of patients with stage IV bladder carcinoma can be cured. The potential for cure is restricted to patients with stage IV disease with involvement of pelvic organs by direct extension or small volume metastases to regional lymph nodes. These patients can receive radical cystectomy with or without preoperative irradiation. Studies suggest that radical cystectomy with preservation of sexual function can be performed in some men and that new forms of urinary diversion can obviate the need for an external urinary appliance.

RECURRENT BLADDER CANCER

The prognosis for any patient with progressive or recurrent invasive bladder cancer is generally poor. Management of recurrence depends on prior therapy, sites of recurrence, and individual patient considerations. Treatment of new superficial or locally invasive tumors that develop in the setting of previous conservative therapy for superficial bladder neoplasia has been discussed earlier in this summary. Recurrent or progressive disease in distant sites or after definitive local therapy has an extremely poor prognosis, and clinical trials should be considered whenever possible.

In patients with recurrent transitional cell carcinoma, combination chemotherapy has produced high response rates with occasional complete responses seen. Results from a randomized trial that compared M-VAC (methotrexate, vinblastine, doxorubicin, and cisplatin) to single-agent cisplatin in advanced bladder cancer show a significant advantage with M-VAC in both response rate and median survival.

Seventeen

Pediatric Oncology

Childhood Brain Tumors

GENERAL INFORMATION

Primary brain tumors are a diverse group of diseases that together constitute the most common solid tumor of childhood. Brain tumors are classified according to histology, but tumor location and extent of spread are important factors that affect treatment and prognosis. Immunohistochemical analysis, cytogenetic and molecular genetic findings, and measures of mitotic activity are increasingly used in tumor diagnosis and classification.

Approximately 50% of brain tumors in children are infratentorial, with three fourths of these located in the cerebellum or fourth ventricle. Common infratentorial (posterior fossa) tumors include the following:

1. Cerebellar astrocytoma (usually pilocytic but also fibrillary and high-grade)
2. Medulloblastoma (primitive neuroectodermal tumor)
3. ependymoma (low-grade or anaplastic)
4. Brain stem glioma (often diagnosed neuroradiologically without biopsy; may be high-grade or low-grade)
5. Atypical teratoid

Supratentorial tumors include those tumors that occur in the sellar or suprasellar region and/ or in the cerebrum or diencephalon. Sellar/ suprasellar tumors comprise approximately 20% of childhood brain tumors and include the following:

1. Craniopharyngioma
2. Diencephalic (chiasm, hypothalamic, and/or thalamic) gliomas generally of low grade
3. Germ cell tumors (germinoma and nongerminomatous)

Other tumors that occur supratentorially include the following:

1. Low-grade astrocytoma or glioma (grade 1 or grade 2)
2. High-grade or malignant astrocytoma (anaplastic astrocytoma, glioblastoma multiforme (grade 3 or grade 4))
3. Mixed glioma (low-grade or high-grade)
4. Oligodendroglioma (low-grade or high-grade)
5. Primitive neuroectodermal tumor (cerebral neuroblastoma)
6. Ependymoma (low-grade or anaplastic)
7. Meningioma

8. Choroid plexus tumors (papilloma and carcinoma)
9. Pineal parenchymal tumors (pineoblastoma, pineocytoma, or mixed pineal parenchymal tumor)
10. Neuronal and mixed neuronal glial tumor (ganglioglioma, desmoplastic infantile ganglioglioma, dysembryoplastic neuroepithelial tumor)
11. Metastasis (rare) from extra neural malignancies.

Spinal Cord Tumors

Primary central nervous system spinal cord tumors comprise approximately 1 to 2% of all childhood nervous system tumors. As is the case for primary brain tumors, such lesions are histologically heterogeneous. Approximately 70% of all intramedullary spinal cord tumors will be low-grade astrocytomas and/or gangliogliomas. Other tumor types which occur include ependymomas, higher-grade glial tumors, and (rarely) primitive neuroectodermal tumors. Myxopapillary ependymomas have a proclivity to develop in the conus and caudae equina region. Symptoms and signs of spinal cord tumors are highly dependent on the location of the tumor and its extent; some low-grade spinal cord tumors are associated with large cysts that extend rostrally and caudally and have been termed holocord astrocytomas. At times, it is impossible to distinguish a tumor which arises in the medulla from a tumor which arises in the upper cervical cord.

Important general concepts that should be understood by those caring for a child who has a brain tumor include the following:

1. Selection of an appropriate therapy can only occur if the correct diagnosis is made and the stage of the disease is accurately determined.
2. Children with primary brain tumors represent a major therapy challenge that, for optimal results, requires the coordinated efforts of pediatric specialists in fields such as neurosurgery, neurology, rehabilitation, neuropathology, radiation oncology, medical oncology, neuroradiology, endocrinology, and psychology, who have special expertise in the care of patients with these diseases.
3. More than one half of children diagnosed with brain tumors will survive 5 years from diagnosis. In some subgroups of patients, an even higher rate of survival and cure is possible. Each child's treatment should be approached with curative intent, and the possible long-term sequelae of the disease and its treatment should be considered before therapy is begun.
4. For the majority of childhood brain tumors, the optimal treatment regimen has not been determined. Children who have brain tumors should be considered for enrollment in a clinical trial when an appropriate study is available. Such clinical trials are being carried out by institutions and cooperative groups.
5. The cause of the vast majority of childhood brain tumors remains unknown.

CELLULAR CLASSIFICATION

The classification of brain tumors is based on both histopathological characteristics and location in the brain. Undifferentiated neuroectodermal tumors of the cerebellum have historically been referred to as medulloblastomas, while tumors of identical histology in the pineal region would be diagnosed as pineoblastomas The nomenclature of pediatric brain tumors is controversial and potentially confusing. Some pathologists advocate abandoning the traditional morphologically-based classifications such as medulloblastoma in favor of a terminology that relies more extensively on the phenotypic characteristics of the tumor. In such a system, medulloblastoma is referred to as primitive neuroectodermal tumor (PNET) and then subdivided on the basis of cellular differentiation. The most recent World Health Organization classification of brain tumors maintains the term "medulloblastoma" for posterior fossa undifferentiated tumors. It also maintains separate categories for primitive neuroectodermal tumors, ependymoblastomas, and pineal small round cell tumors (pineoblastomas). The pathologic classification of pediatric brain tumors is a specialized area that is undergoing evolution; review of the diagnostic tissue by a neuropathologist who has particular expertise in this area is strongly recommended.

Spinal Cord Tumors

The classification of spinal cord tumors is based on histopathologic characteristics of the tumor and does not differ from that of primary brain tumors.

Medulloblastoma

This tumor usually originates in the cerebellum. It may spread contiguously to the cerebellar peduncle, floor of the fourth ventricle, into the cervical spine, or above the tentorium. In addition, it may spread via the cerebrospinal fluid intracranially and/or to the spinal cord. Every patient with medulloblastoma should be evaluated with diagnostic imaging of the entire neuraxis, and when possible, lumbar cerebrospinal fluid analysis for free-floating tumor cells. The most sensitive method available for evaluating spinal cord subarachnoid metastasis is spinal magnetic resonance imaging (MRI) performed with gadolinium. If MRI is used, the entire spine must be imaged in at least 2 planes with contiguous MR slices performed after gadolinium enhancement. Because medulloblastoma occasionally metastasizes outside the central nervous system, especially to bone, a bone scan with plain film correlation as well as a bone marrow aspiration and biopsy may be useful in symptomatic patients or in those with abnormal blood cell counts. Cerebrospinal fluid shunts at the time of surgery have not been shown to increase the risk of leptomeningeal relapse. Until recently, the most commonly used staging system was that proposed by Harisiadis and Chang. This system rates the tumor by an intraoperative evaluation of both size and extent as well as by the presence of metastatic disease. Alternative postoperative staging systems are now being used that are based on surgical impression and postoperative imaging studies. Patients with disseminated disease at diagnosis are clearly at highest risk for disease relapse. Other factors that may portend an unfavorable outcome include younger age at diagnosis, brain stem involvement, subtotal resection, and a nonposterior fossa tumor. The prognostic importance of brain stem involvement is still being debated. These prognostic variables must be evaluated in the context of the treatment received. Biologic markers such as TrkC, C-MYC expression, and HER2, may be independent predictors but have not yet been incorporated into stratification schemas. Two major subclassifications are now being used:

- *Average risk:* Children older than 3 years of age with posterior fossa tumors; tumor is totally or "near-totally" (<1.5 cc's of residual disease) resected; no dissemination.
- *Poor risk:* Children younger than 3 years of age or those with metastatic disease and/or subtotal resection (>1.5 cc's of residual disease) and/or nonposterior fossa location.

TREATMENT OPTION OVERVIEW

Many of the improvements in survival in childhood cancer have been made as a result of clinical trials that have attempted to improve on the best available, accepted therapy. Clinical trials in pediatrics are designed to compare new therapy with therapy that is currently accepted as standard. This comparison may be done in a randomized study of 2 treatment arms or by evaluating a single new treatment and comparing the results with those previously obtained with existing therapy.

Because of the relative rarity of cancer in children, all patients with brain tumors should be considered for entry into a clinical trial. To determine and implement optimum treatment, treatment planning by a multidisciplinary team of cancer specialists who have experience treating childhood brain tumors is required. Radiation therapy of pediatric brain tumors is technically very demanding and should be carried out in centers that have experience in that area in order to ensure optimal results. Less than optimal techniques have resulted in failure at the junction of the brain and spine fields or in the cribriform plate region.Patients should be treated in a center experienced with this therapy.

In the past, treatment has included surgery with radiation therapy. There is evidence to suggest that more extensive surgical resections are related to an improved rate of survival, primarily in children with nondisseminated posterior fossa disease at diagnosis. Chemotherapy has been shown to be active in patients with recurrent medulloblastomas. Prospective, randomized trials and large single-arm trials suggest that adjuvant chemotherapy given during and after radiation therapy may improve overall survival for the subset of children with medulloblastoma who have less favorable prognostic factors, and there has been enthusiasm for exploring the role of chemotherapy in the treatment of childhood brain tumors. Children younger than 3 years of age are particularly susceptible to the adverse effect of radiation on brain development. Debilitating effects on growth and neurologic development have frequently been observed, especially in younger children. For this reason, the role of chemotherapy in allowing a delay in the administration of radiation therapy is under study, and preliminary results suggest that chemotherapy can be used to delay, and sometimes obviate, the need for radiation therapy in children with medulloblastoma. Surveillance testing is presently a part of all ongoing medulloblastoma studies. Secondary tumors have increasingly been diagnosed in long-term survivors.Long-term management of these patients is complex and requires a multidisciplinary approach.

Untreated Childhood Medulloblastoma

Careful evaluation to determine fully the extent of disease must precede the treatment of medulloblastoma. Surgery should be an attempt at maximal tumor reduction; children without disseminated disease at diagnosis have improved progression-free survival if there is minimal residual disease present after surgery. Postoperatively, studies should be conducted to determine if the patient has high risk of relapse. Risk criteria are outlined in the stage information section.Patients with extensive tumor should be considered at "high risk" for relapse and be treated on protocols specifically designed for them.

Treatment Options

Average Risk

The traditional postsurgical treatment for these patients has been radiation therapy consisting of 5,400 to 5,580 cGy to the posterior fossa and approximately 3,600 cGy to the entire neuraxis (i.e., the whole brain and spine). While the standard boost in medulloblastoma is the entire posterior fossa, patterns of failure data suggest that the use of a tumor bed boost might be equally effective, yet associated with reduced toxicity. The minimal dose of radiation therapy needed for disease control is unknown. Attempts to lower the dose of craniospinal radiation therapy to 2,340 cGy without chemotherapy have resulted in an increased incidence of isolated leptomeningeal relapse.Radiation therapy, when coupled with chemotherapy, has been shown to result in disease control in up to 80% of patients and may decrease the severity of neurocognitive sequelae

Long-term survivors who were prepubertal at the time of diagnosis are at high risk for growth failure due to hypothalamic failure and growth hormone replacement therapy has not been shown to increase the likelihood of disease relapse.

Poor Risk

In poor-risk patients, the addition of chemotherapy has improved the duration of disease-free survival. Some studies show that approximately 50 to 60% of such patients will experience long-term disease control. These are patients who, at diagnosis, have locally extensive and often unresectable tumor in the posterior fossa, brain stem involvement at diagnosis, and/or noncontiguous metastatic disease within or outside of the central nervous system. Adjuvant chemotherapy has improved progression-free survival for patients with these "poor-risk" parameters at diagnosis. Such patients should be considered for entry into a clinical trial. Long-term survivors who were prepubertal at the time of diagnosis are at high risk for growth failure due to hypothalamic failure and growth hormone replacement therapy has not been shown to increase the likelihood of disease relapse.

Children Younger Than 3 Years of Age

Some patients younger than 3 years of age with newly diagnosed medulloblastoma will respond, at least partially, to chemotherapy. Some patients, especially those with minimal residual postoperative disease, may have a long-lasting response. Those children treated with chemotherapy alone may have better neurocognitive outcome than those treated with radiation therapy, with or without chemotherapy For this reason, strong consideration should be given to entering patients younger than 3 years of age in studies that use chemotherapy to delay, modify, or possibly obviate the need for radiation therapy. High-dose chemotherapy with autologous bone marrow rescue followed by focal radiation therapy has been used with some success in young children with locally recurrent disease for whom primary chemotherapy has failed. Although chemotherapy is being used to prevent neurologic damage caused by radiation therapy in very young patients, neurologic deficits may be present in children prior to the initiation of therapy, and progressive neurologic damage has been noted during therapy.

RECURRENT CHILDHOOD MEDULLOBLASTOMA

Recurrence is not uncommon and may develop many years after initial treatment. Disease may recur at the primary tumor site or, especially in malignant tumors, at noncontiguous central nervous system sites. Systemic relapse is rare, but may occur. At time of relapse, a complete evaluation for extent of recurrence is indicated for all malignant tumors and, at times, for more benign lesions. Biopsy or surgical resection may be necessary for confirmation of relapse because other entities such as secondary tumor and treatment-related brain necrosis may be clinically indistinguishable from tumor recurrence. The need for surgical intervention must be individualized on the basis of the initial tumor type, the length of time between initial treatment and the reappearance of the lesion, and the clinical picture. Patients with medulloblastoma that recurs after radiation therapy alone should be considered for treatment with known active agents, which include vincristine, cyclophosphamide, cisplatin, carboplatin, lomustine, and etoposide; although response is seen in more than 50% of patients, long-term disease control is rare. Entry into studies of novel therapeutic approaches including high-dose chemotherapy and autologous stem cell rescue at the time of relapse after radiation therapy alone or radiation therapy and chemotherapy should be considered.

CHILDHOOD CEREBELLAR ASTROCYTOMA

Cellular Classification

The classification of brain tumors is based on both histopathologic characteristics and location in the brain. More than 80% of all childhood cerebellar gliomas will be pilocytic astrocytomas, which are also considered to be grade 1 astrocytomas. The majority of the remainder will be diffuse or fibrillary astrocytomas. Malignant gliomas are rare. The pathologic classification of pediatric brain tumors is a specialized area that is undergoing evolution; review of the diagnostic tissue by a neuropathologist who has particular expertise in this area is strongly recommended. These generally low-grade, often cystic astrocytic tumors are localized to the cerebellum. Except for malignant gliomas, contiguous spread or metastasis outside that region is extremely rare. The presence of certain histologic features has been used retrospectively to stratify cerebellar astrocytomas into two distinct groups: pilocytic or Gilles type A tumors and diffuse or Gilles type B tumors; the latter tumors have a poor prognosis. Expert neuropathologic review is important.

Treatment Option Overview

Many of the improvements in survival in childhood cancer have been made as a result of clinical trials that have attempted to improve on the best available, accepted therapy. Clinical trials in pediatrics are designed to compare new therapy with therapy that is currently accepted as standard. This comparison may be done in a randomized study of two treatment arms or by evaluating a single new treatment and comparing the results with those that were previously obtained with existing therapy.

Because of the relative rarity of cancer in children, all patients with brain tumors should be considered for entry into a clinical trial. To determine and implement optimum treatment, treatment planning by a multidisciplinary team of cancer specialists who have experience treating childhood brain tumors is required. Radiation therapy of pediatric brain tumors is technically very demanding and should be carried out in centers that have experience in that area in order to ensure optimal results.

Untreated Childhood Cerebellar Astrocytoma

Surgical resection is the primary treatment for childhood cerebellar astrocytoma Complete or near complete removal can be obtained in 90 to 95% of patients with juvenile pilocytic tumors. Diffuse cerebellar astrocytomas may be less amenable to total resection, and this may account for the poorer outcome. The extent of resection necessary for cure is unknown because patients with microscopic and even gross residual tumor after surgery may experience long-term progression-free survival without postoperative therapy. Following resection, a post-operative MRI is obtained. Surveillance scans are then obtained periodically for 5 years for totally resected tumors, although the value of this is uncertain. The optimal use of radiation therapy is the subject of controversy. Some radiation oncologists advocate the treatment of patients with residual disease, and others withhold treatment until tumor progression has been documented. Chemotherapy may be useful for delaying radiation therapy in the very young child with unresectable, progressive cerebellar astrocytoma.

Recurrent Childhood Cerebellar Astrocytoma

Recurrence may take place in childhood cerebellar gliomas and may develop many years after initial treatment. Disease can be at the primary tumor site or, especially in malignant tumors, at noncontiguous central nervous system sites. Systemic relapse is rare; but may occur. At the time of recurrence, a complete evaluation to determine the extent of relapse is indicated for all patients . Biopsy or surgical resection may be necessary for confirmation of relapse because other entities such as secondary tumor and treatment-related brain necrosis may be clinically indistinguishable from tumor recurrence. The need for surgical intervention must be individualized on the basis of the initial tumor type, the length of time between initial treatment and the reappearance of the mass lesion, and the clinical picture.

Patients with cerebellar astrocytoma (pilocytic or diffuse) who relapse after being treated with surgery alone should be considered for another surgical resection. If this is not feasible, local radiation therapy is the usual treatment. If there is recurrence in an unresectable site after irradiation, chemotherapy should be considered. There is little information regarding the activity of chemotherapy in this disease. Studies of novel therapeutic approaches that are designed to test the activity and toxicity of chemotherapy in recurrent brain tumor patients should be considered.

Childhood Ependymoma

Although there is no formal staging system, ependymomas can be divided into supratentorial and infratentorial tumors. They usually originate in the ependymal linings of ventricles in the posterior fossa or supratentorial region, and have access to the cerebral spinal fluid (CSF) and therefore may occur throughout the entire neuraxis. Thirty percent of ependymomas arise outside of the posterior fossa. Every patient with ependymoma should be evaluated with diagnostic imaging of the spinal cord and whole brain. The most sensitive method available for evaluating spinal cord subarachnoid metastasis is spinal magnetic resonance imaging (MRI) performed with gadolinium. If MRI is used, the entire spine must be imaged in at least 2 planes with contiguous MR slices performed after gadolinium enhancement. While a number of factors have sometimes been associated with an unfavorable outcome (younger age at diagnosis, lower doses of radiation, anaplastic histology, subtotal resection), age and extent of resection have consistently been the most important factor. These prognostic variables must be evaluated in the context of the treatment received.

Treatment Option Overview

Many of the improvements in survival in childhood cancer have been made as a result of clinical trials that have attempted to improve on the best available, accepted therapy. Clinical trials in pediatrics are designed to compare new therapy with therapy that is currently accepted as standard. This comparison may be done in a randomized study of 2 treatment arms or by evaluating a single new treatment and comparing the results with those previously obtained with existing therapy.

Because of the relative rarity of cancer in children, all patients with brain tumors should be considered for entry into a clinical trial. To determine and implement optimum treatment, treatment planning by a multidisciplinary team of cancer specialists who have experience treating childhood brain tumors is required. Radiation therapy of pediatric brain tumors is technically very demanding and should be carried out in centers that have experience in that area in order to ensure optimal results.

In the past, treatment has included surgery with radiation therapy. There is evidence to suggest that more extensive surgical resections are related to an improved rate of survival. Chemotherapy has been shown to be active in patients with ependymoma but a small prospective, randomized trial suggests that its activity is limited. Children younger than 3 years of age are particularly susceptible to the adverse effect of radiation on brain development. Debilitating effects on growth and neurologic development have frequently been observed, especially in younger children. For this reason, the role of chemotherapy in allowing a delay in the administration of radiation therapy is under study. Studies are underway evaluating the role of early radiation therapy for local control in infants. Long-term management of these patients is complex and requires a multidisciplinary approach.

There is evidence that surveillance neuro-imaging in childhood ependymoma will identify tumors that have recurred when the patient is asymptomatic, however, it is unclear whether this detection will change the ultimate prognosis of the patient.

Newly Diagnosed Childhood Ependymoma

In the newly diagnosed patient, careful evaluation to fully determine the extent of disease must precede the treatment of ependymoma. Surgery should be performed in an attempt at maximal tumor reduction; children have improved progression-free survival if there is minimal residual disease present after surgery. Postoperatively, studies such as cerebral spinal fluid (CSF) cytological evaluation should be conducted to determine the extent of residual disease and dissemination. Patients with residual tumor or disseminated disease should be considered at high risk for relapse and should be treated on protocols specifically designed for them. Those with no evidence of residual tumor still have an approximately 20 to 40% relapse risk in spite of postoperative radiation therapy.

Post surgical Treatment Options

- *Surgery alone:* Limited experience with surgery alone for completely resected supratentorial tumors suggest that, in select cases, this may be an option.
- *No residual disease, no disseminated disease:* The traditional postsurgical treatment for these patients has been radiation therapy consisting of 5,400 to 5,580 cGy to the tumor bed. It is not necessary to treat the entire CNS (whole brain and spine) since these tumors usually recur at the local site. When possible, patients should be treated in a center experienced with this therapy. There is no evidence that adjuvant chemotherapy improves the outcome for patients with ependymoma.
- *Residual disease; no disseminated disease:* Consideration of reresection should be made since patients who have complete resections have better disease control. The traditional postsurgical treatment for these patients has been radiation therapy consisting of 5,400 to 5,580 cGy to the tumor bed. It is not necessary to treat the entire CNS (whole brain and spine) since these tumors usually recur at the local site. When possible, patients should be treated in a center experienced with this therapy. There is no evidence that adjuvant chemotherapy, including high-dose chemotherapy with stem cell rescue, is of any benefit.

Children with CNS disseminated disease: In children with disseminated disease, long-term survivors have been reported and aggressive therapy is warranted. Regardless of degree of surgical resection, these patients require radiation therapy to the entire CNS (whole brain and spine) along with boosts to local disease and bulk areas of disseminated disease. The traditional local postsurgical radiation doses in these patients has been 5,400 to 5,580 cGy. Doses of approximately 3,600 cGy to the entire neuraxis (i.e., the whole brain and spine) should also be administered, but may be modulated depending on the age of the patient. Boosts to bulk areas of spinal disease between 4,140 cGy and 5,040 cGy should be administered, with doses depending on the age of the patient and the location of the tumor. When possible, patients should be treated in a center experienced with this therapy. Trials are ongoing to evaluate the possible role of radiation therapy and chemotherapy in these patients.

Postsurgical management of children younger than 3 years of age: Because of the known effects of radiation on growth and neurocognitive development, its use immediately after surgery in children under 3 years of age is limited. Some patients younger than 3 years of age with newly diagnosed ependymoma will respond, at least partially, to chemotherapy. For this reason, strong consideration should be given to entering patients younger than 3 years of age in studies that use chemotherapy to delay the need for radiation therapy. Although chemotherapy is being used to prevent neurologic damage caused by radiation therapy in very young patients, neurologic deficits may be present in children prior to the initiation of therapy, and progressive neurologic damage has been noted during therapy. The need and timing of radiation therapy for children who have successfully completed chemotherapy and have no residual disease is still to be determined.

Recurrent Childhood Ependymoma

Recurrence is not uncommon in both benign and malignant childhood brain tumors and may develop many years after initial treatment. For ependymoma, delays beyond 10 to 15 years have been reported. Disease generally recurs at the primary tumor site even in children with malignant ependymomas. Systemic relapse is extremely rare. At time of relapse, a complete evaluation for extent of recurrence is indicated for all patients. The need for surgical intervention must be individualized on the basis of the extent of tumor, the length of time between initial treatment and the reappearance of the recurrent lesion, and the clinical picture. Patients with recurrent ependymomas who have not previously received radiation therapy and/or chemotherapy, should be considered for treatment with these modalities. Active agents include cyclophosphamide, cisplatin, carboplatin, lomustine, and etoposide.

Central Nervous System Germ Cell Tumor

Germ cell brain tumors usually arise in the pineal or suprasellar regions. Histologic subtypes include teratoma (both mature and immature), germinoma, choriocarcinomas, and nongerminomatous germ cell tumors (i.e., embryonal cell carcinoma, yolk cell tumor, and mixed germ cell tumors). These tumors have a propensity for subarachnoid spread. Every patient with a germinoma or malignant germ cell tumor should be evaluated with diagnostic imaging of the spinal cord and whole brain. The best method for evaluating spinal cord subarachnoid metastasis is MRI with gadolinium enhancement. Cerebrospinal fluid should be examined cytologically and levels of alphafetoprotein (AFP), and human chorionic gonadotropin (HCG) determined. AFP and/or HCG may be elevated in the serum of such patients. Prognosis is related to histology; patients with germinoma have a more favorable outcome than those with nongerminomatous germ cell tumors (nongerminomas).

Childhood Supratentorial Primitive Neuroectodermal Tumors

The classification of brain tumors is based on both histopathologic characteristics and location in the brain. Undifferentiated neuroectodermal tumors of the cerebellum have historically been referred to as medulloblastomas, while tumors of identical histology in the pineal region are diagnosed as pineoblastomas and cortical lesions have been called central neuroblastomas or cortical primitive neuroectodermal tumors. Studies have suggested that there are different molecular genetic aberrations in the tumor cells of medulloblastomas and supratentorial primitive neuroectodermal tumors. This group also includes some tumors formerly called central neuroblastomas. The nomenclature of pediatric brain tumors is controversial and potentially confusing. Some pathologists advocate abandoning the traditional morphologically based classifications such as medulloblastoma in favor of a terminology that relies more extensively on the phenotypic characteristics of the tumor. In such a system, medulloblastoma is referred to as primitive neuroectodermal tumor and then subdivided on the basis of cellular differentiation. The most recent World Health Organization classification of brain tumors maintains the term "medulloblastoma" for posterior fossa undifferentiated tumors. It also maintains separate categories for cerebral primitive neuroectodermal tumors and for pineal small round cell tumors (pineoblastomas). The pathologic classification of pediatric brain tumors is a specialized area that is undergoing evolution; review of the diagnostic tissue by a neuropathologist who has particular expertise in this area is strongly recommended.

Stage Information

Supratentorial primitive neuroectodermal tumor (PNET, cerebral neuroblastoma, and pineoblastoma).

2-year survival rate: 30 to 50%.

Poorly differentiated small round cell tumors of the cerebrum have been referred to as cerebral neuroblastoma and as primitive neuroectodermal tumors. These tumors in the pineal body have classically been called pineoblastomas. Histologically, these tumors may be similar to cerebellar medulloblastoma with varying proportions of features that suggest astrocytic or ependymal differentiation. Genetic aberrations of supratentorial brain tumors appear to be different from those of infratentorial primitive neuroectodermal tumors (PNET, medulloblastoma). Tumors may spread throughout the subarachnoid space. Every patient with a primitive neuroectodermal tumor or with pineoblastoma should be evaluated with diagnostic imaging of the spinal cord and whole brain. The most sensitive method currently available for evaluating spinal cord subarachnoid metastasis is spinal magnetic resonance imaging performed with gadolinium. Cerebrospinal fluid should be examined cytologically for tumor cells. There is no generally accepted staging system for supratentorial primitive neuroectodermal tumors and for pineoblastomas, but the staging system used for medulloblastoma is conventionally used for tumor dissemination. Prognosis is probably related to the extent of disease at diagnosis and after surgery. Patients with cystic tumors may fare better.

Treatment Option Overview

Supratentorial primitive neuroectodermal and pineal tumors (pineoblastoma).

Many of the improvements in survival in childhood cancer have been made as a result of clinical trials that have attempted to improve on the best available, accepted therapy. Clinical trials in pediatrics are designed to compare new therapy with therapy that is currently accepted as standard. This comparison may be done in a randomized study of 2 treatment arms or by evaluating a single new treatment and comparing the results with those previously obtained with existing therapy.

Because of the relative rarity of cancer in children, all patients with brain tumors should be considered for entry into a clinical trial. To determine and implement optimum treatment, treatment planning by a multidisciplinary team of cancer specialists who have experience treating childhood brain tumors is required. Radiation therapy, if needed, is technically very demanding and should be carried out in centers that have experience in that area to ensure optimal results.

In the past, treatment has included surgery with radiation therapy. There is evidence to suggest that more extensive surgical resections are related to an improved rate of survival for patients with medulloblastoma without dissemination at diagnosis, primarily in children with nondisseminated posterior fossa disease at diagnosis. This has not yet been proven for childhood supratentorial primitive neuroectodermal and pineal (pineoblastoma) tumors. Chemotherapy has been shown to be active in patients with recurrent supratentorial primitive neuroectodermal tumors, and there has been enthusiasm for exploring the role of chemotherapy in the treatment of all childhood brain tumors. The results of prospective, randomized trials and large single-arm trials have suggested that adjuvant chemotherapy given during and after radiation therapy may improve overall survival for a subset of children with medulloblastoma. There is no evidence that preradiation chemotherapy is of benefit in this tumor. A number of nonrandomized trials suggest potential benefit of post-radiation chemotherapy Children younger than 3 years of age are particularly susceptible to the adverse effect of radiation on brain development. Debilitating effects on growth and neurologic development have frequently been observed, especially in younger children. For this reason, the role of chemotherapy in allowing a delay in the administration of radiation therapy is under study, and preliminary results suggest that chemotherapy can be used to delay, if not obviate, the need for radiation therapy in some children less than 3 years of age with primitive neuro-ectodermal tumors.

Childhood Craniopharyngioma

Treatment Options

Therapies for craniopharyngioma include surgery and conventional external radiation therapy, and in selected cases, stereotactic radiosurgery or intracavitary irradiation. In general, each of these modalities, either alone or in combination, can give a high rate of long-term disease control in the majority of patients. Debate centers on the relative morbidity of the different approaches. Treatment of cystic tumors with intracavitary chemotherapy has also been reported.

Childhood Acute Lymphoblastic Leukemia

General Information

ALL is the most common cancer occurring in children, representing 23% of cancer diagnoses among children younger than 15 years and occurring at an annual rate of approximately 30 to 40 per million There is a sharp peak in ALL incidence among children ages 2 to 3 years (>80 per million per year), with rates decreasing to 20 per million for ages 8 to 10 years. The incidence of ALL among children ages 2 to 3 years is approximately 4-fold greater than that for infants and is nearly 10-fold greater than that for children who are 19 years old. There are few identified factors associated with increased risk of ALL. The primary accepted nongenetic risk factors for ALL are prenatal exposure to x-rays and postnatal exposure to high doses of radiation (e.g., therapeutic radiation as previously used for conditions such as tinea capitis and thymus enlargement). *Children with Down syndrome have increased risk for developing both ALL and acute myeloid leukemia (AML),* with a cumulative risk for developing leukemia of approximately 2.1% by age 5 years and 2.7% by age 30 years. Approximately two thirds of the cases of acute leukemia in children with Down syndrome are ALL. Increased occurrence of ALL is also associated with certain genetic conditions, including neurofibromatosis, Shwachman syndrome Bloom syndrome and ataxia telangiectasia

Certain cases of ALL that develop in children may have a prenatal origin. Evidence in support of this comes from the observation that the immunoglobulin or T-cell receptor antigen rearrangements that are unique to each patient's leukemia cells can be detected in blood samples obtained at birth. Similarly, there are data that patients with ALL characterized by specific chromosomal translocations have blood cells carrying the translocation at the time of birth.

Seventy-five percent to 80% of children with ALL attain remission and survive free of leukemia recurrence at least 5 years from diagnosis with current treatments that incorporate systemic therapy (e.g., combination chemotherapy) and specific central nervous system (CNS) preventive therapy (i.e., intrathecal chemotherapy with or without cranial irradiation). Ten-year event-free survival of multiple large prospective trials conducted in different countries for children treated primarily in the 1980s is approximately 70%.

Cellular Classification and Prognostic Variables

Children with acute lymphoblastic leukemia (ALL) are usually treated according to risk groups defined by both clinical and laboratory features. The intensity of treatment required for favorable outcome varies substantially among subsets of children with ALL. Risk-based treatment assignment is utilized for children with ALL so that those children who have a very good outcome with modest therapy can be spared more intensive and toxic treatment, while a more aggressive (and thus more toxic) therapeutic approach can be provided for patients who have a lower probability of long-term survival.

Risk-based treatment assignment requires the availability of prognostic factors that reliably predict outcome. For children with ALL, a number of clinical and laboratory features have demonstrated prognostic value, some of which are described below. The factors described are grouped into the following categories: clinical and laboratory features at diagnosis; leukemic cell characteristics at diagnosis; and response to initial treatment. As in any discussion of prognostic factors, it is critical to remember that the relative order of significance and the interrelationship of the variables are often treatment dependent and require multivariate analysis to determine which factors operate independently as prognostic variables. Because prognostic factors are treatment dependent, improvements in therapy may diminish or abrogate the significance of any of these presumed prognostic factors. For example, a report from the Children's Cancer Group (CCG) showed that the adverse prognostic significance of slow early response disappears when these patients receive intensified postinduction chemotherapy.

A subset of the prognostic factors discussed below is used for the initial stratification of children with ALL for treatment assignment, and at the end of this section there are brief descriptions of the prognostic groupings currently applied to clinical trials in the United States.

Clinical and Laboratory Features at Diagnosis

1. *Age at diagnosis:* Age at diagnosis has strong prognostic significance, reflecting the different underlying biology of ALL in different age groups.

   Infants with ALL have a particularly high risk of treatment failure, with the risk of treatment failure being greatest for young infants (younger than 3 months) and those with poor early-response to prednisone. Rearrangement of the *MLL* gene at chromosome band 11q23 can be detected in the leukemia cells of a large percentage of infants with ALL, and the poor outcome for infants with ALL is strongly associated with the presence of the *MLL* gene rearrangement. Infants *lacking MLL gene rearrangements* tend to be older than 6 months of age, have lower white blood cell

(WBC) counts, and have a better prognosis than infants possessing *MLL* gene rearrangements ALL in infants is also associated with a constellation of other characteristics associated with poor outcome, including elevated WBC count, central nervous system leukemia, lack of CD10 (cALLa antigen) expression, and poor response to initial treatment. The recent association of increased *FLT3* expression in infant ALL with *MLL* rearrangements has provided a potentially important growth and survival receptor to target therapeutically.

Young children (1-9 years) have a favorable outcome in comparison to either older children and adolescents or in comparison to infants.

2. *WBC count at diagnosis:* Higher WBC counts at diagnosis represent an increased risk for treatment failure in patients with B-precursor ALL. A WBC count of 50,000/μL is generally used as an operational cut point between better and poorer prognosis although the relationship between WBC count and prognosis is a continuous rather than a step function. Elevated WBC count is often associated with other high-risk prognostic factors, including unfavorable chromosomal translocations such as t(4;11) and t(9;22) (see below).
3. *Central nervous system status at diagnosis:* Central nervous system (CNS) status at diagnosis has prognostic significance. Patients who have a nontraumatic diagnostic lumbar puncture may be placed into 3 categories according to their CNS status:
   - *CNS1:* CSF <5 WBC/μL with cytospin negative for blasts.
   - *CNS2:* CSF <5 WBC/μL with cytospin positive for blasts.
   - *CNS3:* CSF >/= 5 WBC/μL with cytospin positive for blasts.

   Children with ALL who present with CNS disease at diagnosis (i.e., CNS3) are at higher risk for treatment failure (both within the CNS and systemically) compared to patients not meeting the criteria for CNS disease at diagnosis. Patients with small numbers of leukemic cells in the cerebrospinal fluid at diagnosis that are below those required for a diagnosis of CNS disease (i.e., CNS2) may be at increased risk of CNS relapse, although this observation may not apply to all treatment regimens. Any increased risk associated with CNS2 status on overall outcome can apparently be overcome by more intensive intrathecal therapy. A traumatic lumbar puncture which includes blasts at diagnosis appears to be associated with increased risk of CNS relapse and indicates an overall poorer outcome.
4. *Gender:* The *prognosis for girls with ALL is slightly better* than for boys with ALL. One reason for the superior prognosis for girls is the occurrence of testicular relapses among boys, but boys also appear to be at increased risk for bone marrow and CNS relapse for reasons that are not well understood.

Leukemic Cell Characteristics

1. *Morphology: In the past, ALL lymphoblasts were classified using the French-American-British (FAB) criteria* as having L1 morphology, L2 morphology, or L3 morphology. Due to the lack of independent prognostic significance and the subjective nature of this classification system, it is no longer used in the United States. Most cases of ALL which show L3 morphology express surface immunoglobulin and have a *C-MYC* gene translocation identical to the findings for Burkitt's lymphoma (e.g., t[8;14]). The treatment of this specific, rare form of ALL (B-cell ALL) is completely different than for other forms of childhood ALL. Cases with L3 morphology that do not express surface immunoglobulin and do not show *C-MYC* translocation, should be treated as B-precursor

ALL. Conversely, patients with *C-MYC* translocations and L3 morphology who do not express surface immunoglobulin should be treated as B-cell ALL/Burkitt's lymphoma.

2. *Immunophenotype:*
   - *B-precursor ALL:* B-cell precursor (or B-lineage) ALL, defined by the expression of CD19, HLA-DR, CD10 *(cALLa)*, and other B-cell associated antigens, represents 80% to 85% of childhood ALL. Approximately 80% of B-precursor ALL express the cALLa, CD10 antigen. The lack of cALLa expression has also been shown in some series to be associated with a worse prognosis. For example, CD10 negativity is observed in a higher proportion of infants with B-precursor ALL and is associated with poor outcome.
   - *Stage of B-cell maturation:* There are 3 major subtypes of B-lineage ALL:
     - § Early pre-B (no surface or cytoplasmic immunoglobulin).
     - § Pre-B (presence of cytoplasmic immunoglobulin).
     - § B-cell (presence of surface immunoglobulin).

   Approximately three quarters of patients with B-precursor ALL have the early pre-B phenotype and have the best prognosis. The leukemic cells of patients with pre-B ALL contain cytoplasmic immunoglobulin (cIg), an intermediate stage of B-cell differentiation. Twenty-five percent of patients with pre-B ALL have the t(1;19) translocation (see below). Approximately 3% of patients have transitional pre-B ALL expression of surface immunoglobulin heavy chain without light chain, without *C-MYC* gene involvement or L3 morphology. Patients with this phenotype respond well to therapy used for B-cell precursor ALL. Approximately 2% of patients present with B-cell ALL (surface Ig expression, generally with FAB L3 morphology and *C-MYC* gene translocation). B-cell ALL is a systemic manifestation of Burkitt's and Burkitt's-like non-Hodgkin's lymphoma, and its treatment is completely different from that for other forms of childhood ALL. Rare cases of ALL that express surface Ig but lack *C-MYC* gene translocations are appropriately treated as B-precursor ALL rather than B-cell ALL.
   - *T-cell ALL:* T-cell ALL is defined by the leukemic cell expression of the T-cell-associated antigens CD2, CD7, CD5, or CD3 and is frequently associated with a constellation of clinical features including male sex, older age, leukocytosis, and mediastinal mass Approximately 12% of children with newly diagnosed ALL have the T-cell phenotype. With appropriately intensive therapy, however, children with T-cell ALL have an outcome similar to that for children with B-precursor ALL. Cytogenetic abnormalities common in B-cell lineage ALL (e.g., hyperdiploidy) are uncommon in T-cell ALL Neither presence of a mediastinal mass, nor rapidity of radiographic response of the mass to therapy, is associated with an adverse outcome in T-cell ALL
   - *Myeloid antigen expression:* Up to one third of childhood ALL cases have leukemia cells that express myeloid-associated surface antigens. Myeloid-associated antigen expression appears to be associated with specific ALL subgroups, notably those with *MLL* gene rearrangements and those with the *TEL-AML1* gene rearrangement There is no independent adverse prognostic significance for myeloid surface antigen expression

3. *Cytogenetics*
   - *Chromosome number:*
     - § *Hyperdiploidy:* Hyperdiploidy (>50 chromosomes per cell or DNA index

>1.16) is the presence of additional copies of whole chromosomes and occurs in 20% to 25% of cases of B-precursor ALL but very rarely in cases of T-cell ALL. Hyperdiploidy can be evaluated by measuring the DNA content of cells (DNA index) or by karyotyping. Hyperdiploidy generally occurs in cases with favorable prognostic factors (age 1-9 years and low WBC count), and is itself associated with favorable prognosis However, outcome of children with hyperdiploidy is heterogeneous and depends on age, sex, and specific trisomies Hyperdiploid leukemia cells are particularly susceptible to undergoing apoptosis, and accumulate methotrexate and high levels of its active polyglutamate metabolites,which may explain the favorable outcome commonly observed for these cases.

§ *Trisomies:* For the treatment approaches utilized by both the former Pediatric Oncology Group (POG) and the former Children's Cancer Group (CCG), *extra copies of certain chromosomes appear to be specifically associated with favorable prognosis among hyperdiploid* ALL cases. In POG studies, patients whose leukemia cells have extra copies of both chromosome 4 and chromosome 10 appear to have particularly favorable outcome. In CCG studies, children with *trisomies of chromosomes 10 and 17 have an excellent prognosis.* In new Children's Oncology Group (COG) trials, the presence of trisomies for 4, 10, and 17 will be utilized to define a potentially favorable (low)-risk group.

§ *Hypodiploidy:* Approximately 1% of children with ALL have leukemia cells showing hypodiploidy with less than 45 chromosomes. These patients are at high risk for treatment failure. There is a significant trend for progressively worse outcome with a decreasing chromosome number, such that cases with 24 to 28 chromosomes (near haploidy) have the worst outcome.

- *Chromosomal translocations:* Recurring chromosomal translocations can be detected in a substantial number of cases of childhood ALL, and some of these translocations, as described below, have prognostic significance.

TEL-AML1 (t(12;21) cryptic translocation): Fusion of the *TEL* (*ETV6*) gene on chromosome 12 to the *AML1* (*CBFA2*) gene on chromosome 21 can be detected in 20 to 25% of cases of B-precursor ALL, but is rarely observed in T-cell ALL. Children with the t(12;21) cryptic translocation resulting in the *TEL-AML1* fusion are generally 2 to 9 years of age Patients with the *TEL-AML1* fusion have an excellent outcome There is controversy about whether ultimate event-free survival (EFS) is actually superior to that of other patients with B-precursor ALL, or whether the ultimate EFS is similar but the timing of relapse is significantly later for patients with the *TEL-AML1* fusion compared to other patients with B-precursor ALL Patients with *TEL AML1* fusion seem to have a better outcome after relapse than other patients, although, because of small numbers, the difference statistically is not significantly different

The Philadelphia chromosome t(9;22) is present in approximately 3% of pediatric ALL patients and confers an unfavorable prognosis, especially when it is associated with either a high WBC count or slow early response to initial therapy Philadelphia-positive ALL is more common in older patients with B-precursor ALL and high WBC count.

Translocations involving the *MLL* (11q23) gene occur in approximately 8% of childhood ALL cases, and are generally associated with increased risk for treatment failure The t(4;11) is the most common translocation involving the *MLL* gene in children with ALL and occurs in approximately 2% of cases Patients with t(4;11) generally present in infancy with high WBC count, and they are more likely than other children with ALL to have CNS disease and to have a poor response to initial therapy While both infants and adults with the t(4;11) are at high risk for treatment failure, children with the t(4;11) appear to have a better outcome than either infants or adults Irrespective of the type of 11q23 abnormality, infants with leukemia cells having 11q23 abnormalities had a worse treatment outcome than older patients whose leukemia cells had an 11q23 abnormality Of interest, the t(11;19) occurs in approximately 1% of cases and occurs in both B-precursor and T-cell ALL Outcome for infants with t(11;19) is poor, but outcome appears relatively favorable for children with T-cell ALL and the t(11;19) translocation.

The t(1;19) translocation occurs in 5% to 6% of childhood ALL, and involves fusion of the *E2A* gene on chromosome 19 to the *PBX1* gene on chromosome 1 The t(1;19) may occur as either a balanced translocation or as an unbalanced translocation and is primarily associated with pre-B ALL (cytoplasmic immunoglobulin positive). Its presence was initially associated with inferior outcome in the context of antimetabolite-based therapy Studies have shown that the poorer prognosis associated with t(1;19) can be largely overcome by more intensive therapy Some studies suggested that cases with a balanced translocation t(1;19) had a worse outcome than did those with an unbalanced translocation der(19) t(1;19), but this finding is not consistent in other studies.

4. *Early Response to Treatment:* The rapidity with which leukemia cells are eliminated following onset of treatment is also associated with outcome. Because treatment response is influenced by the drug sensitivity of leukemic cells and host pharmacodynamics and pharmacogenomics, this measure should have strong prognostic significance. Various ways of evaluating the leukemia cell response to treatment have been utilized, including:

1. *Day 7 and day 14 bone marrow responses:* Patients who have a rapid reduction in the leukemia cells in their bone marrow within 7 or 14 days following initiation of multiagent chemotherapy have a more favorable prognosis than do patients who have slower clearance of leukemia cells from the bone marrow. This "response to treatment" prognostic factor initially used by the CCG, will also be utilized in new COG ALL trials to stratify patients into prognostic categories for treatment assignment.

2. *Peripheral blood response to steroid prephase:* Patients with a reduction in peripheral blast count to less than 1,000/μL after a 7-day induction prephase with prednisone and 1 dose of intrathecal methotrexate ("good prednisone response") have a more favorable prognosis than patients whose peripheral blast counts remain above 1,000/μL ("poor prednisone response") Treatment stratification for protocols of the German Berlin-Frankfurt-Munster clinical trials group is based on early response to the prednisone 7-day induction prephase. Patients whose blast counts are less than 1,000/μL at diagnosis have a slightly better outcome compared to other prednisone good responders.

3. *Peripheral blood response to multiagent induction therapy:* Patients with persistent circulating leukemia cells at 7 to 10 days after the initiation of multiagent chemotherapy are at increased risk of relapse

compared to patients who have clearance of peripheral blasts within 1 week of therapy initiation. Rate of clearance of peripheral blasts has been found to be of prognostic significance in T-lineage as well as B-lineage ALL.

TREATMENT OPTION OVERVIEW

Risk-based treatment assignment is an important therapeutic strategy utilized for children with acute lymphoblastic leukemia (ALL). This approach allows children who historically have a very good outcome to be treated with modest therapy and to be spared more intensive and toxic treatment, while allowing children with a historically lower probability of long-term survival to receive more intensive therapy that may increase their chance of cure A subset of the known prognostic factors (e.g., age, white blood cell (WBC) count at diagnosis, presence of specific cytogenetic abnormalities) are used for the initial stratification of children with ALL into treatment groups with varying degrees of risk for treatment failure. Event-free survival (EFS) rates for children meeting "good risk" age and WBC criteria exceed 80%, while for children meeting "high risk" criteria, EFS rates are approximately 70%. Application of biological factors (e.g., specific chromosomal translocations, and hypodiploidy) can identify patient groups with expected outcome survival rates ranging from less than 40% to greater than 85%.

UNTREATED CHILDHOOD ACUTE LYMPHOBLASTIC LEUKEMIA

Induction Chemotherapy

Three-drug induction therapy using vincristine, prednisone/dexamethasone, plus L-asparaginase in conjunction with intrathecal therapy (IT), results in complete remission rates of greater than 95%. For patients at high risk for treatment failure, a more intense induction regimen (4 or 5 agents) may result in improved event-free survival (EFS) and "high risk" patients generally receive induction therapy that includes an anthracycline (e.g., daunomycin) in addition to vincristine, prednisone/dexamethasone, plus L-asparaginase. For patients who are at standard or low risk of treatment failure, 4-drug induction therapy does not appear necessary for favorable outcome provided that adequate postremission intensification therapy is administered. Because of the likelihood of increased toxicity with 4-drug induction therapy, most centers treat standard or lower risk patients with dexamethasone, vincristine, and L-asparaginase and reserve the use of induction regimens using 4 or more agents for higher risk patients.

In general, patients will achieve a complete remission within the first 4 weeks. Patients who require more than 4 weeks to achieve remission have a poor prognosis.

The early institution of adequate CNS sanctuary therapy is critical in preventing CNS relapse. A current goal of ALL therapy design is to achieve effective CNS sanctuary therapy while minimizing neurotoxicity. Every patient with ALL receives intrathecal chemotherapy with methotrexate alone or methotrexate with cytarabine plus hydrocortisone. Intrathecal therapy may also have a significant systemic effect that could result in a decrease in marrow relapse rate. Significant control of bone marrow relapse did not occur until CNS sanctuary therapy was instituted. The long-term deleterious effects of cranial radiation when used for CNS prophylaxis, particularly at doses greater than 1,800 cGy, have been recognized for years. Childhood Acute Lymphoblastic Leukemia in Remission

Consolidation/Intensification

Once remission has been achieved, systemic treatment in conjunction with central nervous system (CNS) sanctuary therapy follows. The intensity of the postinduction chemotherapy varies considerably, but all patients receive some form of intensification following achievement of remission and before beginning continuous maintenance therapy. Intensification may involve the use of intermediate- or high-dose methotrexate,] the use of similar drugs as those used to achieve remission the use of different drug combinations with little known cross resistance to the induction therapy drug combination,the extended use of high-dose L-asparaginase, or combinations of the above.

Maintenance

The backbone of maintenance therapy in most protocols includes daily oral mercaptopurine and weekly oral methotrexate. If the patient has not had cranial radiation, intrathecal chemotherapy for CNS sanctuary therapy is generally given during maintenance therapy. Clinical trials generally call for giving *oral mercaptopurine* in the evening, which is supported by evidence that this practice may improve event-free survival (EFS) Pulses of *vincristine and prednisone/dexamethasone* are often added to the standard maintenance regimen. Maintenance chemotherapy generally continues until 2 to 3 years of continuous complete remission. Extending the duration of maintenance therapy to 5 years does not improve outcome.

Postinduction Treatment for Childhood Acute Lymphoblastic Leukemia Subgroups

T-cell Acute Lymphoblastic Leukemia

Protocols of the former Pediatric Oncology Group (POG) treated children with T-cell acute lymphoblastic leukemia (ALL) distinctly from children with B-precursor ALL. The POG protocol for patients with T-cell ALL was designed to evaluate the role of high-dose methotrexate and the role of the cardioprotectant dexrazoxane.

Infants With Acute Lymphoblastic Leukemia

Because of their distinctive biological characteristics and their high risk for leukemia recurrence, infants with ALL are treated on protocols specifically designed for this patient population.

Treating infants with and without *MLL* gene rearrangements with different treatment protocols has been evaluated in a Japanese study. A favorable outcome was obtained with antimetabolite-based therapy for *MLL*-negative patients, while outcome remained unfavorable, despite intensive chemotherapy, for infants with *MLL* gene rearrangements. This raises the question as to whether infants with precursor-B immunophenotype and germline *MLL* configuration should be treated on the same protocols as similar patients older than one year.

For infants with t(4;11), the role of bone marrow transplantation was evaluated in a retrospective analysis of 256 patients initially treated between 1983 and 1995. No benefit was observed for any type of allogeneic stem cell transplant compared to intensive chemotherapy without transplant.

Recurrent Childhood Acute Lymphoblastic Leukemia

Standard Treatment Options

The prognosis for a child with acute lymphoblastic leukemia (ALL) whose disease recurs depends on the time and site of relapse If the recurrence occurs in the bone marrow either during front-line therapy or within 6 months of discontinuation of initial therapy, the prognosis for long-term survival is poor with a less than 10% likelihood of long-term survival using chemotherapy alone However, if relapse occurs more than a year after discontinuation of initial therapy, the prognosis is better with 30 to 40% of these patients achieving long-term, disease-free survival in large studies using aggressive salvage chemotherapy Children with T-cell ALL who relapse at any time also have survival rates less than 20%. There are preliminary data that minimal residual disease (MRD) status after induction of second remission is of prognostic significance in patients with late-relapsing disease. Targeted therapies specific for ALL are being developed, including monoclonal antibody-based therapies and using drugs that inhibit signal transduction pathways required for leukemia cell growth and survival. Information about ongoing clinical trials is available from the.........

Childhood Acute Myeloid Leukemia/Other Myeloid Malignancies

General Information

AML is the most common type of myeloid malignancy of childhood. Between 75% and 85% of children with AML can achieve a complete remission following appropriate induction chemotherapy. Children with newly diagnosed AML have an event-free 5-year survival rate of approximately 50% The most consistent prognostic factor across studies of AML in children is white blood cell (WBC) count at diagnosis. Children who have a WBC count greater than $100,000/ml^3$ have a poor prognosis. Additional factors that have been associated with a poor prognosis are secondary AML and monosomy 7 karyotype. Children with leukemia cell chromosomal abnormalities t(8;21) and inv 16 have a high likelihood of achieving remission and a decreased likelihood of relapse. Translocations of chromosomal band !1q23, including most AML secondary to epipodophyllotoxin, are less favorable in most studies. One exception to the poor prognostic significance of translocations at chromosome band 11q23 may be the t(9;11). In some reports, outcome has been relatively favorable for patients whose leukemia cells have t(9;11), although favorable outcome has not been observed in other series *Children with Down syndrome have an increased risk of leukemia with a ratio of ALL to AML typical for childhood acute leukemia, except during the first 3 years of life when AML (especially M7) predominates. Neonates with Down syndrome may manifest a transient myeloproliferative syndrome (TMS). This disorder mimics congenital AML but improves spontaneously within 4 to 6 weeks.* The myelodysplastic syndromes *(MDS)* represent a heterogeneous group of disorders of hematopoiesis leading to variable degrees of pancytopenia and often AML. In adults, MDS have been classified by the FAB group into distinct categories. The FAB MDS classification is not an adequate classification for the syndromes that occur in children. The World Health Organization (WHO) has developed a modified classification schema for MDS. Previously MDS were classified as having less than 30% blasts. *The WHO has changed the MDS classification to having less than 20% blasts.* The optimal management of MDS in children has not been well-studied in prospective trials.

Juvenile myelomonocytic leukemia (JMML), formerly termed juvenile chronic myeloid leukemia (JCML), is a rare hematopoietic malignancy of childhood accounting for less than 1% of all childhood leukemias. A number of clinical and laboratory features distinguish JMML from adult-type chronic myeloid leukemia, a disease noted only occasionally in children. Few approaches other than hematopoietic stem cell transplantation have resulted in long-term survival for this disease. Children with neurofibromatosis 1 (NF1) and Noonans syndrome are at increased risk for developing JMML and up to 14% of cases of JMML occur in children with NF1.

Cellular Classification

FAB classification for childhood acute myeloid leukemia

The most comprehensive morphologic-histochemical classification system for acute myeloid leukemia (AML) was developed by the French-American-British (FAB) Cooperative Group. This classification system categorizes AML into the following major subtypes:

- *M0: acute myeloblastic leukemia without localized differentiation.*

  Note: Recognition of M0 AML requires reactivity with either monoclonal antibody CD13 or CD33 or myeloperoxidase (MPO) expression by immunohistochemistry. To be categorized as M0, the leukemic blasts must not display specific morphologic or histochemical features of either AML or acute lymphocytic leukemia (ALL).]
- M1: acute myeloblastic leukemia without maturation.
- M2: acute myeloblastic leukemia with maturation.
- M3: acute promyelocytic leukemia (AProL or APL with 15;17 translocation).

  Note: Identifying this subtype is critical since the risk of fatal hemorrhagic complication prior to or during induction is high and the appropriate therapy is different.]
- M4: acute myelomonocytic leukemia (AMML).
- M5: acute monocytic leukemia (AMoL).
- M5a: AMoL without differentiation (monoblastic).
- M5b: AMoL with differentiation.
- M6: acute erythroleukemia.
- M7: acute megakaryocytic leukemia.

Note: Diagnosis of M7 can be difficult without the use of flow cytometry as the blasts can be morphologically confused with lymphoblasts. Characteristically, the blasts display cytoplasmic blebs. Marrow aspiration can be difficult due to myelofibrosis, and marrow biopsy with reticulin stain can be helpful].

Other extremely rare subtypes of AML include acute eosinophilic leukemia and acute basophilic leukemia.

Fifty percent to 60% of children with AML can be classified as having M1, M2, M3, M6, or M7 subtypes; approximately 40% have M4 or M5 subtypes. About 80% of children younger than 2 years with AML have a M4 or M5 subtype. The response to cytotoxic chemotherapy among children with the different subtypes of AML is relatively similar. One exception is FAB subtype M3, for which all-*trans* retinoic acid plus chemotherapy achieves remission and cure in most children with AML.

Histochemical Evaluation

The treatment for children with AML differs significantly from that for ALL. As a consequence, it is crucial to distinguish AML from ALL. Special histochemical stains should be performed on bone marrow specimens of all children with acute leukemia to confirm their diagnosis. The stains most commonly used include myeloperoxidase, PAS, Sudan Black B, and esterase. In most cases the staining pattern with these histochemical stains will distinguish AML from AMML and ALL (see below).

	M0	*AML,APL (M1-M3)*	*AMML (M4)*	*AMoL (M5)*	*AEL (M6)*	*AMKL (M7)*	*ALL*
* *[Note: These reactions are inhibited by fluoride.]*							
Myeloperoxidase	–	+	+	–	–	–	–
Nonspecific esterases							
Chloracetate	–	+	+	–/+	–	–	–
Alpha-naphthol acetate	–	–	+*	+*	–	–/+*	–
Sudan Black B	–	+	+	–	–	–	–
PAS	–	–	–/+	–/+	+	–	+

The use of monoclonal antibodies to determine cell surface antigens of AML cells is helpful to reinforce the histologic diagnosis. Various "lineage-specific" monoclonal antibodies that detect antigens on AML cells should be used at leukemia diagnosis, along with a battery of lineage-specific T- and B-lymphocyte markers to help distinguish AML from ALL and mixed-lineage or biphenotypic or biclonal leukemias. Various cluster designations (CD) that are currently thought to be relatively lineage-specific for AML include CD33, CD13, CD14, CDw41 (or platelet antiglycoprotein IIB/IIIA), CD15, CD11B, CD36, and antiglycophorin A. Lineage-associated B-lymphocytic antigens CD10, CD19, CD20, CD22, and CD24 may be present in 10 to 20% of AMLs, but monoclonal surface immunoglobulin and cytoplasmic immunoglobulin heavy chains are usually absent; similarly, CD2, CD3, CD5, and CD7 lineage-specific T-lymphocytic antigens are present in 20 to 40% of AMLs. The expression of lymphoid-associated antigens by AML cells is relatively common but has no prognostic significance.

Immunophenotyping can also be helpful in distinguishing some FAB subtypes of AML. Testing for the presence of HLA-DR can be helpful in identifying APL. Overall, HLA-DR is expressed on 75 to 80% of AMLs but rarely expressed on APL. In addition, APL cases with PML-RARalpha were noted to express CD34/CD15 and demonstrate a heterogenous pattern of CD13 expression. Testing for the presence of glycoprotein Ib, glycoprotein IIB/IIIa, or Factor VIII antigen expression is helpful in making the diagnosis of M7 (megakaryocytic leukemia). *Glycophorin expression is helpful in making the diagnosis of M6 (erythroleukemia).*

Cytogenetic Evaluation

Chromosomal analyses should be performed on children with AML because they are important diagnostic and prognostic markers. Clonal chromosomal abnormalities have been identified in the blasts of about 75% of children with AML and are useful in defining subtypes with particular characteristics (e.g., t(8;21) with M2, t(15;17) with M3, inv 16 with M4 eo, 11q23 abnormalities with M4 and M5, t(1;22) with M7).

Molecular probes and newer cytogenetic techniques (e.g., fluorescence in situ hybridization (FISH)) can detect cryptic abnormalities that were not evident by standard cytogenetic banding studies. This is clinically important when optimal therapy differs, as in APL. Use of these techniques can identify cases of APL when the diagnosis is suspected but the t(15;17) is not identified by routine cytogenetic evaluation. The presence of the Philadelphia chromosome in children with AML most likely represents chronic myelogenous leukemia (CML) that has transformed to AML rather than de novo AML.

Classification of Myelodysplastic Syndromes in Children

The FAB classification of myelodysplastic syndromes (MDS) is not completely applicable to children. In adults, MDS is divided into several distinct categories based on the presence of myelodysplasia, types of cytopenia, specific chromosomal abnormalities, and the percentage of myeloblasts.

A modified classification schema for MDS and myeloproliferative disorders has been developed by the World Health Organization (WHO). The primary WHO classification changes include:

- Cases with 20 to 29% blasts should be called AML, thus eliminating refractory anemia with excess blasts in transformation (RAEB-T).
- RAEB is now divided into RAEB-1 (5-9% bone marrow (BM) blasts) and RAEB-2 (10-19% BM blasts).
- Multilineage dysplasia will be highlighted under refractory anemia with ringed sideroblasts (RARS) or refractory anemia (RA).

- Juvenile myelomonocytic leukemia (JMML) and proliferative chronic myelomonocytic leukemia (CMML) will be under MDS/MPD (myeloproliferative disorder).
- MDS unclassified, will include severe myelofibrosis.
- MDS associated with isolated del(5q) will be a separate category.
- Monocytosis (under 13,000 monocytes) will be listed under the other subtypes rather than a separate category.

RARS is rare in children. RA and RAEB are more common. The WHO classification schema has a new subgroup that includes JMML (formerly, Juvenile Chronic Myeloid Leukemia), CMML, and Philadelphia chromosome-negative (Ph-) chronic myelogenous leukemia. This group can show mixed myeloproliferative and sometimes myelodysplastic features. JMML shares some characteristics with adult CMML but is a distinct syndrome (see below). The Infantile Monosomy 7 Syndrome includes children less than 4 years of age at diagnosis with any type of myelodysplasia and monosomy 7. This entity shares many characteristics with JMML and may be best considered a subset of this disease. Older children with monosomy 7 and characteristics of MDS should be classified by the FAB MDS classification. An alternative classification schema in children has been proposed.

Diagnostic Classification of Juvenile Myelomonocytic Leukemia

JMML, is a rare leukemia that accounts for less than 1% of childhood leukemia cases. JMML typically presents in young children (median age approximately 1 year) and occurs more commonly in boys (male to female ratio approximately 2.5:1). Common clinical features at diagnosis include hepatosplenomegaly (97%), lymphadenopathy (76%), pallor (64%), fever (54%), and skin rash (36%). In children presenting with clinical features

WHO classification of myelodysplastic syndromes

	RA	*RARS*	*RCMD*	*RCMD-RS*	*RAEB-1*	*RAEB-2*	*MDS-U*	*5q*
Anemia	+	+	+/-	+/-	+/-	+/-	+/-	+
Granulocytopenia			+/-	+/-	+	+	+	
Thrombocytopenia			+/-	+/-	+	+	+	
Marrow dysplasia								
erythroid	+	+			+/-	+/-		
myeloid			>/= 10% in 2 or more myeloid cell lines	>/= 10% in 2 or more myeloid cell lines	+/-	+/-	+ in one myeloid cell line	
megakaryocytic	+/-	+/-		+/-				
Auer's rods			None	None	None	+/-	None	None
Ringed sideroblasts	<15%	>or = 15%	<15%	>or = 15%				
Peripheral blasts	Rare or none	None	Rare or none	Rare or none	<5%	5-19%	Rare or none	<5%
Bone marrow blasts	<5%	<5%	<5%	<5%	5-9%	10-19%	<5%	<5%
Peripheral monocytosis (>1 × 10⁹/L)			No	No	No	No		

RA= refractory anemia (Includes only erythroid dysplasia); RARS= refractory anemia with ringed sideroblasts (Includes only erythroid dysplasia); RCMD= refractory cytopenia with multilineage dysplasia; RCMD-RS= refractory cytopenia with multilineage dysplasia and ringed sideroblasts; RAEB-1= refractory anemia with excess blasts-1: 5-9% marrow blasts; RAEB-2= refractory anemia with excess blasts-2: 10-19% marrow blasts; MDS-U= myelodysplastic syndrome-unclassified; 5q= myelodysplastic syndrome associated with isolated del(5q) suggestive of JMML, a definitive diagnosis requires the following:

Category	*Item*
Minimal Laboratory criteria (all 3 have to be fulfilled)	1. No Ph chromosome, no bcr-abl rearrangement
	2. Peripheral blood monocyte count > 1 × 10^9/L
	3. Bone marrow blasts < 20%
Criteria for definite diagnosis (at least 2 must be fulfilled)	1. Hemoglobin F increased for age
	2. Myeloid precursors on peripheral blood smear
	3. White blood count > 10 × 10^9/L
	4. Clonal abnormality (including monosomy 7)
	5. GM-CSF hypersensitivity of myeloid progenitors in vitro

While the majority of children with JMML have no detectable cytogenetic abnormalities, a minority show loss of chromosome 7 in bone marrow cells. Children with myelodysplastic syndrome and monosomy 7 have sometimes been considered to have *"Monosomy 7 Syndrome,"* defined by age younger than 4 years and by loss of chromosome 7.However, data provide limited support for the concept of monosomy 7 as a distinct syndrome, and instead support considering children with clinical features of JMML as having 1 disorder without regard to the presence or absence of chromosome 7.

Treatment Option Overview

Many of the improvements in survival for children and adolescents with acute myeloid leukemia (AML) have been made using new therapies that have attempted to improve on the best available therapy. The mainstay of the therapeutic approach is systemically administered combination chemotherapy. Future approaches involving risk group stratification and biologically targeted therapies are being tested to improve antileukemic treatment while sparing normal tissues Optimal treatment of AML requires control of bone marrow and systemic disease. Treatment of the central nervous system, usually with intrathecal medication, is a component of most pediatric AML protocols but has not yet been shown to contribute directly to an improvement in survival.

Treatment is ordinarily divided into 2 phases: (1) induction (to attain remission) and (2) post-remission consolidation/intensification. Post-remission therapy may consist of varying numbers of courses of intensive chemotherapy and/or allogeneic bone marrow transplantation (BMT). For example, the Children's Cancer Group (CCG) trial (CCG-2961) uses induction therapy followed by 2 courses of chemotherapy, 1 utilizing high-dose cytarabine. A pediatric AML regimen developed by the United Kingdom Medical Research Council (MRC) utilizes 3 or 4 courses of chemotherapy following remission induction chemotherapy

Maintenance therapy is not part of most pediatric AML protocols with the exception of the Berlin-Frankfurt-Munster (BFM) protocols. In aggressively treated AML, maintenance therapy does not appear to be of value. Treatment of AML is usually associated with severe and protracted myelosuppression along with other associated complications. Treatment with hematopoietic growth factors (G-CSF, GM-CSF) has been used in an attempt to reduce the toxicity associated with severe myelosuppression but does not influence ultimate outcome. Virtually all adult randomized trials of hematopoietic growth factors (G-CSF, GM-CSF) have demonstrated significant reduction in the time to neutrophil recovery but varying degrees of reduction in morbidity and little if any effect on mortality.

Untreated Childhood Acute Myeloid Leukemia and Other Myeloid Malignancies

The general principles of therapy for children and adolescents with acute myeloid leukemia (AML)

are discussed below, followed by a more specific discussion of the treatment of children with acute promyelocytic leukemia (APL), Down syndrome, myelodysplastic syndrome (MDS), and juvenile myelomonocytic leukemia (JMML).

Induction Chemotherapy for Acute Myelogenous Leukemia

Contemporary effective pediatric AML protocols result in 75 to 90% complete remission (CR) rates. Of those patients who do not go into remission, about one half have resistant leukemia and one half die from the complications of the disease or its treatment. To achieve a complete remission, inducing profound bone marrow aplasia (with the exception of the M3 APL subtype) is usually necessary. Because induction chemotherapy produces severe myelosuppression, morbidity and mortality from infection or hemorrhage during the induction period may be significant.

The two most effective drugs used to induce remission in children with AML are cytarabine and an anthracycline. Commonly used pediatric induction therapy regimens use cytarabine and an anthracycline in combination with other agents such as etoposide and/or thioguanine. For example, the Children's Cancer Group (CCG) intensively-timed DCTER regimen utilizes cytarabine, daunorubicin, dexamethasone, etoposide, and thioguanine and is given as 2 4-day treatments separated by 6 days. The German Berlin-Frankfurt-Munster (BFM) Group has studied cytarabine and daunorubicin plus etoposide (ADE) given over 8 days, and the United Kingdom Medical Research Council (MRC) has studied a similar ADE regimen given over 10 days. The MRC has also studied cytarabine and daunorubicin given with thioguanine (DAT). A randomized trial that included both children and adults comparing either etoposide or thioguanine given with cytarabine and daunorubicin (i.e., ADE versus DAT) showed no difference between the thioguanine and etoposide arms in remission rate or disease-free survival

The anthracycline that has been most used in induction regimens for children with AML is daunorubicin although idarubicin has also been used. A randomized study in children with newly diagnosed AML comparing daunorubicin and idarubicin (each given with cytarabine and etoposide) observed a trend favoring idarubicin, but the small benefit for idarubicin in terms of remission rate and event-free survival was not statistically significant. Similarly, studies comparing idarubicin and daunorubicin in adults with AML have not produced compelling evidence that idarubicin is more efficacious than daunorubicin. In the absence of convincing data that another anthracycline produces superior outcome to daunorubicin when given at an equitoxic dose, daunorubicin remains the anthracycline most commonly used during induction therapy for children with AML.

Randomized trials evaluating hematopoietic growth factors during induction therapy for patients with AML have not been performed in children, and so the potential benefit of these agents for children with AML must be extrapolated from the adult experience. Hematopoietic growth factors such as granulocyte-macrophage colony-stimulating factor (GM-CSF) or granulocyte colony-stimulating factor (G-CSF) during AML induction therapy have been evaluated in multiple placebo-controlled studies in attempts to reduce the toxicity associated with prolonged myelosuppression. Treatment with hematopoietic growth factor generally begins within a day or 2 following the completion of cytotoxic therapy and continues until granulocyte recovery. A reduction of several days in the duration of neutropenia with the use of either G-CSF or GM-CSF has been observed Most, but not all, randomized studies showed statistically significant reductions in the duration of hospitalization and antibiotic use in patients receiving hematopoietic growth factors. However, significant effects on treatment-related mortality or overall survival were rarely observed

Central Nervous System Prophylaxis

Although the presence of central nervous system (CNS) leukemia at diagnosis (i.e., clinical neurologic features and/or leukemic cells in cerebral spinal fluid on cytocentrifuge preparation) is more common in childhood AML than in childhood acute lymphoblastic leukemia (ALL), reduction in overall survival directly attributable to CNS involvement is presently less common in childhood AML. This finding is perhaps related to both the higher doses of chemotherapy used in AML (with potential crossover to the CNS) and the fact that marrow disease has not yet been as effectively brought under long-term control in AML as in ALL. Children with M4 and M5 AML have the highest incidence of CNS leukemia (especially those with inv 16 or 11q23 chromosomal abnormalities). The use of some form of CNS treatment (intrathecal chemotherapy with or without cranial irradiation) is now incorporated into most protocols for the treatment of childhood AML and is considered a standard part of the treatment for this disease.

Acute Promyelocytic Leukemia

Acute promyelocytic leukemia (APL) is a distinct subtype of AML and is treated differently than other types of AML. The characteristic chromosomal abnormality associated with APL is t(15;17). This translocation involves a chromosome breakpoint that includes the retinoid acid receptor and that leads to production of the PML-RARalpha fusion protein. Clinically, APL is characterized by a severe coagulopathy often present at the time of diagnosis. Mortality during induction due to bleeding complications is more common in this subtype than other French-American-British (FAB) classifications. Due to the extremely low incidence of CNS disease in patients with APL, a lumbar puncture is not required at the time of diagnosis and prophylactic intrathecal chemotherapy is not administered. Studies have demonstrated that the absence of PML-RARalpha RNA chimeric transcript expression at the end of therapy, as detected by RT-PCR monitoring, predicts a low risk of relapse.

The leukemia cells from patients with APL are especially sensitive to the differentiation-inducing effects of *all-trans retinoic acid (ATRA).* The basis for the dramatic efficacy of ATRA against APL is the ability of pharmacologic doses of ATRA to overcome the repression of signaling caused by the PML-RARalpha fusion protein at physiologic ATRA concentrations. Restoration of signaling leads to differentiation of APL cells and then to postmaturation apoptosis. Most patients with APL achieve a complete remission when treated with ATRA, although single agent ATRA is generally not curative. A series of randomized clinical trials have defined the benefit for combining ATRA with chemotherapy during induction therapy and also the utility of employing ATRA as maintenance therapy. With the use of ATRA and chemotherapy, the 2-year survival rates for patients with APL have improved from approximately 40% to between 50 and 80%. Induction therapy for the current nationwide trial for children and adults with APL utilizes ATRA with standard-dose cytarabine and daunorubicin, and consolidation therapy employs ATRA with daunorubicin. *Arsenic trioxide* has also been identified as an active agent in patients with APL, with 70 to 90% of patients achieving remission following treatment with this agent.

Children with Down syndrome

Children with Down syndrome have an increased risk of developing leukemia, particularly AML

M7 and myelodysplastic syndrome. Most children with AML and Down syndrome can be cured of their leukemia. Appropriate therapy for these children is less intensive than current AML therapy and bone marrow transplantation (BMT) is not indicated in first remission

Transient Myeloproliferative Disorder (TMD): is a disorder primarily found in Down syndrome patients during the newborn period. It is characterized by an uncontrolled proliferation of myeloblasts. These blasts are frequently of megakaryocytic origin with varying degrees of differentiation and are clonal in nature. Information regarding the presentation and natural course of this disease is lacking. TMD can be distinguished from congenital AML primarily by its spontaneous resolution. Thus, TMD is managed with supportive care only during the first few months of life.

Myelodysplastic Syndromes

Studies have attempted to retrospectively classify and analyze the outcome of children with MDS. This continues to be problematic. The FAB classification of adult MDS is only partially helpful in the categorization of children with MDS. Children with MDS present with FAB subtypes of refractory anemia (RA), refractory anemia with excess blasts (RAEB), and refractory anemia with excess blasts in transformation (RAEB-T). The related syndromes of JMML and Infantile Monosomy 7 can also be classified as MDS but will be discussed below. The optimal therapy for childhood MDS is controversial. The CCG #2891 trial, which accrued patients between 1989 to 1995, included children with myelodysplastic syndrome. Children with RA/RAEB do not respond to AML induction therapy as well as patients with AML. Because failure rates after BMT are lower in this group when treated at diagnosis, strong consideration should be given for such treatment, especially when a 5/6 or 6/6 matched family donor is available. The optimum therapy for patients with RA/RAEB without matched family donors is unknown. Some of these patients require no therapy for years and have indolent diseases. However, alternative forms of BMT, utilizing matched unrelated donors, or perhaps cord blood should be considered in an exploratory fashion when treatment is required, usually for severe cytopenia. An analysis of 37 children with MDS treated on AML-BFM 83, 87, and 93 protocols confirmed the induction response of 74% for patients with RAEB-T, and suggested transplantation was beneficial

Juvenile Myelomonocytic Leukemia

Historically, more than 90% of juvenile myelomonocytic leukemia patients died despite the use of chemotherapy. Patients appeared to follow 3 distinct clinical courses: (1) rapidly-progressive disease and early demise; (2) transiently-stable disease followed by progression and death; and (3) clinical improvement which lasted up to 9 years before progression or, rarely, long-term survival. A more recent retrospective review from the United Kingdom described 31 children (19 JMML; 12 monosomy 7 [Mo 7]) in which chemotherapy (nonintensive and intensive) and marrow-ablative therapy with marrow reconstitution from a sibling or unrelated, HLA-matched donor was used. The projected 5-year survival rate was 5% in patients with JMML and 40% in those with Mo 7.

Based upon these laboratory observations, 12 patients with JMML were evaluated in a pilot study using *cis*-retinoic acid (C-RA). Of 10 evaluable patients, responses were as follows: 2 CR, 3 partial responses (PR), 1 minimal response (MR), 4 progressive disease (PD). Toxicity was minimal. Responses were relatively slow and most children who experienced progressive disease did so within a few weeks of C-RA treatment. Transplantation seems to offer the best chance of cure for JMML

CHILDHOOD HODGKIN'S LYMPHOMA

General Information

Childhood Hodgkin's lymphoma is one of the few pediatric malignancies that shares aspects of its biology and natural history with an adult cancer. When treatment approaches for children were modeled after those used for adults, substantial morbidities (primarily musculoskeletal growth inhibition) resulted from the unacceptably high irradiation doses. Thus, new strategies utilizing chemotherapy and lower-dose radiation were developed. Approximately 90 to 95% of children with Hodgkin's lymphoma can be cured, prompting increased attention to devising nonmorbid therapy for these patients. Contemporary treatment programs use a risk-adapted approach in which patients receive multiagent chemotherapy (with intensity varying by stage) and low-dose involved-field irradiation.

Hodgkin's lymphoma comprises 6% of childhood cancers. *A striking male:female predominance is found among young children, with a ratio of 4:1 for 3- to 7-year-olds, and 3:1 for 7- to 9-year-olds. For patients older than 10 years, the ratio is 1.3:1 (a ratio more similar to that of adults).* In the United States, Hodgkin's lymphoma is uncommon in children younger than 10 years. Younger children have a higher incidence of lymphocyte-predominant and mixed cellularity histology and a lower incidence of nodular-sclerosing histology than adolescents and adults. The incidence of Hodgkin's lymphoma continues to increase during the early teen and adolescent years.

Hodgkin's lymphoma is characterized by a variable number of characteristic multinucleated giant cells (Reed-Sternberg [R-S] cells) or large mononuclear cell variants (Hodgkin's cells) in an inflammatory milieu. This inflammatory milieu consists of small lymphocytes, histiocytes, epithelioid histiocytes, neutrophils, eosinophils, plasma cells, and fibroblasts in different proportions depending on the histologic subtype. It has been conclusively shown that R-S cells and/or Hodgkin's cells represent a clonal population. Almost all cases of Hodgkin's lymphoma arise from preapoptotic germinal center B cells that cannot synthesize immunoglobulin. The R-S cell appears to be resistant to apoptotic stimuli. Deregulation of the nuclear transcription factor NFkB in the R-S cells may explain the resistance to apoptosis.

Epstein-Barr virus (EBV) genetic material can often be detected in R-S or Hodgkin's cells. In the United States, EBV positivity is most common in children younger than 10 years. EBV positivity is most commonly found in tumors with mixed cellularity histology and is extremely rare in patients with lymphocyte-predominant histology. The incidence of EBV tumor cell positivity is only 15 to 20% in adolescents and young adults. EBV serologic status is not a prognostic factor for outcome in pediatric Hodgkin's lymphoma.] *Although rare, Hodgkin's lymphoma can be familial.*

Approximately 80% of patients present with painless adenopathy, commonly in the supraclavicular or cervical area. Enlarged nodes are generally firm and have a rubbery texture. Many patients have some degree of mediastinal involvement at presentation. Approximately 25% of patients may have systemic symptoms such as fever, night sweats, and weight loss that are secondary to release of lymphokines and cytokines by R-S or Hodgkin's cells. Approximately 20% of patients will have a mediastinal mass whose maximum diameter is greater than one third of the chest diameter and/or a node or nodal aggregate >10 cm. Approximately 80 to 85% of children and adolescents with Hodgkin's lymphoma have involvement of lymph nodes and/or the spleen only (stages I-III). The remaining

15 to 20% of patients will have noncontiguous extranodal involvement (stage IV). The most common sites of extranodal involvement are the lung, liver, bones, and bone marrow.

Cellular Classification and Biologic Correlates

Hodgkin's lymphoma can be divided into 2 broad pathologic classes:
- Classical Hodgkin's lymphoma.
- Nodular lymphocyte predominant Hodgkin's lymphoma (NLPHL).

Classical Hodgkin's Lymphoma

Classical Hodgkin's lymphoma is divided into 4 subtypes:
- Lymphocyte-rich Classical Hodgkin's lymphoma (LRCHL).
- Nodular sclerosis Hodgkin's lymphoma (NSHL).
- Mixed cellularity Hodgkin's lymphoma (MCHL).
- Lymphocyte-depleted Hodgkin's lymphoma (LDHL).

These subtypes are defined according to the number of Reed-Sternberg (R-S) cells, characteristics of the inflammatory milieu, and the presence or absence of fibrosis.

The hallmark of classic Hodgkin's lymphoma is the R-S cell. This is a binucleated or multinucleated giant cell which is often characterized by a bilobed nucleus, with 2 large nucleoli, giving an "owl's eye" appearance to the cells. A striking characteristic is the rarity (about 1%) of the malignant R-S cell in specimens and the abundant reactive cellular infiltrate of lymphocytes, macrophages, granulocytes, and eosinophils. R-S or *Hodgkin's cells generally do not express B-cell antigens such as CD-45, CD-19, and CD-79A. Almost all patients express CD-30 and more than 80% of patients express CD-15. CD-20 is expressed in approximately 30 to 40% of cases.* R-S/Hodgkin's cells show constitutive activation of the nuclear factor kappa B pathway, which may prevent apoptosis and provide a survival advantage. Most cases of classic Hodgkin's lymphoma are characterized by expression of tumor necrosis factor receptors (TNF-R) and their ligands, as well as an unbalanced production of Th2 cytokines and chemokines. Activation of TNF-R results in constitutive activation of nuclear factor kappa B.

The histologic features and clinical symptoms of Hodgkin's lymphoma have been attributed to the numerous cytokines secreted by the R-S cells, which include interleukin-1 and interleukin-6, and tumor necrosis factor. Interleukin-5 could be responsible for the eosinophilia in MCHL, and transforming growth factor-b for the fibrosis in the NSHL subtype. These cytokines also enable the cells to evade immunologic surveillance as well as promote their own replication.
- NSHL histology accounts for approximately 80% of Hodgkin's lymphoma cases in older children and adolescents, but only 45% of cases in younger children. This subtype is distinguished by the presence of collagenous bands that divide the lymph node into nodules, which often contain an R-S cell variant called the lacunar cell. Some pathologists subdivide nodular sclerosis into 2 subgroups (NS-1 and NS-2) on the basis of the number of R-S cells present.
- MCHL histology is more common in younger children (about 35%) than in adolescents or adults (10 to 20%). R-S cells are frequent in a background of abundant normal reactive cells (lymphocytes, plasma cells, eosinophils, histiocytes). This subtype can be confused with peripheral T-cell lymphoma.
- LRCHL may have a nodular appearance, but immunophenotypic analysis allows distinction between this form of Hodgkin's lymphoma and nodular lymphocyte-predominant disease. LRCHL cells express CD-15 and CD-30 while NLPHL almost never expresses CD-15.

Patients with completely resected stage I LRCHL require chemotherapy with or without radiotherapy, while patients with completely resected stage I NLPHL may be followed without postsurgical chemotherapy or radiation therapy.

Nodular Lymphocyte Predominant Hodgkin's Lymphoma

This pathologic class of Hodgkin's lymphoma is characterized by large cells with multi-lobed nuclei, referred to as "popcorn" cells. These cells express B-cell antigens such as CD-19, CD-20, CD-22 and CD-79A, and are negative for CD-15. These cells may or may not express CD-30. The OCT-2 and BOB.1 oncogenes are both expressed in NLPHL; they are not expressed in the cells of patients with classical Hodgkin's lymphoma. It is sometimes difficult to distinguish NLPHL from progressive transformation of germinal centers and/or T-cell-rich B-cell lymphoma. NLPHL is most common in males younger than 10 years. Patients with NLPHL generally present with localized, nonbulky disease. Almost all patients are asymptomatic.

Prognostic factors in Hodgkin's Lymphoma

As the treatment of Hodgkin's lymphoma has improved, factors that influence outcome have diminished in importance. However, several factors continue to influence the success and choice of therapy. These factors are interrelated in the sense that disease stage, bulk, and biologic aggressiveness are frequently codependent. Further complicating the determination of prognostic factors is that relevant variables may differ on the basis of staging evaluation and treatment.

Pretreatment factors associated with an adverse outcome include advanced stage of disease, the presence of "B" symptoms, the presence of bulk disease, extranodal extension, male sex, and elevated erythrocyte sedimentation rate. In a multivariate analysis , "B" symptoms, histology, and male sex were significantly adverse prognostic factors for event-free survival (EFS) There is some controversy as to whether histology is an important prognostic factor. Serum markers that have been associated with an adverse outcome include soluble vascular cell adhesion molecule-1, tumor necrosis factor, soluble CD-30, BETA-2 microglobulin, transferrin, and serum IL-10 level. High levels of caspase 3 in Reed-Sternberg (R-S) cells has been associated with a favorable outcome.

On univariate analysis, stage IV, nodular-sclerosing histology (NSHL), "B" symptoms, white blood cell (WBC) =11,500/mm^3, hemoglobin =11.0 g/dL, bulky mediastinal disease, extranodal disease, and erythrocyte sedimentation rate (ESR) =50 mm/hr were significant for inferior disease-free survival (DFS) and overall survival (OS).

The rapidity of response to initial therapy is an important prognostic variable in many forms of cancer, including Hodgkin's lymphoma. In certain Hodgkin's lymphoma studies, rapidity of response to chemotherapy is used to determine subsequent therapy. Positron emission tomography (PET) scanning may be a very good method to assess early response in Hodgkin's lymphoma.

Although prognostic factors will continue to be influenced by choice of therapy, parameters such as disease stage, bulk, number of involved sites, and systemic symptomatology are likely to remain relevant to outcome. Nonetheless, as therapy becomes increasingly tailored to prognostic factors and therapeutic response, overall outcome should become less affected by these parameters.

Staging and Diagnostic Evaluation

Stage is a critical determinant in the selection of treatment. Evaluation of the child with Hodgkin's lymphoma includes history, physical examination, imaging (including chest X-rays; computed tomographic (CT) scans of chest, abdomen, and pelvis; gallium scan and/or positron emission tomography (PET) scan) and laboratory studies. The postero-anterior (PA) and lateral chest radiograph remains important since the criterion for bulky mediastinal lymphadenopathy is defined by the ratio of the measurement of the mediastinal lymph nodes to the maximal measurement of the chest cavity on an upright chest radiograph; mediastinal ratios that equal or exceed 33% are considered bulky. CT scans help delineate the status of intrathoracic lymph node groups (including the hila and cardiophrenic angle), lung parenchyma, pericardium, pleura, and the chest wall, demonstrating abnormalities in about one half of patients with unremarkable chest radiographs. Definition of disease involvement of intrathoracic tissues by CT will often dictate more aggressive therapy than would otherwise have been administered. Distinguishing normal (or hyperplastic) thymus from nodes in children can be problematic. Bone marrow aspiration and biopsy should be performed in patients with advanced disease (stage III or IV) and/or symptoms (fever, weight loss, or night sweats) Bone scans are performed in patients with bone pain or elevated alkaline phosphatase. In the past, lymphangiograms were commonly used to evaluate involvement of the abdominal lymph nodes in patients with Hodgkin's lymphoma; however, more false-positives occur in children than in adults, and the studies are technically more difficult to perform. Lymphangiography is no longer used in the staging of children. *Fluorodeoxyglucose (FDG)-PET has advantages over gallium-67 because the scan is a 1-day procedure with higher resolution, better dosimetry, and less intestinal activity and has a quantitation potential; however, its false-positive and false-negative rates are still under investigation in childhood Hodgkin's lymphoma.* When standard dose radiation therapy was an acceptable treatment strategy for patients with early stage Hodgkin's lymphoma, exploratory laparotomy with splenectomy was performed to determine the presence and extent of abdominal involvement. Since all pediatric patients with Hodgkin's lymphoma receive chemotherapy, staging laparotomies are no longer routinely performed.

Patients with large mediastinal masses are at risk of cardiac or respiratory arrest during general anesthesia or heavy sedation. Although this is less likely to be problematic in Hodgkin's lymphoma than in non-Hodgkin's lymphoma, appropriate planning of the surgical approach is essential. After a careful physiologic and radiographic evaluation of the patient has been carried out, the least invasive procedure should be used to establish the diagnosis of lymphoma. If a significant pleural effusion is present, a thoracentesis should be considered, although cytologic diagnosis is rarely made in Hodgkin's lymphoma. If at all possible, the diagnosis of Hodgkin's lymphoma should be established by lymph node biopsy. Aspiration cytology alone is not recommended because of the lack of stromal tissue, the small number of cells present in the specimen, and the difficulty of classifying Hodgkin's lymphoma into one of the subtypes. When the diagnostic procedures described above are not fruitful, a CT or ultrasound-guided core needle biopsy should be considered. This procedure can frequently be carried out using light sedation and local anesthesia, before more invasive procedures are undertaken. Mediastinoscopy, anterior mediastinotomy, or thoracoscopy are the procedures of choice when other diagnostic modalities fail to establish the diagnosis. A formal thoracotomy is rarely indicated for the diagnosis of Hodgkin's lymphoma. If a diagnostic operative procedure cannot be performed because of the risk of general anesthesia or heavy sedation and if needle biopsy is not feasible, then preoperative treatment with localized radiation therapy should be considered. Because preoperative treatment may hinder an accurate tissue diagnosis, a diagnostic biopsy should be obtained as soon as the risks of general anesthesia or heavy sedation are thought to be alleviated.

The staging classification currently used for Hodgkin's lymphoma was adopted at the Ann Arbor Conference held in 1971 and revised in 1989.

Subclassification of Stage

Hodgkin's lymphoma can be subclassified into A and B categories: "A" for those patients who are asymptomatic and "B" for those patients with any of the following specific symptoms:

- Unexplained loss of more than 10% of body weight in the 6 months before diagnosis.
- Unexplained fever with temperatures above 38° C for more than 3 days.
- Drenching night sweats.

Extralymphatic disease resulting from direct extension of an involved lymph node region is designated "E." Extralymphatic disease presents confusing problems in staging. The designation "E" is not appropriate for cases of widespread disease, which should be considered stage IV. If pathologic proof of noncontiguous involvement of 1 or more extralymphatic sites has been documented, the symbol for the site of involvement, followed by a plus sign (+), is listed. Current practice is to assign a clinical stage on the basis of findings of the clinical evaluation; however, pathologic confirmation of noncontiguous extralymphatic involvement is strongly suggested for assignment to stage IV.

Stage I

Involvement of a single lymph node region or, in the case of stage I(E), direct extension from that node to an adjacent extralymphatic region.

Stage II

Involvement of 2 or more lymph node regions (number to be stated) on the same side of the diaphragm, or extension from any one of these lymph nodes to an extralymphatic adjacent organ, or stage II(E).

Stage III

Involvement of lymph node regions on both sides of the diaphragm, which may also be accompanied by extension to an adjacent extralymphatic organ, [stage III(E)], involvement of the spleen [stage III(S+)], or both [stage III(E+S)].

Stage IV

Noncontiguous involvement of 1 or more extralymphatic organs or tissues with or without associated lymph node involvement.

End of Chemotherapy Re-evaluation

Restaging is carried out at the end of chemotherapy. The purpose of restaging is to assess the degree of response to initial chemotherapy. Although complete response can be defined as absence of disease by clinical examination and/or imaging studies, complete response in Hodgkin's lymphoma trials is often defined by more than a 70 to 80% reduction of disease and a change from initial positivity to negativity on either gallium or PET scanning. This definition is necessary in Hodgkin's lymphoma because fibrotic residual is common, particularly in the mediastinum.

Recently, many centers have switched functional imaging from gallium to PET scanning.

Treatment Approach for Children and Adolescents with Hodgkin's Lymphoma

In general, the use of combined chemotherapy and radiation broadens the spectrum of potential toxicities, while reducing the severity of individual drug- or radiation-related toxicities. Current approaches use chemotherapy alone with or without low-dose involved-field radiation therapy (LD-IFRT). The volume of radiation and the intensity/duration of chemotherapy are determined by prognostic factors at presentation, including presence of constitutional symptoms, disease stage, and bulk.

Devising the ideal therapeutic approach for children with Hodgkin's lymphoma is complicated by their increased risk for late adverse effects. In particular, radiotherapy doses used in adults can cause profound musculoskeletal growth retardation and increase the risk for cardiovascular disease and secondary solid malignancies in children. Further complicating the treatment of children are gender-specific differences in chemotherapy-induced gonadal injury. The desire to cure young children with minimal side effects has stimulated attempts to reduce the intensity of chemotherapy (particularly alkylating agents) and radiation dose and volume. Because of differences in age-related child developmental status and the gender-related sensitivity to chemotherapy, no single treatment approach is ideal for all pediatric and young adult patients.

Pediatric oncologists agree that standard-dose radiotherapy, particularly applied to the mantle field, has unacceptable toxicity, including growth disturbance in prepubertal children, increased risk for breast cancer in young females, and cardiovascular complications. Therefore, all children and adolescents treated in pediatric cancer centers generally receive combination chemotherapy as initial treatment. Intensity and duration of initial chemotherapy is generally based on anatomic disease stage and the presence or absence of symptoms at diagnosis and the presence or absence of bulk disease.

The following strategies have been utilized to treat children and adolescents with Hodgkin's lymphoma:

- Chemotherapy and LD-IFRT for all patients.
- Chemotherapy alone for selected patients; chemotherapy and LD-IFRT for other patients.
- Initial chemotherapy intensity (number of cycles) determined by early response assessment followed by no further therapy or LD-IFRT.

Chemotherapy for Childhood/ Adolescent Hodgkin's Lymphoma

Drugs utilized as front-line therapy for children and adolescents with Hodgkin's lymphoma include:

- Cyclophosphamide
- Procarbazine
- Vincristine and/or vinblastine
- Prednisone or dexamethasone
- Doxorubicin or epirubicin
- Bleomycin
- Dacarbazine
- Etoposide
- Methotrexate
- Cytosine arabinoside

Radiation Therapy for Children and Adolescents with Hodgkin's Lymphoma

As discussed in the previous sections, most newly diagnosed children will be treated with risk-adapted chemotherapy alone or in combination with LD-IFRT. LD-IFRT involves the use of meticulous and judiciously designed fields to achieve local control of disease and to minimize damage to normal tissue.

Low-Risk Disease (stages I-IIA; no bulk; no "B" symptoms):

- VAMP × 4 plus LD-IFRT.
- COPP/ABV hybrid × 4 plus LD-IFRT.
- DBVE × 2 (complete response) or × 4 (partial response) and LD-IFRT.
- OEPA (males) or OPPA (females) × 2 and LD-IFRT.

Table 17.1: Chemotherapy regimens and their corresponding agents

Chemotherapy regimens	*Corresponding agents*
ABVD	Doxorubicin (Adriamycin), bleomycin, vinblastine, dacarbazine
ABVE (DBVE)	Doxorubicin (Adriamycin), bleomycin, vincristine, etoposide
VAMP	Vincristine, doxorubicin (Adriamycin), methotrexate, prednisone
OPPA +/– COPP (females)	Vincristine (Oncovin), prednisone, procarbazine, doxorubicin (Adriamycin), cyclophosphamide, vincristine (Oncovin), prednisone, procarbazine
OEPA +/- COPP (males)	Vincristine (Oncovin), etoposide, prednisone, doxorubicin (Adriamycin), cyclophosphamide, vincristine (Oncovin), prednisone, procarbazine
COPP/ABV	Cyclophosphamide, vincristine (Oncovin), prednisone, procarbazine, doxorubicin (Adriamycin), bleomycin, vinblastine
BEACOPP (advanced stage)	Bleomycin, etoposide, doxorubicin (Adriamycin), cyclophosphamide, vincristine (Oncovin), prednisone, procarbazine
Cytarabine/etoposide	
COPP	Cyclophosphamide, vincristine (Oncovin), prednisone, procarbazine
CHOP	Cyclophosphamide, doxorubicin (Adriamycin), vincristine (Oncovin), prednisone
ABVE-PC (DBVE-PC)	Doxorubicin (Adriamycin), bleomycin, vincristine, etoposide, prednisone, cyclophosphamide

Intermediate-Risk Disease (all stage I and II patients not classified as early stage; stage IIIA; stage IVA):

- COPP/ABV × 6 plus LD-IFRT.
- DBVE-PC × 3 (complete response after 3) or × 5 (partial response after 3) plus LD-IFRT.
- OPPA/OEPA × 2; COPP × 2 plus LD-IFRT.

High-Risk Disease (stages IIIB, IVB):

- Intensive chemotherapy with cytarabine/etoposide, COPP/ABV or CHOP (2 cycles of each) plus LD-IFRT.
- Escalated dose BEACOPP × 6 plus LD-IFRT.
- OPPA/OEPA × 2; COPP × 4 plus LD-IFRT.

Nodular Lymphocyte Predominant Hodgkin's Lymphoma

Current standard therapy for children with nodular lymphocyte predominant Hodgkin's lymphoma (NLPHL) is chemotherapy plus LD-IFRT. There have been a number of reports in the literature of patients with completely resected stage I NLPHL who received no further therapy. In a series of 31 patients treated with surgery alone, there were 7 deaths (median follow-up, 7 years), but only 1 death resulted from Hodgkin's lymphoma.

Treatment Strategies Under Clinical Investigation for Childhood/Adolescent Hodgkin's Lymphoma

Intermediate-Risk Disease

The new Children's Oncology Group (COG) Intermediate Risk Trial (stages I and II with either "B" symptoms or bulk, stage II AE, stage III and IVA) will evaluate early response after 2 cycles of ABVE-PC to determine subsequent treatment:

- Patients who achieve a rapid response to 2 cycles of ABVE-PC will receive an additional 2 cycles of chemotherapy. Complete responders will then be randomized to receive or not receive LD-IFRT. Partial responders will receive LD-IFRT. The hypothesis is that rapid response will delineate a subgroup of patients who will not require LD-IFRT.

- Patients who show a slow response to 2 cycles of ABVE-PC will be randomized to receive 2 additional cycles of ABVE-PC or 2 cycles of ABVE-PC and 2 cycles of a noncross-resistant combination (dexamethasone, etoposide, cisplatin, cytarabine [ARA-C]-{DECA}) prior to LD-IFRT. The hypothesis is that additional noncross-resistant chemotherapy prior to LD-IFRT will improve EFS for patients with slow initial disease resolution.

Nodular Lymphocyte Predominant Hodgkin's Lymphoma

- A proposed COG study will evaluate surgery alone for patients with stage I completely resected NLPHL. Other patients with stage I or stage II disease will receive 4 cycles of VAMP chemotherapy. Patients showing a complete response will receive no further therapy; other patients will receive LD-IFRT. Patients with advanced-stage disease will be treated on stage-appropriate protocols which include all histologies.

The designations in PDQ that treatments are "standard" or "under clinical evaluation" are not to be used as a basis for reimbursement determinations.

PRIMARY PROGRESSIVE/RECURRENT HODGKIN'S LYMPHOMA IN CHILDREN AND ADOLESCENTS

Treatment failure in children and adolescents with Hodgkin's lymphoma can be divided into 3 groups:

- Primary progressive disease.
- Relapse limited to the site(s) of initial involvement (in patients treated with chemotherapy alone).
- Other relapse.

The presence of "B" symptoms and extranodal disease at the time of relapse are adverse prognostic features. In the German Pediatric Oncology and Hematology Group (GPOH) and Children's Cancer Group (CCG) Hodgkin's lymphoma trials, most relapses occurred in patients who received chemotherapy alone as primary treatment, and most of the relapses were limited to sites of initial involvement. Patients with favorable disease at diagnosis (i.e., stage IA or stage IIA; no bulk; no "B" symptoms) with relapse confined to an area of initial involvement after chemotherapy and no radiation can generally be salvaged with further chemotherapy and low-dose involved-field radiation therapy (LD-IFRT).

A number of chemotherapy drugs not generally used in the initial treatment of Hodgkin's lymphoma have documented activity against recurrent Hodgkin's lymphoma including:

- Moderate or high-dose cytarabine.
- Carboplatin/cisplatin
- Ifosfamide
- Etoposide
- Vinorelbine
- Gemcitabine
- Vinblastine

Combination regimens used in the treatment of progressive/recurrent Hodgkin's lymphoma include:

- ICE (ifosfamide, carboplatin, etoposide)
- DECAL (dexamethasone, etoposide, cisplatin, cytarabine, L-asparaginase]
- Ifosfamide and vinorelbine
- Vinorelbine/gemcitabine

The most commonly utilized preparative regimen for peripheral blood stem cell transplant is the BEAM regimen (carmustine [BCNU], etoposide, cytarabine, melphalan). Carmustine may produce significant pulmonary toxicity. Other non-carmustine-containing preparative regimens include thiotepa and etoposide, combined with either cyclophosphamide, carboplatin, or melphalan. Busulfan has also been utilized in certain preparative regimens.

EWING'S FAMILY OF TUMORS

General Information

EFTs occur most frequently in the second decade of life and account for 4% of childhood and adolescent malignancies. The incidence in boys is slightly higher than in girls (ratio of 1.1:1). ETB(Ewing's Tumor of Bone) is estimated to be 60% of the EFTs. The sites of origin for ETB are: distal (27%) and proximal extremities (25%); pelvis (20%); chest (20%); and spine and skull (9%).

Major prognostic factors include site, tumor volume, and the presence of metastases. Clinical and biological factors for ETB and, to some extent EOE, are discussed below.

- *Site, size, age, and sex:* In ETB the most favorable sites are distal extremities. Central location (e.g., skull, clavicle, vertebrae, and ribs), proximal extremities and the pelvis are associated with a much less favorable prognosis. Size is also significant, but larger lesions tend to occur in the more unfavorable sites. Younger children have better event-free survival than older adolescents and young adults Girls with ETB have a better prognosis than boys.
- *Clinical findings:* The presence of fever, anemia, or an elevated lactic dehydrogenase (LDH) are poor prognostic signs for patients with ETB. Increased serum LDH levels prior to treatment correlate with metastatic disease and shorter disease-free survival
- *Surgical resectability:* Surgical resection for ETB, EOE, and for PNET is an important variable. This applies to both complete resection or incomplete resection with only microscopic residual disease.
- *Chemotherapy:* Approximately 20 to 30% of the patients with ETB have overt metastases at the time of diagnosis. For EOE, 13% have overt metastases at diagnosis. Less than 20% of children with localized ETB survive their disease with only local therapy, i.e., a complete surgical excision and/or intensive radiation therapy. The overall survival markedly improved when multiagent intensive chemotherapy was added to radiation therapy, and the 5-year survival is up to 70% in many large studies, and 10-year event-free survival is approximately 50%.
- *Metastases:* Although the prognosis is thought to be poor, it has been observed that with intensive therapy, survival in patients with ETB who have only pulmonary metastases is slightly higher than for patients with bone or bone marrow metastases.
- *Routine histopathology:* Traditionally, a major distinction has been made between classical Ewing's sarcoma (which shows minimal evidence of differentiation) and PNET (which shows evidence of neural differentiation), however, the degree of neural differentiation does not influence outcome.
- *Biological features:* Reverse transcription polymerase chain reaction (RT-PCR) of the fusion transcripts from 112 patients with ETB and EOE revealed that the type I EWS-FL1 transcript was an important favorable prognostic feature in patients with localized primary tumors. In a study of a relatively small number of patients, overexpression of the p53 protein was a highly unfavorable prognostic feature. The presence of additional cytogenetic abnormalities, in particular loss of 16q, may be unfavorable. RT-PCR can be used to examine bone marrow for the presence of detectable translocation transcripts. In a single retrospective study among patients who did not have clinically detectable metastatic disease, positive RT-PCR for fusion

transcripts was associated with a greater risk of recurrence after treatment.

- *Response to preoperative therapy:* Multiple studies have shown that patients with minimal or no residual tumor after presurgical chemotherapy have a significantly better event-free survival compared to patients with larger amounts of viable tumor. Massive tumor necrosis after induction chemotherapy is a very favorable sign.

CELLULAR CLASSIFICATION

Ewing's tumors of bone and soft tissues belong to the group of neoplasms commonly referred to as "small round blue cell tumors of childhood." The *MIC2* gene product (*CD99*) is a surface membrane protein that is expressed in most cases of Ewing's sarcoma/primitive neuroectodermal tumor (PNET) family of tumors and is useful in the diagnosis of these tumors when the results are interpreted in the context of clinical and pathologic parameters. *MIC2* is not pathognomic for Ewing's sarcoma, and positivity by immunochemistry is found in several other tumors including synovial sarcoma.

Ewing's Tumor of Bone and Extraosseous Ewing's

The individual cells of Ewing's tumor of bone (ETB) and extraosseous Ewing's tumor of bone (EOE) (i.e., classical Ewing's) contain round to oval nuclei with fine dispersed chromatin without nucleoli. Occasionally, cells with smaller, more hyperchromatic (and probably degenerative) nuclei are present giving a "light cell/dark cell" pattern. The cytoplasm varies in amount, but in the classic case it is clear and contains glycogen, which can be highlighted with a periodic acid-Schiff (PAS) stain. The tumor cells are tightly packed and grow in a diffuse pattern without evidence of structural organization. Many pathologists no longer make a distinction between EOE and PNET.

Primitive Neuroectodermal Tumor (PNET)

The histologic appearance of the PNET differs somewhat from ETB and EOE. These tumors are typically composed of round to ovoid hyperchromatic cells with minimal cytoplasm. The tumor cells are typically arranged in nests and trabeculae with variable rosette formation. The rosettes may have a central lumen, but are often ill-defined, composed of tumor cells arranged around an empty space. The classic lobular growth pattern is best appreciated at low power, and differs from the typical diffuse growth seen in classical Ewing's. Occasionally, groups of cytologically uniform, round cells with dispersed chromatin resembling those in classical Ewing's are seen interspersed in an otherwise typical PNET. This overlap of features lends confidence to the concept that these tumors are indeed the same tumor with a spectrum of differentiation. PNETs also show variable staining with some neural markers including neuron-specific enolase, Leu-7, synaptophysin, neurofilament, and S100. The demonstration of neurosecretory granules by electron microscopy enhances the pathologist's ability to make the diagnosis of PNET.

Cytogenetic studies of the EFTs have identified a consistent alteration of the *EWS* locus on chromosome 22 band q12 that may involve other chromosomes, including 11 or 21. Characteristically, the amino terminus of the *EWS* gene is juxtaposed with the carboxy terminus of another gene. In the majority of cases (90%), the carboxy terminus is provided by *FLI1*, a member of the Ets family of transcription factors gene located on chromosome 11 band q24. Other Ets family members which may combine with the *EWS* gene in order of frequency are *ERG* (located on chromosome 21), *ETV1* (located on chromosome 7), and *E1AF* (located on chromosome 17), which result in the following translocations: t(21:22), t(7;22), and t(17;22) respectively. Besides these consistent aberrations involving the *EWS* gene at 22q12, additional numerical and structural aberrations have been observed in EFTs, including gains of chromosomes 2, 5, 7, 8, 9, and 12, the nonreciprocal translocation t(1;16) (q12; q11.2), and deletions at the short arm of chromosome 1. A molecular test (RT-PCR and restriction analysis of PCR products), currently available on a research basis only, now offers the opportunity of markedly simplifying the definition of the EFTs. The molecular assay can be performed on relatively small amounts of tissue obtained by minimally invasive biopsies and is capable of providing results faster than cytogenetic analysis.

STAGE INFORMATION

Localized: For Ewing's tumor of bone, the tumor is defined as localized when, by clinical and imaging techniques, it has not spread beyond the primary site or regional lymph nodes. There may be contiguous extension into adjacent soft tissue. Extraosseous Ewing's has been grouped using the rhabdomyosarcoma staging system shown below:

- Group I : Completely excised.
- Group II : Microscopic residual.
- Group III : Gross residual.

Metastatic: These tumors have spread to distant sites, most commonly lung, bone, and/or bone marrow. Lymph node and, in particular, central nervous system metastases are less common. By other staging systems in common use, this is stage 4 or group IV.

TREATMENT OPTION OVERVIEW

It is important for patients to be evaluated by all disciplines (e.g., radiologist, chemotherapist, pathologist, surgeon or orthopedic oncologist, and radiation oncologist) as early as possible. The surgeon or orthopedic oncologist who will perform the definitive surgery should be involved during the biopsy so that the incision can be placed in an acceptable location. This is especially important if it is thought that the lesion can be totally excised or if a limb salvage procedure may be attempted. The radiation oncologist and pathologist should be consulted prior to biopsy/surgery in order to be sure that the incision will not compromise the radiation port and so that multiple types of tissue samples are obtained (e.g., tissue culture for cytogenetics, imprints, frozen tissue, as well as formalin-fixed tissue). Diagnostic scans (chest x-ray, chest computed tomography (CT), magnetic resonance imaging (MRI), or CT of the primary) should be performed prior to any procedure that requires anesthesia because anesthesia-induced abnormalities in the chest may be difficult to assess. Other studies such as a bone scan and bone marrow biopsy may be obtained preoperatively if the index of suspicion is high.

The successful treatment of patients with tumors of the Ewing's family (EFTs) requires the use of multidrug chemotherapy, in addition to radiation therapy and/or surgical therapy to the primary tumor. Many patients with metastatic disease at diagnosis respond well to the therapy given to patients with localized disease; however, in most cases the disease is only partially controlled or recurs. Patients with only lung metastases have a better event-free survival than those with metastases to bone and/or bone marrow.

Improved survival was suggested in small nonrandomized groups at high risk of relapse using very high doses of chemotherapy with radiation therapy and possibly surgery with or without autologous bone marrow transplant. A larger study which accounted for all patients from initial diagnosis failed to show benefit for high-dose therapy with autologous stem cell reconstitution used as consolidation therapy. The risk of secondary leukemia may be increased with dose-intensive regimens.

Patients treated for EFTs have a risk for developing second malignancies which is significantly higher than the general population. Treatment-related acute myeloblastic leukemia (t-AML) and myelodysplastic syndrome (t-MDS) have been reported in 1 to 2% of survivors of EFT. Treatment-related acute myeloblastic leukemia and t-MDS arise most commonly from 2 to 4 years following diagnosis and are more common in patients whose initial treatment included etoposide. It is very rare to develop treatment-related leukemia more than 5 to 6 years from diagnosis. Patients remain at increased risk for developing a second solid tumor for life. By 6 years from diagnosis, the risk approaches 3%. The risk appears to be greater in patients treated with radiation therapy.

LOCALIZED TUMORS OF THE EWING'S FAMILY

Current standard chemotherapy in the United States includes *vincristine, doxorubicin, and cyclophosphamide (VAdriaC)* alternating with ifosfamide and etoposide. The importance of doxorubicin has been demonstrated in randomized, comparative trials.

Local control can be achieved by surgery and/or radiation. Surgery is generally the preferred approach if the lesion is resectable. Radiation therapy should be delivered in a setting in which stringent planning techniques are applied by those experienced in the treatment of the Ewing's family of tumors. Such an approach will result in local control of the tumor with acceptable morbidity in a majority of patients. The radiation dose may be adjusted depending upon the extent of residual disease after the initial surgical procedure. Radiation therapy is generally administered in fractionated doses totaling approximately 5,580 cGy to the prechemotherapy tumor volume. The current recommendations of the Intergroup Ewing's Sarcoma Study (IESS) for patients with gross residual disease is 4,500 cGy to original disease site plus a 1,080 cGy boost to gross residual disease. For those with microscopic residual disease, the recommendation is 4,500 cGy plus a 540 cGy boost. *No radiation therapy is recommended for those who have no evidence of microscopic residual disease following surgical resection.*

METASTATIC TUMORS OF THE EWING'S FAMILY

Prognosis of patients with metastatic disease is poor.

Childhood Liver Cancer

General Information

Liver cancer, a rare malignancy in children and adolescents, is divided into 2 major histologic subgroups: *hepatoblastoma and hepatocellular carcinoma.* The age of onset of liver cancer in children is related to the histology of the tumor. *Hepatoblastomas usually occur before 3 years of age, whereas the incidence of hepatocellular carcinoma in the United States varies little with age between 0 and 19 years.* The overall survival rate for children with hepatoblastoma is 70% but is only 25% for hepatocellular carcinoma.

The majority of patients with either hepatoblastoma or hepatocellular carcinoma have a serum tumor marker, alpha-fetoprotein, that parallels disease activity. Lack of a significant decrease of alpha-fetoprotein levels with treatment may predict a poor response to therapy Absence of elevated alpha-fetoprotein may be a poor prognostic sign in hepatoblastoma; it is associated with the small-cell (anaplastic) histologic variant, which responds very poorly to therapy. Occasionally hepatoblastomas produce beta-human chorionic gonadotropin resulting in isosexual precocity. Severe osteopenia is not uncommon. Hepatoblastoma is part of the constellation of findings associated with the Beckwith-Wiedemann syndrome. Loss of the allele of maternal origin at the 11p15.5 familial Beckwith-Wiedemann syndrome locus occurs in many hepatoblastomas. Thus, the genetic abnormality that results in Beckwith-Wiedemann may be directly involved in the pathogenesis in some cases of hepatoblastoma, and imprinting may play a role. About 2% of children with hepatoblastoma have hemihypertrophy. Less than 1% of children with hemihypertrophy are at increased risk for developing hepatoblastoma within the first several years of life. There is a clear association between hepatoblastoma and familial adenomatous polyposis (FAP); children in families that carry the FAP gene are at an increased risk for hepatoblastoma, although it occurs in less than 1% of FAP family members. Childhood hepatoblastomas frequently have mutations in the beta-catenin gene, the function of which is closely related to FAP A relationship between very low birth weight and hepatoblastoma has been reported.

Hepatocellular carcinoma is associated with hepatitis B and C infection especially in children with perinatally acquired virus. Therefore, widespread hepatitis B immunization may decrease the incidence of hepatocellular carcinoma. *Compared to adults, the incubation period from hepatitis virus infection to the genesis of hepatocellular carcinoma is extremely short in some children with perinatally acquired virus.* Mutations in the Met/hepatocyte growth factor gene occur in childhood hepatocellular carcinoma, and this could be the mechanism that results in a shortened incubation period Several specific types of nonviral liver injury and cirrhosis in children are associated with hepatocellular carcinoma: tyrosinemia, biliary cirrhosis, and alpha-1-antitrypsin deficiency.

Cellular Classification

The cells of the "adult"-type hepatocellular carcinoma are epithelial compared with a less differentiated embryonal appearance of hepatoblastoma. Hepatocellular carcinoma also differs from hepatoblastoma in that it often arises in a previously abnormal, cirrhotic liver. However, hepatocellular carcinomas in children, unlike adults, do not arise from cirrhotic livers. Both histologic types more commonly arise in the right lobe of the liver. The hepatocellular nature of the tumor cells may be demonstrated by the finding of AFP or alpha-1-antitrypsin. Analysis of patients with resectable hepatoblastoma has suggested that tumors characterized as having pure "fetal" histology have a better prognosis when compared with those having an admixture of more primitive and rapidly dividing embryonal components or other undifferentiated tissues. In addition, a distinctive histologic variant of hepatocellular carcinoma has been described in the noncirrhotic livers of older children and young adults. Termed fibrolamellar carcinoma, it has been associated with an improved prognosis.

Stage Information

Postsurgical Staging

A staging system based on postsurgical extent of tumor and surgical resectability has been used in the United States to group children with liver cancer. This staging system is used to determine treatment. Children diagnosed with stage I and II hepatoblastoma have a cure rate of greater than 90% compared to 60% for stage III and approximately 20% for stage IV. In children diagnosed with hepatocellular carcinoma, those with stage I have a good outcome. Stage II is too rarely seen to predict outcome, and stages III and IV are usually fatal. The fibrolamellar variant of hepatocellular carcinoma may have a better prognosis.

Stage I:

- No metastases, tumor completely resected

Stage II:

- No metastases, tumor grossly resected with microscopic residual disease (i.e., positive margins); or tumor rupture, or tumor spill at the time of surgery.

Stage III:

- No distant metastases, tumor unresectable or resected with gross residual tumor, or positive lymph nodes.

Stage IV:

- Distant metastases regardless of the extent of liver involvement.

Treatment Option Overview

Many of the improvements in survival in childhood cancer have been made using new therapies that have attempted to improve on the best available, accepted therapy. Clinical trials in pediatrics are designed to compare potentially better therapy with therapy that is currently accepted as standard. This comparison may be done in a randomized study of two treatment arms or by evaluating a single new treatment, comparing the results with those previously obtained with standard therapy.

Because of the relative rarity of cancer in children, all children with liver cancer should be considered for entry into a clinical trial. Treatment planning by a multidisciplinary team of cancer specialists with experience treating tumors of childhood is required to determine and implement optimum treatment. Involvement of surgeons with experience in pediatric liver resection is critical.

Historically, resection of the primary tumor has been required to cure malignant liver tumors in children. Preoperative chemotherapy can convert a nonresectable tumor to a resectable one. Chemotherapy in some cases is able to eradicate pulmonary metastases completely and eliminate multinodular tumor foci in the liver. *Chemotherapy has been much more successful in the treatment of hepatoblastoma than in hepatocellular carcinoma.* In recent years, virtually all children with hepatoblastoma have been treated with chemotherapy, and in some centers, even children with resectable hepatoblastoma are treated with preoperative chemotherapy, which may reduce the incidence of surgical complications at the time of resection. Following chemotherapy, complete resection was obtained in about 70% of children. This strategy resulted in an overall survival of 75% at 5 years after diagnosis for all children entered on the study In contrast, the current Intergroup protocol for treatment of children with hepatoblastoma does not treat stage I tumors of purely fetal histology with chemotherapy unless they develop progressive disease, and resection at the time of diagnosis is encouraged for all tumors amenable to resection without undue risk. Further study will be needed to determine whether presurgical chemotherapy is preferable to resection followed by chemotherapy.

Surgical resection of distant disease has also contributed to the cure of children with hepatoblastoma. Resection of pulmonary metastases is recommended when the number of metastases is limited and is often performed at the same time as resection of the primary tumor. When possible, resection of areas of locally invasive disease, such as in the diaphragm, and of isolated brain metastasis is recommended.

Radiation therapy, even in combination with chemotherapy, has not cured children with nonresectable tumors. However, there may be a role for radiation therapy in the management of incompletely-resected hepatoblastoma. The dose of radiation that can be safely delivered immediately following resection is limited by its impairment of liver regeneration.

Liver transplantation has recently been associated with significant success in the treatment of children with unresectable hepatic tumors. Post transplant survival rates as high as 80% have been reported for children with hepatoblastomas. Intravenous invasion, positive lymph nodes and contiguous spread did not have a significant adverse effect on outcome. For children with hepatocellular carcinoma the overall five-year disease-free survival rate was approximately 60%. Due to the poor prognosis in patients with hepatocellular carcinoma, liver transplant should be considered early in the course for disorders such as tyrosinemia and familial intrahepatic cholestasis prior to the development of liver failure and malignancy. The fibrolamellar variant of hepatocellular carcinoma may have a better outcome with liver transplant than other hepatocellular carcinomas.

Stage I and II Childhood Liver Cancer

Postsurgically staged, stage I and II and presurgically staged, PRETEXT stage 1, 2, and 3 hepatoblastoma.

Combination chemotherapy has been demonstrated to have significant benefit in children with hepatoblastoma. Cisplatin-based chemotherapy has resulted in a survival rate of greater than 90% for children with stage I and stage II disease. Comparable results were obtained in an international study in which children were treated with doxorubicin/cisplatin chemotherapy prior to attempted resection of the liver tumor. In this study, 88% of the children in whom complete resection was achieved following the well-tolerated chemotherapy survived event-free 5 years after diagnosis.

Treatment Options

Complete surgical excision followed by four courses of combination chemotherapy with cisplatin, vincristine, and fluorouracil or comparable combination chemotherapy. Completely excised tumor of purely fetal histology may be treated with doxorubicin alone or carefully followed without further therapy.

Stage I and II Hepatocellular Carcinoma

Treatment Options

In a randomized trial, 7 of 7 patients with stage I hepatocellular carcinoma survived, disease-free, after adjuvant cisplatin-based chemotherapy. In a survey of childhood liver tumors treated prior to the consistent use of chemotherapy only 12 of 33 patients with hepatocellular carcinoma who had complete excision of the tumor survived It is probable that adjuvant chemotherapy does benefit children with completely resected hepatocellular carcinoma. Treatment with cisplatin and doxorubicin may be recommended as adjuvant therapy since these are active agents in the treatment of hepatocellular carcinoma. Studies in adults in China suggest that hepatic arterial chemoembolization before surgery may improve the outcome of subsequent hepatectomy

Stage III Childhood Liver Cancer

Postsurgically staged, stage III and presurgically staged, PRETEXT stage 4 hepatoblastoma.

Standard Treatment Options

In approximately 75% of children and adolescents with initially unresectable hepatoblastoma, tumors can be rendered resectable with cisplatin-based preoperative chemotherapy, and 60 to 65% will survive disease-free. A randomized clinical trial has demonstrated similar efficacy with cisplatin/vincristine/fluorouracil, or cisplatin/doxorubicin in the treatment of hepatoblastoma; the combination of cisplatin/vincristine/fluorouracil, however, resulted in considerably less toxicity. However, another chemotherapy regimen including doxorubicin/cisplatin at different doses and schedules demonstrated comparable results with less toxicity. A combination of ifosfamide, cisplatin, and doxorubicin has also been successfully used in the treatment of advanced-stage disease. Patients whose tumors remain unresectable should be considered for alternative chemotherapy, such as high-dose cisplatin with etoposide, radiation therapy, direct hepatic infusion of chemotherapeutic agents, or orthotopic liver transplantation.

Treatment Options Under Clinical Investigation

Combination chemotherapy with cisplatin/carboplatin.

Stage III Hepatocellular Carcinoma

In a randomized trial, cisplatin/vincristine/fluorouracil with or without doxorubicin given by continuous infusion was ineffective in adequately treating unresectable hepatocellular carcinoma. Therapy failed in 23 of 26 patients with stage III disease. No particular treatment for unresectable hepatocellular carcinoma has proved especially effective in the pediatric age group. Occasional patients may benefit from treatment with cisplatin/doxorubicin therapy, especially if localized hepatic tumor shrinks adequately to allow resection of disease.

Stage IV Childhood Liver Cancer

Stage IV Hepatoblastoma

The outcome for hepatoblastoma that is metastatic at diagnosis is not good, but cure is possible in 25 to 30% of patients In a study employing a well-tolerated regimen of doxorubicin/cisplatin chemotherapy, over 50% of patients with metastases at presentation survived 5 years from diagnosis. Half of these survivors developed progressive disease that was successfully treated with surgery and other interventions If possible, stage IV patients with resected primary tumor should have any remaining pulmonary metastases surgically removed. A randomized clinical trial has demonstrated equal efficacy with cisplatin/vincristine/fluorouracil and cisplatin/doxorubicin in the treatment of hepatoblastoma; the combination of cisplatin/vincristine/fluorouracil, however, resulted in considerably less toxicity. A combination of ifosfamide, cisplatin, and doxorubicin has also been successfully used in the treatment of advanced-stage disease. Patients whose tumors remain unresectable should be considered for alternative chemotherapy, such as high-dose cisplatin with etoposide, radiation therapy direct hepatic infusion of chemotherapeutic agents, or, if metastatic disease is controlled, orthotopic liver transplantation.

Standard Treatment Options

Four courses of cisplatin/vincristine/fluorouracil or doxorubicin/cisplatin combination chemotherapy followed by attempted complete tumor resection. If the tumor is completely removed, 2 postoperative courses of the same chemotherapy should be given. If the tumor is not resectable after 4 courses of chemotherapy, alternative therapies should be considered.

Treatment options under clinical investigation: Cisplatin/carboplatin combination chemotherapy.

Alternative therapies:

- Chemotherapy with high-dose cisplatin/etoposide or continuous infusion of doxorubicin.
- Radiation therapy followed by re-exploration if metastatic disease is controlled.
- Chemoembolization by hepatic arterial infusion.
- Orthotopic liver transplantation if metastatic disease is controlled.
- Phase I or II clinical trials of chemotherapy.

Stage IV Hepatocellular Carcinoma

In a randomized trial, cisplatin/vincristine/fluorouracil with or without doxorubicin given by continuous infusion was ineffective in adequately treating unresectable hepatocellular carcinoma. Therapy failed in 12 of 13 patients with stage IV disease. No particular treatment for unresectable hepatocellular carcinoma has proved especially effective in the pediatric age group. Occasional patients may benefit from treatment with cisplatin/doxorubicin therapy, especially if localized hepatic tumor shrinks adequately to allow resection of disease.

Neuroblastoma

General Information

Neuroblastoma is predominantly a tumor of early childhood, with two thirds of the cases presenting in children younger than 5 years of age. In rare cases, neuroblastoma can be discovered prenatally by fetal ultrasonography Neuroblastoma originates in the adrenal medulla or the paraspinal sites where sympathetic nervous system tissue is present. The most common symptoms are due to a tumor mass or to bone pain from metastases. *Proptosis and periorbital ecchymosis are common and arise from retrobulbar metastasis. Extensive bone marrow metastasis may result in pancytopenia.* Abdominal distention with respiratory compromise due to massive liver metastases occurs in infants. Because they originate in paraspinal ganglia, neuroblastomas may invade through neural foramina and compress the spinal cord, causing paralysis. Fever, anemia, and hypertension are found occasionally. Multifocal neuroblastoma occurs rarely, usually in infants, and generally has a good prognosis. Rarely, children may have severe watery diarrhea due to the secretion of vasoactive intestinal peptide by the tumor.

Children with neuroblastoma rarely present with paraneoplastic neurologic findings including cerebellar ataxia or *opsoclonus/myoclonus*. The opsoclonus/myoclonus syndrome appears to be caused by an immunologic mechanism that is not yet fully defined Unlike other neuroblastomas, the primary tumor usually is diffusely infiltrated with lymphocytes. Patients who present with this syndrome often have neuroblastomas with favorable biologic features and are likely to survive, although tumor-related deaths have been reported. Neurologic dysfunction is most often a presenting symptom but may arise after removal of the tumor. Opsoclonus/myoclonus is frequently associated with pervasive and permanent neurologic and cognitive deficits, including psychomotor retardation. Some patients may clinically respond to removal of the neuroblastoma, but improvement may be slow and partial; symptomatic treatment is often necessary. Adrenocorticotropic hormone (ACTH) treatment is thought to be effective, but some patients do not respond to ACTH. Various drugs, plasmapheresis, and intravenous gamma-globulin have been reported to be effective in selected cases. It has been suggested that the long-term neurologic outcome may be superior in patients treated with chemotherapy, possibly by means of its immunosuppressive effects.

The diagnosis of neuroblastoma requires the involvement of pathologists who are familiar with childhood tumors. Some neuroblastomas cannot be discriminated from other small round-blue cell tumors of childhood (such as lymphomas, primitive neuroectodermal tumor, and rhabdomyosarcoma) by conventional light microscopy. Evidence for sympathetic neuronal differentiation may be demonstrated by immunohistochemistry, electron microscopy, or by finding elevated levels of serum catecholamines (dopamine, norepinephrine) or urine catecholamine metabolites: vanillylmandelic acid (VMA) or homovanillic acid (HVA).

The minimum criterion for a diagnosis of neuroblastoma that has been established by international agreement is based on 1 of the following: (1) An unequivocal pathologic diagnosis made from tumor tissue by light microscopy (with or without immunohistology, electron microscopy, or increased levels of serum catecholamines or urinary catecholamine metabolites); (2) The combination of bone marrow aspirate or trephine biopsy containing unequivocal tumor cells (e.g., syncytia or immunocytologically-positive clumps of cells) and increased levels of serum catecholamines or urinary catecholamine metabolites as described above.

Approximately 70% of all patients with neuroblastoma have metastatic disease at diagnosis. The prognosis for patients with neuroblastoma is related to their age at diagnosis, clinical stage of disease, and (in patients older than 1 year of age) regional lymph node involvement.

Children of any age with localized neuroblastoma and infants younger than 1 year of age with advanced disease and favorable disease characteristics have a high likelihood of long-term, disease-free survival. Older children with advanced-stage disease, however, have a significantly decreased chance for cure despite intensive therapy. As an example, aggressive multiagent chemotherapy has resulted in a 2-year survival rate of approximately 20% in older children with stage IV neuroblastoma. Neuroblastoma in the adolescent or adult has a worse long-term prognosis regardless of stage or site and, in many cases, a more prolonged course

A number of biologic variables have been studied in children with this tumor. Of particular importance are Shimada histology, aneuploidy of tumor DNA, and amplification of the *N-myc* oncogene within tumor tissue, since treatment decisions may be based on these factors. An open biopsy is usually needed to obtain adequate tissue for determination of these biological characteristics. *Hyperdiploid tumor DNA is associated with a favorable prognosis especially in infants with neuroblastoma, while N-myc amplification is associated with a poor prognosis regardless of patient age.* In contrast to N-myc gene amplification, the degree of expression of the N-myc gene in the tumor does not predict prognosis. Amplification of N-myc is associated with *deletion of chromosome 1p and gain of the long arm of chromosome 17(17q), the latter of which independently predicts a poor prognosis.* A higher proportion of proliferating tumor cells may independently predict poor prognosis. *Expression of the gene encoding one of the high-affinity neurotrophin receptors (termed TRK-A), is associated with good prognosis tumors.. Increased levels of telomerase RNA, elevated serum ferritin, elevated serum lactate dehydrogenase, and the persistence of neuroblastoma cells in bone marrow during or after chemotherapy are each associated with poor prognosis.* Biologic staging consisting of N-myc copy number and age is useful in defining prognosis and treatment of stage III neuroblastoma. Neuroblastoma has been categorized into 3 biological groups. One type expresses the TRK-A neurotrophin receptor, is hyperdiploid, and tends to spontaneously regress. Another type expresses the TRK-B neurotrophin receptor, has gained an additional chromosome, 17q, has loss of heterozygosity of 14q, and is genomically unstable. In a third type, chromosome 1p is lost and the N-myc gene becomes amplified.

Many of the improvements in survival in childhood cancer have been made using new therapies that have attempted to improve on the best available, accepted therapy. Clinical trials in pediatrics are designed to compare potentially better therapy with therapy that is currently accepted. This may be done in a randomized study of 2 treatment arms or by evaluating a single new treatment and comparing the results with those previously obtained with standard therapy.

Spontaneous regression of neuroblastoma has been well described in infants, especially in those with the 4S pattern of metastatic spread. Regression generally occurs only in tumors with a near triploid number of chromosomes that also lack N-myc amplification and loss of chromosome 1p. *Features associated with spontaneous regression include the lack of expression of telomerase, expression of Ha-ras, and expression of the neurotrophin receptor TrkA, a nerve growth factor receptor. Recent studies have suggested that selected infants who appear to have asymptomatic, small, low-stage neuroblastoma detected by screening, often have tumors that spontaneously regress and may be observed safely without surgical intervention or tissue diagnosis.*

Cellular Classification

One clinicopathologic staging system involves evaluation of tumor specimens for the amount of stromal development, the degree of neuroblastic maturation, and the mitosis-karyorrhexis index of the neuroblastic cells. Favorable and unfavorable prognoses are defined on the bases of these histologic parameters and on patient age. The prognostic significance of this classification system, and of related systems using similar criteria, has been confirmed in several studies. Neuroblastomas containing many differentiating cells, termed ganglioneuroblastomas, tend to have favorable biological properties and have a better prognosis.

Stage Information

The treatment section of this document is organized to correspond to the Children's Oncology Group (COG) risk-based schema for treatment of neuroblastoma. This schema is based on 3 factors: patient age at diagnosis, certain biological characteristics of the patient's neuroblastoma tumor, and the stage of the tumor as defined by the International Neuroblastoma Staging System (INSS). The INSS has replaced the previously used Children's Cancer Group (CCG) and Pediatric Oncology Group (POG) staging systems. The INSS is described below, and the COG risk-based treatment schema is described in Table 17.1.

A thorough evaluation for metastatic disease should be performed prior to therapy initiation. The following investigations are recommended:

1. Bone marrow should be assessed by bilateral posterior iliac crest marrow aspirates and trephine (core) bone marrow biopsies to exclude bone marrow involvement. To be considered adequate, core biopsy specimens must contain at least 1 cm of marrow (excluding cartilage).
2. Bone should be assessed by metaiodobenzylguanidine (*MIBG*) scan (applicable to all sites of disease) and by technetium 99 scan if the results of the MIBG scan are negative or unavailable. Plain radiographs of positive lesions are recommended.
3. Palpable lymph nodes should be clinically examined and histologically confirmed. Nonpalpable lymph nodes should be assessed by computerized tomography (CT) scan with three-dimensional (3D) measurements.
4. The abdomen and liver should be assessed by CT scan and/or magnetic resonance imaging (MRI). Ultrasound is considered suboptimal for accurate 3D measurements.
5. The chest should be examined by anteroposterior and lateral chest radiography. CT scans and/or MRI are necessary if the results are positive or if abdominal disease extends into the chest.
6. Lumbar puncture should be avoided as CNS metastasis at diagnosis is rare and lumbar puncture may be associated with an increased incidence of subsequent development of CNS metastasis.

International Neuroblastoma Staging System

The International Neuroblastoma Staging System (INSS) combines certain features of the previously used POG and CCG systems. It has been shown to identify distinct prognostic groups.

- *Stage 1*: Localized tumor with complete gross excision, with or without microscopic residual disease; representative ipsilateral lymph nodes negative for tumor microscopically (nodes attached to and removed with the primary tumor may be positive).
- *Stage 2A*: Localized tumor with incomplete gross excision; representative ipsilateral nonadherent lymph nodes negative for tumor microscopically.
- *Stage 2B*: Localized tumor with or without complete gross excision, with ipsilateral nonadherent lymph nodes positive for tumor. Enlarged contralateral lymph nodes must be negative microscopically.
- *Stage 3*: Unresectable unilateral tumor infiltrating across the midline, with or without regional lymph node involvement; or localized unilateral tumor with contralateral regional lymph node involvement; or midline tumor with bilateral extension by infiltration (unresectable) or by lymph node involvement. The midline is defined as the vertebral column. Tumors originating on 1 side and crossing the midline must infiltrate to or beyond the opposite side of the vertebral column.
- *Stage 4*: Any primary tumor with dissemination to distant lymph nodes, bone, bone marrow, liver, skin, and/or other organs (except as defined for stage 4S).
- *Stage 4S*: Localized primary tumor (as defined for stage 1, 2A, or 2B), with dissemination limited to skin, liver, and/or bone marrow (limited to infants less than 1 year of age). Marrow involvement should be minimal (<10% of total nucleated cells identified as malignant by bone biopsy or by bone marrow aspirate). More extensive bone marrow involvement would be considered to be stage 4 disease. The results of the MIBG scan (if performed) should be negative for disease in the bone marrow.

Treatment Option Overview

This risk-based neuroblastoma treatment plan assigns each patient to a low-, intermediate-, or high-risk group. In patients without metastatic disease, initial surgery is performed to establish the diagnosis, to resect as much of the primary tumor as safely possible, to accurately stage disease through sampling of regional lymph nodes that are not adherent to the tumor, and to obtain adequate tissue for biologic studies.

Low Risk

Treatment for patients categorized as low risk (Table 17.1) consists most commonly of surgery alone but in some cases surgery combined with 6 to 12 weeks of chemotherapy. Chemotherapy is reserved for patients who are symptomatic, such as from spinal cord compression or, in 4S, respiratory compromise secondary to hepatic infiltration. The chemotherapy consists of carboplatin, cyclophosphamide, doxorubicin, and etoposide. The cumulative dose of each agent is kept low in order to minimize permanent injury from the chemotherapy regimen.

Intermediate Risk

Patients categorized as intermediate risk (Table 17.1) are treated with surgery and 12 to 24 weeks of the same chemotherapy regimen described above.

High Risk

In contrast, patients categorized as high risk (Table 17.1) are generally treated with aggressive multiagent chemotherapy consisting of very high doses of the drugs listed above but often also including ifosfamide and high-dose cisplatin. After a response to chemotherapy, resection of the primary tumor should be attempted, followed by myeloablative chemotherapy, sometimes total-body irradiation, and autologous stem cell transplantation. Irradiation of residual tumor and original sites of metastases is often performed before, during, or after myeloablative therapy. After recovery, patients are treated with oral 13-cis-retinoic acid for 6 months. Both myeloablative therapy and retinoic acid improve outcome in patients categorized as high risk.

Radiation

Radiation therapy is reserved for patients with symptomatic life- or organ-threatening tumor that does not respond rapidly enough to chemotherapy, or for intermediate-risk patients whose tumor has responded incompletely to both chemotherapy and attempted resection and also has unfavorable biologic characteristics. Radiation therapy to the primary site is recommended for high-risk patients even in cases of complete resection.

Relapse Therapy for Low and Intermediate Risk Patients

As part of the COG treatment plan, specific relapse therapy is defined for low- and intermediate-risk patients determined by patient age at recurrence, stage and biology of the recurrence.

Urgent Chemotherapy

Immediate treatment should be undertaken for symptomatic spinal cord compression. Neurologic recovery is more likely the less the severity of compromise and the shorter the duration of symptoms. Neurologic outcome appears to be similar whether cord compression is treated with chemotherapy, radiation therapy, or surgical laminectomy. However, laminectomy may result in later scoliosis, and chemotherapy is often needed whether or not surgery or radiation is used.

Treatment of Low Risk Neuroblastoma

Patients with low-risk neuroblastoma have a cure rate greater than 90%. The following tumors are categorized as low risk.

1. INSS stage 1 tumors in patients of any age. Stage 1 is defined as gross complete resection.
2. INSS stage 2A and 2B tumors in infants.
3. INSS stage 2A and 2B tumors in children over 1 year of age and in whom the tumor demonstrates either favorable Shimada histopathology or nonamplification of *N-myc*.
4. INSS stage 4S tumors in infants less than 1 year of age with all favorable biological features (i.e., *N-myc* not amplified, favorable Shimada histopathology, and hyperdiploid DNA).

Low-risk neuroblastomas are generally treated with surgical resection and observation or observation alone.

Stage 2 low-risk tumors are treated with chemotherapy only if less than 50% of the tumor has been resected. In the other low-risk patients, chemotherapy is recommended only for life- or organ-threatening symptoms that cannot be relieved by safe surgical resection of the mass. Such symptoms include respiratory distress, renal or bowel ischemia, spinal cord compression, gastrointestinal or genitourinary obstruction, or coagulopathy. Chemotherapy is given for 6 to 24 weeks and consists of moderate doses of carboplatin, cyclophosphamide, doxorubicin, and etoposide. The cumulative dose of each agent is kept low in order to minimize permanent injury from the chemotherapy regimen. Radiation therapy is reserved for patients with symptomatic life- or organ-threatening tumor that does not respond rapidly enough to chemotherapy.

The treatment of children with low-risk stage 4S disease is dependent on clinical presentation. Children who are clinically stable with this special pattern of neuroblastoma may not require therapy. The development of complications, such as functional compromise from massive hepatomegaly, is an indication for intervention, especially in infants younger than 2 to 3 months of age.

Treatment of Intermediate Risk Neuroblastoma

Patients with Intermediate-Risk neuroblastoma generally have a cure rate of 70% to 90%. The following patients are categorized as intermediate risk:

1. INSS stage 3 tumors in infants less than 1 year of age and in whom the tumor lacks N-myc gene amplification.
2. INSS stage 3 tumors in children 1 year of age or older and in whom the tumor lacks N-myc gene amplification and has favorable Shimada histopathology.
3. INSS stage 4 tumors in infants less than 1 year of age and in whom the tumor lacks N-myc gene amplification.
4. INSS stage 4S tumors in infants less than 1 year of age and in whom the tumor lacks N-myc gene amplification and has either unfavorable Shimada histopathology or is near diploid in chromosome number, or both.

There is considerable variation in outcome, and, therefore, in treatment for children with stage 3 disease (tumor involving both sides of the midline by virtue of either invasion into normal tissues or lymph node metastasis). Infants younger than 1 year of age have a greater than 80% chance of cure while older children have a cure rate of 50 to 70% with current relatively intensive therapy.

Patients classified as intermediate risk with stage 3 tumors with favorable or unfavorable Shimada histology are treated with 12 weeks and 24 weeks of chemotherapy respectively. In patients classified as intermediate risk with favorable biology, radiation therapy is reserved for patients with symptomatic life- or organ-threatening tumor that does not respond rapidly enough to chemotherapy. In patients classified as intermediate risk with unfavorable biologic features, radiation therapy is given if residual viable tumor remains after 24 weeks of chemotherapy and second-look surgery.

Treatment of High Risk Neuroblastoma

The following patients are considered to have high-risk neuroblastoma:

1. INSS stage 2A/2B tumors in children over 1 year of age and in whom the tumor has both unfavorable Shimada histology and N-myc gene amplification.
2. INSS stage 3 tumors in infants less than 1 year of age and in whom the tumor demonstrates N-myc gene amplification.
3. INSS stage 3 tumors in children over 1 year of age and in whom the tumor demonstrates either *N-myc* gene amplification or unfavorable Shimada histology.
4. INSS stage 4 tumors in infants less than 1 year of age at diagnosis and in whom the tumor demonstrates *N-myc* gene amplification.
5. INSS stage 4 tumors in children over 1 year of age.
6. INSS stage 4S tumors in infants less than 1 year of age at diagnosis and in whom the tumor demonstrates *N-myc* gene amplification.

For children with high-risk neuroblastoma, long-term survival ranges from 10 to 40%. Children with aggressively treated, high-risk neuroblastoma may develop late recurrences, some more than 5 years after completion of therapy. A randomized study was performed comparing high-dose therapy with purged autologous bone marrow transplantation versus 3 cycles of intensive consolidation chemotherapy.

Standard Treatment

Patients classified as high risk receive treatment with an aggressive regimen of combination chemotherapy consisting of very high drug doses.

Drugs often used include cyclophosphamide, ifosfamide, cisplatin, carboplatin, vincristine, doxorubicin, and etoposide. After a response to chemotherapy, resection of the primary tumor should be attempted, followed by myeloablative chemotherapy and stem cell rescue (bone marrow and/or peripheral blood stem cell transplantation). The use of purged stem cells is under investigation. Radiation to the primary tumor site should be undertaken whether or not a complete excision was obtained. Radiation of sites of metastatic disease is determined on an individual case basis. After recovery, patients are treated with oral 13-cis-retinoic acid for 6 months. Both myeloablative therapy and postchemotherapy retinoic acid improve outcome in patients categorized as high risk.

Under Clinical Evaluation

- Monoclonal antibody therapy with or without GM-CSF following chemotherapy.
- Targeted radiation therapy with 131I-metaiodobenzylguanidine (131I-MIBG).
- Tandem myeloablation and stem cell transplantation.
- Inclusion of myeloablative doses of 131I MIBG prior to stem cell transplantation.

Childhood Rhabdomyosarcoma

General Information

Childhood rhabdomyosarcoma, a soft tissue malignant tumor of skeletal muscle origin, accounts for approximately 3.5% of the cases of cancer among children 0 to 14 years and 2% of the cases among adolescents and young adults 15 to 19 years of age. It is a curable disease in most children with localized disease who receive combined modality therapy, with more than 70% surviving 5 years after diagnosis. The most common primary sites for rhabdomyosarcoma are the head and neck (e.g., parameningeal, orbit, pharyngeal, etc.), the genitourinary tract, and the extremities. Other less common primary sites include the trunk, chest wall, the abdomen (including the retroperitoneum and biliary tract), and the perineal/anal region.

Most cases of rhabdomyosarcoma occur sporadically with no recognized predisposing factor or risk factor although a small proportion are associated with genetic conditions. These conditions include Li-Fraumeni cancer susceptibility syndrome (with germline *p53* mutations) neurofibromatosis type I and Beckwith-Wiedemann syndrome (although Wilms' tumor and hepatoblastoma are more commonly associated with this latter syndrome).

The prognosis for a child or adolescent with rhabdomyosarcoma is related to the site of origin, resectability, presence of metastases, number of metastatic sites, and histopathology. There are also preliminary data describing the possible prognostic significance of age and unique biological characteristics of rhabdomyosarcoma tumor cells. Examples of both clinical and biological factors with proven or possible prognostic significance are briefly described below.

- Primary sites with more favorable prognoses include the orbit and nonparameningeal head and neck, paratestis and vagina (nonbladder, nonprostate genitourinary) and the biliary tract.
- Tumor burden at diagnosis has prognostic significance. Patients with smaller tumors (< 5 cm) have improved survival compared to children with larger tumors, while children with metastatic disease at diagnosis have the poorest prognosis. The prognostic significance of metastatic disease is modified by tumor histology (embryonal favorable) and by the number of metastatic sites. Similarly, patients with metastatic genitourinary (nonbladder, nonprostate) primary tumors have a more favorable outcome compared to patients with metastatic disease and primary tumors at other

sites. In addition, patients with otherwise localized disease but with proven regional lymph node involvement have a poorer prognosis than patients without regional nodal involvement.

- The extent of disease following the primary surgical procedure (i.e., the clinical group) is also correlated with outcome In the Intergroup Rhabdomyosarcoma Study (IRS) III, patients with gross residual disease after initial surgery (Clinical Group III) had a 5-year survival rate of approximately 70% compared with a greater than 90% 5-year survival rate for patients with no residual tumor after surgery (Clinical Group I) and an approximately 80% 5-year survival rate for patients with microscopic residual tumor following surgery (Clinical Group II).
- The *alveolar subtype is more prevalent among patients* with less favorable clinical features (e.g., younger than 1 or older than 10 years, extremity primaries, and metastatic disease), and is generally associated with a worse outcome. In the IRS-I and IRS-II studies, the alveolar subtype was associated with a less favorable outcome even in patients whose primary site was completely resected (Clinical Group I). Statistically significant differences in survival for histopathologic subtype were not, however, noted when all patients with rhabdomyosarcoma were analyzed, nor were differences noted by histologic subtype in a large group of German children with rhabdomyosarcoma.
- Tumor expression of the *P-glycoprotein* gene and its association with multidrug resistance and outcome are under investigation. The available data are discordant.

Because treatment and prognosis depend, in part, on the histology of the tumor, it is necessary that the tumor tissue be reviewed by pathologists with experience in the evaluation and diagnosis of tumors in children. Additionally, the diversity of primary sites, the distinctive surgical and radiation therapy treatments for each primary site, and the subsequent site-specific rehabilitation underscore the importance of treating children with rhabdomyosarcoma in medical centers with appropriate experience in all therapeutic modalities.

Rhabdomyosarcoma can be divided into several histologic subsets: embryonal, botryoid, and spindle cell subtypes of embryonal rhabdomyosarcoma, alveolar, and pleomorphic.] The embryonal subtype is the most frequently observed subtype in children, accounting for approximately 60 to 70% of rhabdomyosarcomas of childhood. Tumors with embryonal histology typically arise in the head and neck region or in the genitourinary tract, although they may occur at any primary site. Botryoid tumors represent about 10% of all rhabdomyosarcoma cases and are embryonal tumors that arise under the mucosal surface of body orifices such as the vagina, bladder, nasopharynx, and biliary tract. The spindle cell variant of embryonal rhabdomyosarcoma is most frequently observed at the paratesticular site. *Both the botryoid and the spindle cell subtypes are associated with very favorable outcome.*

Stage Information

- *Group I:* Localized disease that is completely resected with no regional nodal involvement. Approximately 13% of all patients are in this group.
- *Group II:*
  - § *IIA:* Localized, grossly resected tumor with microscopic residual disease but no regional nodal involvement.
  - § *IIB:* Loco-regional disease with tumor-involved lymph nodes with complete resection and no residual disease.
  - § *IIC:* Loco-regional disease with involved nodes, grossly resected, but with evidence

of microscopic residual tumor at the primary site and/or histologic involvement of the most distal regional node (from the primary site).

Approximately 20% of all patients are in groups IIA + B + C.

- *Group III:* Localized, gross residual disease including incomplete resection, or biopsy only of the primary site. Approximately 48% of all patients are in this group.
- *Group IV:* Distant metastatic disease present at the time of diagnosis. Approximately 18% of all patients are in this group.
- *Stage 1:* Localized disease involving the orbit or head and neck (excluding parameningeal sites), or genitourinary region (excluding bladder/prostate sites), or biliary tract (favorable sites).
- *Stage 2:* Localized disease of any other primary site not included in the stage 1 category (unfavorable sites). Primary tumors must be less than or equal to 5 cm in diameter, and there must be no clinical regional lymph node involvement by tumor.
- *Stage 3:* Localized disease of any other primary site. These patients differ from stage 2 patients by having primary tumors greater than 5 cm and/or regional node involvement.
- *Stage 4:* Metastatic disease at diagnosis.
- *Low risk:* patients with localized embryonal rhabdomyosarcoma occurring at favorable sites (i.e., Stage 1) and patients with embryonal rhabdomyosarcoma occurring at unfavorable sites with either completely resected disease (i.e., Group I) or microscopic residual disease (i.e., Group II). In addition, patients with orbital Group III are also considered low risk.
- *Intermediate risk:* patients with embryonal rhabdomyosarcoma occurring at unfavorable sites with gross residual disease (i.e., Group III), patients with metastatic embryonal rhabdomyosarcoma who are younger than 10 years, and patients with nonmetastatic alveolar rhabdomyosarcoma or undifferentiated sarcoma at any site.
- *High risk:* patients with metastatic rhabdomyosarcoma or undifferentiated sarcoma at presentation excepting embryonal cases in children younger than 10 years.

Treatment Option Overview

All children with rhabdomyosarcoma require multimodality therapy. This entails surgical resection, if possible, followed by chemotherapy, followed by second-look surgery for some patients with initially unresected tumors, and, depending on original histologic type, extent of disease, extent of resection, and radiation therapy.

Before biopsy of a suspected tumor mass, imaging studies of the mass and baseline laboratory studies should be obtained. After the diagnosis of rhabdomyosarcoma has been made, an extensive evaluation to determine the extent of the disease should be done prior to instituting therapy. This evaluation should include a chest X-ray, computed tomography (CT) scan of the chest, bone marrow biopsy and aspirate, magnetic resonance imaging (MRI) of the base of the skull base and brain (if it is a parameningeal primary), and CT scan of the abdomen and pelvis (for lower extremity or genitourinary (GU) primaries).

Surgical Management

Treatment Options

The basic principle for the initial surgical treatment of children with rhabdomyosarcoma is complete resection of the primary tumor with a surrounding margin of normal tissue and lymph node sampling of the draining nodal basin. Important exceptions to the rule of normal margin exist (e.g., tumors of the orbit and of the genitourinary region). The principle of wide and complete resection of the primary tumor is less applicable to patients known to have metastatic disease at the initial operation, but is a reasonable concept if easily accomplished. Patients with microscopic residual tumor following their initial excisional procedure appear to have improved prognoses if a second operative procedure consisting of re-excision of the primary tumor bed, prior to initiation of chemotherapy, can achieve complete removal of tumor. Because rhabdomyosarcoma can arise from so many primary muscle and mesenchymal sites, surgical care must be tailored to the unique aspects of each site.

Head and Neck

For head and neck tumors that are superficial and nonorbital, wide excision of the primary tumor (when feasible) and ipsilateral neck lymph node sampling of clinically involved nodes are appropriate. Narrower resection margins (<1 mm) are acceptable because of anatomic restrictions.

Extremity Sites

The definitive surgical procedure involves wide local excision with removal en bloc of a cuff of normal tissue. Primary re-excision may be appropriate in patients whose initial surgical procedure leaves microscopic residual disease that is resectable by a second procedure. Amputation may be indicated for selected patients with extracompartmental lesions involving major neural and/or vascular structures in addition to the muscle of origin. Due to the significant incidence of nodal spread for extremity primary tumors (often without clinical evidence of involvement), and because of the prognostic and therapeutic implications of nodal involvement, extensive pretreatment assessment for regional nodal involvement is warranted.

Truncal Sites

The surgical management of patients with lesions of the chest wall or abdominal wall should follow the same guidelines as for lesions of the extremities, that being wide local excision and an attempt to achieve negative microscopic margins.

Genitourinary System

Primary sites for childhood rhabdomyosarcoma within the genitourinary system include the paratesticular area, bladder, prostate, vagina, and uterus.

Lesions adjacent to the testis or spermatic cord should be removed by orchiectomy and resection of the entire spermatic cord, utilizing an inguinal incision with proximal vascular control (i.e., radical orchiectomy).] Resection of hemiscrotal skin is required when there is tumor fixation or invasion, or when a previous trans-scrotal biopsy has been performed. Paratesticular tumors have been found to have a relatively high incidence of lymphatic spread (26% in Intergroup Rhabdomyosarcoma Study (IRS) I and IRS-II studies),and all patients with paratesticular primary tumors should have thin-cut abdominal and pelvic computerized tomographic (CT) scans with contrast to evaluate nodal involvement. Bladder salvage is an important goal of therapy for patients with tumors arising in the prostate and bladder. In rare cases the tumor is confined to the dome of the bladder and can be completely resected.

Metastatic Sites

Primary resection of metastatic disease is rarely indicated except for isolated pulmonary metastases. Persistent metastatic disease in the lung following radiation and chemotherapy should be resected when possible to render patients disease-free, provided adequate pulmonary function can be preserved.

Chemotherapy Treatment Options

All children with rhabdomyosarcoma should receive chemotherapy, with the quantity and duration of therapy dependent on appropriate risk factor analysis.

Standard Treatment Options

Low-risk Patients

- For children with the most favorable prognosis, an important consideration is maintaining high survival rates (>90%) while minimizing the long-term consequences of chemotherapy. As discussed in the general information and staging sections of this summary, favorable prognosis is defined as patients with embryonal rhabdomyosarcoma occurring in favorable sites (i.e., Stage 1) and embryonal rhabdomyosarcoma with either completely resected disease (i.e., Group I) or microscopic residual disease (i.e., Group II) occurring at unfavorable sites. One subgroup of the favorable-prognosis population has achieved high survival rates with a chemotherapy regimen using only vincristine (VCR) with dactinomycin (DACT).

Intermediate-risk Patients

- Patients with intermediate prognosis have survival rates ranging from 55 to 70%. This category includes patients with embryonal rhabdomyosarcoma at unfavorable sites who have gross residual disease (i.e., Group III), patients with metastatic embryonal rhabdomyosarcoma who are younger than 10 years, and patients with nonmetastatic alveolar rhabdomyosarcoma at any site. For patients with intermediate prognosis, VAC (VCR, DACT, and cyclophosphamide) is the standard chemotherapy treatment.

High-risk Patients

- Patients with metastatic disease at diagnosis (Stage 4) have a poor prognosis with current therapy, and new approaches to treatment are needed to improve survival in this group In the IRS-IV study, 3 combinations of drug pairs were studied in an up-front window: ifosfamide/etoposide (IE), vincristine/melphalan (VM), and ifosfamide/doxorubicin (ID)

UNUSUAL CANCERS OF CHILDHOOD

General Information

Head and Neck Cancers

Head and neck cancers include nasopharyngeal carcinoma, esthesioneuroblastoma, thyroid tumors, mouth cancer, salivary gland cancer, and laryngeal carcinoma. The prognosis, diagnosis, classification, and treatment of these head and neck cancers are discussed below.

Nasopharyngeal Carcinoma

Nasopharyngeal cancer arises in the lining of the nasal cavity and pharynx. This tumor accounts for about one third of all cancers of the upper airways. The incidence of this tumor is approximately 1 in 100,000 persons under the age of 20 in the United States. There is a higher frequency of this tumor in North Africa and Southeast Asia.

Nasopharyngeal carcinoma occurs in association with Epstein-Barr virus (EBV), the virus associated with infectious mononucleosis. The virus can be detected in biopsy specimens of these cancers, and tumor cells can have EBV antigens on their cell surface. Three histologic subtypes are recognized by the World Health Organization. Type 1 is squamous cell carcinoma, type 2 is nonkeratinizing carcinoma, and type 3 is undifferentiated carcinoma.

This cancer most frequently spreads to lymph nodes in the neck, which may alert the patient, parent, or physician to the presence of this tumor. The tumor may also spread to the nose, mouth, and pharynx, causing snoring, epistaxis, obstruction of the eustachian tubes, or hearing loss; it may also invade the base of the skull, causing cranial nerve palsy or difficulty with movements of the jaw (trismus). Distant metastatic sites may include the bones, the lungs, and the liver. The location of the primary tumor can be made by direct inspection of the nasopharynx. A diagnosis can be made from a biopsy of the primary tumor or of enlarged lymph nodes of the neck. Nasopharyngeal carcinomas must be distinguished from all other cancers that can present with enlarged lymph nodes and from other types of cancer in the head and neck area. Thus, diseases such as thyroid cancer, rhabdomyosarcoma, non-Hodgkin's lymphoma, Hodgkin's lymphoma, and Burkitt's lymphoma must be considered, as should benign conditions such as nasal angiofibroma (which presents with epistaxis) and infections draining into the lymph nodes of the neck.

Diagnostic tests should determine the extent of the primary tumor and whether there are metastases. Visualization of the nasopharynx by an ear-nose-throat specialist using a mirror, examination by a neurologist, and magnetic resonance imaging (MRI) of the head and neck can be used to determine the extent of the primary tumor. Evaluation of the chest and abdomen by computed tomography (CT) and bone scan should also be performed to determine whether there is metastatic disease. The levels of EBV and antibody to EBV should also be measured.

Tumor staging is done by the tumor-node-metastasis (TNM) classification system of the American Joint Committee on Cancer. Various reports have indicated an overall survival rate of at least 75% for patients with early-stage disease; there is a lower survival rate for patients with higher-stage disease. No factors other than extent of tumor have correlated with prognosis. New criteria for TNM staging of nasopharyngeal carcinoma has been defined by the American Joint Commission of Cancer (AJCC) and appear to correlate better with outcome than prior staging systems.

Treatment combines the use of surgery, radiation therapy, and chemotherapy. Nasopharyngeal carcinoma generally has spread to the bones of the skull and to lymph nodes in the neck at the time of diagnosis; thus, the principal role of surgery is to obtain adequate diagnostic material from a biopsy of the involved lymph node or the primary site. Combined modality therapy with radiation and chemotherapy appears to be the most effective treatment for this tumor. Chemotherapy approaches include neoadjuvant and/or adjuvant therapy with cisplatin, 5-fluorouracil, and methotrexate. Radiation dose to the tumor should be greater than 60 Gy. An overall survival rate of 78% has been reported with this approach.

Esthesioneuroblastoma

Esthesioneuroblastoma (olfactory neuroblastoma) is a very rare, small round-cell tumor arising from the nasal neuroepithelium that is distinct from primitive neuroectodermal tumors (PNET). Most children present with a nasopharyngeal mass which may have local extension into the orbits, sinuses, or frontal lobe, with associated symptoms. There appears to be a male predominance and the average age of presentation is in adolescence. The youngest child reported with this diagnosis was 2 years old. Metastatic disease is uncommon. The mainstay of treatment has been surgery and radiation, although recent reports indicate increasing use of neoadjuvant chemotherapy. Chemotherapy regimens that have been used with efficacy include VAC (vincristine + actinomycin D + cyclophosphamide)-Adria, ifosfamide/etoposide, and cisplatin plus etoposide or doxorubicin. The long-term survival rate appears to be approximately 60-80%. Local recurrences may occur late.

Thyroid Tumors

Tumors of the thyroid are classified as adenomas or carcinomas. Adenomas are benign growths that may cause enlargement of all or part of the gland, which extends to both sides of the neck and can be quite large. Some of these tumors may secrete hormones. Transformation to a malignant carcinoma may occur in some cells, which then may grow and spread to lymph nodes in the neck or to the lungs.

Most thyroid carcinomas occur in girls. Although rare, these cancers represent about 1.5% of all tumors seen in the pediatric age group. There is an excessive frequency of thyroid adenoma and carcinoma in patients who previously received irradiation to the neck. Thyroid cancer may be associated with the development of other types of malignant tumors, such as the multiple endocrine neoplasia (MEN) syndromes. Thyroid carcinomas are differentiated tumors, meaning that they tend to grow slowly and are not highly malignant. Thyroid radionuclide scans do not demonstrate the uptake of radioisotope into the area of the suspected neoplasm.

Various histologies account for the general diagnostic category of carcinoma of the thyroid. Papillary carcinoma represents 60 to 75% of these tumors, follicular carcinoma 10 to 20%, medullary carcinoma 5 to 10%, and anaplastic carcinoma less than 1%. Follicular carcinomas may be sporadic or familial. Follicular carcinoma and papillary carcinoma generally have a benign course, with an approximately 80% 10-year survival rate. Fifty percent of medullary thyroid carcinomas, which may be familial, have hematogenous metastases at diagnosis. Follicular carcinoma may also have a high incidence of metastases, whereas papillary carcinomas often have multicentric origin. Patients with medullary carcinoma of the thyroid have a guarded prognosis, unless they have very small tumors ("microcarcinoma," defined as less than 1.0 cm in diameter), which carry a good prognosis.

Surgery is the treatment required for all thyroid neoplasms. Total thyroidectomy is recommended for medullary cancer, and the resected parathyroid glands generally are autotransplanted to other sites such as the forearm. A more conservative approach is recommended for papillary carcinoma, with lymph node dissection leading to near-total thyroidectomy. Over the 4 to 6 weeks following surgery, patients may develop hypothyroidism. A radioactive iodine scan is performed to search for residual neoplasm in the functioning thyroid tissue. After the thyroid scan, radioactive iodine (I-131) treatment is given at a dose of 100 to 150 mCu, and the patient is kept in a safe area overnight or until the kidney clears virtually all of the radioactive component. In the postoperative period, hormone replacement therapy must be given to compensate for the lost thyroid hormone. I-131 is usually successful in suppressing thyroid function, after which the patient is treated with synthetic thyroid hormones for life. Periodic evaluations are required to determine whether there is metastatic disease involving the lungs. Lifelong follow-up is necessary. Thyroglobulin levels, T4, and TSH levels should be evaluated periodically to determine whether replacement hormone is appropriately dosed. Patients with thyroid cancer generally have an excellent survival with relatively few side effects. Recurrence is common, however, and is seen more often in children younger than 10 years old.

Oral Cancers

Cancer of the mouth in children or in adolescents is extremely rare This cancer primarily occurs in adults older than 50 years who have used tobacco for many years; however, it can occur in survivors of other childhood tumors who have had radiation therapy to this area. Evidence suggests that oral cancer at younger ages primarily results from the use of smokeless tobacco products among preadolescent boys. Changes in the texture, color, and shape of the mucosal lining of the mouth have been seen, together with degenerative changes of the gingiva, in more than half of all teenagers who use smokeless tobacco. Precancerous lesions are common among children. Squamous cell carcinoma, the most frequent type of cancer in these sites, must be distinguished from benign tumors of the pharynx and neck, e.g., dermoid cysts, lipomas, myofibromas, cystic hygroma, and teratomas. Other tumors in this area may include ameloblastoma or adamantinoma, a rare tumor that may arise in the mandible or the maxilla, as well as in the long bones. The treatment of ameloblastoma is surgical resection, if possible. Ameloblastoma may be benign or malignant; pulmonary metastases may be discovered many years after treatment for this tumor.

Salivary Gland Cancers

Many salivary gland cancers arise in the parotid gland. About 15% of these tumors may arise in the submandibular glands or in the minor salivary glands under the tongue and jaw. These tumors are most frequently benign, but on very rare occasions, may be malignant. The malignant lesions include adenocarcinoma, undifferentiated carcinoma, acinic cell carcinomas, and mucoepidermoid carcinoma. These tumors may occur after radiation therapy is given for treatment of primary leukemia or solid tumors. Radical surgical removal is the treatment of choice, whenever possible, with additional use of radiation therapy and chemotherapy for high-grade tumors or tumors that have spread from their site of origin. Prognosis for patients with these tumors is generally good.

Laryngeal Carcinoma

Benign and especially malignant tumors of the larynx are rare. Malignant tumors may be associated with benign tumors such as *polyps and papillomas*. These tumors may cause hoarseness, difficulty swallowing, and enlargement of the lymph nodes of the neck. Rhabdomyosarcoma is the most common malignant tumor of the larynx in the pediatric age group. Squamous cell carcinoma of the larynx should be managed in the same manner as in adults with carcinoma at this site, with surgery and radiation. Laser surgery may be the first type of treatment utilized for these lesions.

Papillomatosis of the larynx is a benign overgrowth of tissues lining the larynx, associated with the human papillomavirus. This condition is not cancerous and may be treated with interferon. These tumors can cause hoarseness because of their association with wart-like nodules on the vocal cords and may extend into the lung, producing significant morbidity

Thoracic Cancers

Thoracic cancers include breast cancer, bronchial adenomas, bronchial carcinoid tumors, pleuropulmonary blastoma, esophageal tumors, thymomas, tumors of the heart, and mesothelioma. The prognosis, diagnosis, classification, and treatment of these thoracic cancers are discussed below.

Breast Cancer

Most tumors that involve the breast during childhood are benign, yet carcinomas have been reported in both males and females younger than 21 years. There is an increased lifetime risk of breast cancer in female survivors of Hodgkin's lymphoma who were treated with radiation to the chest area. Carcinomas are more frequent than sarcomas. Mammograms should start at age 25 for any patient who has had radiation therapy to the chest. Treatment options include radiation, chemotherapy, and surgery for children and adolescents with breast cancer. Breast tumors may also occur as metastatic deposits from leukemia, rhabdomyosarcoma, or other sarcomas.

Bronchial Adenomas/Carcinoids

Bronchial adenomas, which are slow-growing neoplasms, are also called carcinoid tumors. Primary treatment of these tumors is surgical resection. For bronchial carcinoid tumors, nuclear scans may demonstrate uptake of radioactivity by the tumor or lymph nodes, suggesting metastatic spread. Neither chemotherapy nor radiation therapy is indicated for bronchial carcinoid, unless evidence of metastasis is documented.

Esophageal Tumors

Esophageal cancer is rare in the pediatric age group, although it is relatively common in older adults Symptoms are related to difficulty in swallowing and associated weight loss. Most of these tumors are squamous cell carcinomas, although sarcomas can also arise in the esophagus. The most common benign tumor is leiomyoma. Diagnosis is made by histologic examination of biopsy tissue.

Treatment options for esophageal carcinoma include either external beam, intracavitary radiation therapy, or chemotherapy with the platinum derivatives, paclitaxel, and etoposide, agents commonly used to treat carcinomas. Prognosis generally is poor for this cancer, which rarely can be completely resected.

Thymomas

A cancer of the thymus is not considered a thymoma unless there are neoplastic changes of the epithelial cells that cover the organ. Other tumors that involve the thymus gland include lymphoma, germ cell tumors, carcinomas, carcinoid, and thymoma. Hodgkin's lymphoma and non-Hodgkin's lymphoma may also involve the thymus and must be differentiated from true thymomas.

Thymomas are rare in adults and children. *Various diseases and syndromes are associated with thymoma, including myasthenia gravis, polymyositis, systemic lupus erythematosus, rheumatoid arthritis, thyroiditis, and pure red-cell aplasia. Endocrine (hormonal) disorders including hyperthyroidism, Addison's disease, and panhypopituitarism can also be associated with a diagnosis of thymoma.*

Thymomas are usually located in the front part of the chest, and are usually discovered during a routine chest x-ray. Symptoms can include cough, difficulty with swallowing, tightness of the chest, chest pain, and shortness of breath although non-specific symptoms may occur. These tumors generally are slow-growing, but are potentially invasive, with metastases to distant organs or lymph nodes. Staging is related to invasiveness. Surgery is performed with the goal of a complete resection.

Radiation therapy is necessary for patients with invasive thymoma, whether or not there has been a complete resection. Chemotherapy is usually reserved for patients with advanced-stage disease who have not responded to radiation therapy or corticosteroids. Agents that have been effective include doxorubicin, cisplatin, and paclitaxel. The prognosis for patients with invasive thymoma usually is poor, although significantly higher rates of survival have been reported for patients with tumors that are not locally invasive. Thymic carcinoma, which microscopically resembles undifferentiated nasopharyngeal carcinoma, is associated with Epstein-Barr virus infection, as is nasopharyngeal carcinoma. *This tumor is responsive to chemotherapy and is potentially curable.*

Tumors of the Heart

The most common tumors of the heart are benign and include myxomas and neurofibromas, i.e., tumors of the nerves that innervate the muscles.

Other tumors of the heart can include metastatic spread of rhabdomyosarcoma, melanoma, leukemia, and carcinoma of other sites. Primary tumors of the heart may include benign and malignant teratoma, rhabdomyosarcoma, hemangioma, and chondrosarcoma. Symptoms include abnormalities of heart rhythm, enlargement of the heart, fluid in the pericardial sac, and congestive heart failure. Successful treatment requires surgery, which may include transplantation, and chemotherapy appropriate for the type of cancer that is present.

Mesothelioma

This tumor can involve the membranous coverings of the lung, the heart, or the abdominal organs. These tumors can spread over the surface of organs, without invading far into the underlying tissue, and may spread to regional or distant lymph nodes. Mesothelioma may develop after successful treatment of an earlier cancer, especially after treatment with radiation. In adults, these tumors have been associated with exposure to asbestos, which was used as building insulation. The amount of exposure required to develop cancer is unknown, and there is no information about the risk for children exposed to asbestos.

Benign and malignant mesotheliomas cannot be differentiated using histologic criteria. A poor prognosis is associated with lesions that are diffuse and invasive or for those that recur. In general, the course of the disease is slow, and long-term survival is common. Treatment with various chemotherapeutic agents used for carcinomas or sarcomas may result in partial responses. Pain is an infrequent symptom; however, radiation therapy may be used for palliation of pain.

Papillary serous carcinoma of the peritoneum is sometimes mistaken for mesothelioma. This tumor generally involves all surfaces lining the abdominal organs, including the surfaces of the ovary. Treatment includes surgical resection whenever possible and use of chemotherapy with agents such as cisplatin, carboplatin, and paclitaxel.

Abdominal Cancers

Abdominal cancers include adrenocortical tumors, renal cell carcinoma, carcinoma of the stomach, cancer of the pancreas, colorectal carcinoma, carcinoid tumors, and multiple endocrine neoplasia syndrome. The prognosis, diagnosis, classification, and treatment of these abdominal cancers are discussed below.

Carcinoma of the Adrenal Cortex

Adrenocortical tumors are classified as carcinomas and adenomas. Adrenocortical tumors may be hormonally active or inactive. Adenomas are generally benign, whereas adrenocortical carcinomas frequently secrete hormones and may cause the patient to develop masculine traits, irrespective of the patient's gender. Pediatric patients with adrenocortical carcinoma often have Li-Fraumeni syndrome, which is an inherited condition that predisposes family members to multiple cancers, including breast cancer, rhabdomyosarcoma, and osteosarcoma. Children with Beckwith-Wiedemann Syndrome or hemihypertrophy are at increased risk of developing carcinoma of the adrenal cortex (as well as Wilms' tumor, hepatoblastoma, and other rare cancers) in the first several years of life.

These tumors spread locally to the lymph nodes and can also involve the kidneys, lungs, and bones. Surgical removal should be attempted but may not always be possible if the tumor has spread widely. Additional treatment may include the use of an artificial hormone that blocks the masculinizing effects of the tumor or chemotherapy using cisplatin, 5-fluorouracil, and etoposide. The prognosis for patients who have small, completely resected tumors generally is excellent, but prognosis can be poor for patients who have large primary tumors or metastatic disease at diagnosis.

Renal Cell Carcinoma

Renal cell carcinoma is the most common primary malignancy of the kidney in adults; however, it occurs rarely in children. The annual incidence rate is approximately 4 per 1 million children, compared to an incidence of Wilms' tumor of the kidney that is at least 29-fold higher. Renal cell carcinoma may be associated with von Hippel-Lindau disease, a hereditary condition in which blood vessels within the retina and cerebellum grow excessively. The gene for von Hippel-Lindau is on chromosome 3p14 and is a tumor-suppressor gene whose function is lost in patients with the syndrome. Renal cell carcinoma has also been associated with tuberous sclerosis, a hereditary disease characterized by benign fatty cysts in the kidney. Familial renal cell carcinoma has been associated with an inherited chromosome translocation involving chromosome 3. A high incidence of chromosome 3 abnormalities has also been demonstrated in nonfamilial renal tumors. There is a subset of tumors previously considered to be renal cell carcinoma in young people that appears to be genetically related to alveolar soft part sarcoma.

Renal cell carcinoma may present with an abdominal mass, abdominal pain, or hematuria. In a series of 41 children with renal cell carcinoma, the median age was 124 months with 46% presenting with localized stage I and II, 29% with stage III, and 22% with stage IV disease using the Robson classification system. Sites of metastases were the lungs, liver, and lymph nodes. Event-free survival (EFS) and overall survival was about 55% at 20 years. Patients with stage I and stage II disease had an 89% overall survival rate, while those with stage III and stage IV disease had a 23% overall survival rate at 20 years.

The primary treatment includes total surgical removal of the kidney and associated lymph nodes. Consideration should also be given to treatment with irradiation, chemotherapy, or both. Treatment of metastatic disease is presently unsatisfactory but usually includes the use of immune system modulators such as interferon-alfa and interleukin-2

Carcinoma of the Stomach

The frequency and death rate from stomach cancer has declined worldwide over the past 50 years with the introduction of food preservation practices such as refrigeration. The tumor must be distinguished from other conditions such as non-Hodgkin's lymphoma, malignant carcinoid, leiomyosarcoma, and various benign conditions or tumors of the stomach. Symptoms include vague upper abdominal pain, which can be associated with poor appetite, and weight loss. Many individuals become anemic but otherwise show no symptoms before the development of metastatic spread. Other symptoms may include nausea, vomiting, change in bowel habits, poor appetite, weakness, and Helicobacter pylori infection. Fiberoptic endoscopy can be used to visualize the tumor or to take a biopsy sample to ensure the correctness of diagnosis. Confirmation can also involve an X-ray examination of the upper gastrointestinal tract.

Treatment should include surgical excision with wide margins. For individuals who cannot have a complete surgical resection, radiation therapy may be used along with chemotherapeutic agents such as 5-fluorouracil and irinotecan. Other agents that may be of value are the nitrosoureas, with or without cisplatin, etoposide, doxorubicin, or mitomycin C.

Prognosis depends on the extent of the disease at the time of diagnosis and the success of treatment that is appropriate for the clinical situation. Because of the rarity of stomach cancer in the pediatric age group, little information regarding the treatment outcomes of children exists.

Cancer of the Pancreas

Pancreatic tumors are rare in children and adolescents. Tumors included in the general category can arise at any site within the pancreas. Cancers of the pancreas may be classified as adenocarcinoma, squamous cell carcinoma, acinic cell carcinoma, liposarcoma, lymphoma, papillary-cystic carcinoma, pancreaticoblastoma, malignant insulinoma, glucagonoma, and gastrinoma. Several cases of primitive neuroectodermal tumor (PNET) of the pancreas have been reported in children and young adults. Most pancreatic tumors do not secrete hormones, although some tumors secrete insulin, which can lead to symptoms of weakness, fatigue, hypoglycemia, and coma. If the tumor interferes with the normal function of the islet cells, patients may have watery diarrhea or abnormalities of salt balance. Both carcinoma of the pancreas and pancreaticoblastoma can produce active hormones and can be associated with abdominal mass, wasting, and pain. At times, there is obstruction of the head of the pancreas, which is associated with jaundice and gastrointestinal bleeding. Elevation of alpha-fetoprotein (AFP) has been seen in pancreatoblastoma.

The diagnosis is usually established by biopsy, using laparotomy or a minimally invasive surgery (laparoscopy). A diagnosis can only be achieved after ruling out various benign and cancerous lesions. Treatment includes various surgical procedures to remove the pancreas and duodenum or removal of part of the pancreas. Complete resection is usually possible and long-term survival is likely, although pancreatoblastoma has a high recurrence rate. For pediatric patients, the effectiveness of radiation therapy is not known. Chemotherapy may be useful for treatment of localized or metastatic pancreatic carcinoma. The combination of cisplatin and doxorubicin has produced responses in pancreatoblastoma prior to tumor resection. Other agents that may be of value include 5-fluorouracil, streptozotocin, mitomycin C, carboplatin, gemcitabine, and irinotecan. Response rates and survival rates generally are not good.

Colorectal Carcinoma

Carcinoma of the large bowel is rare in the pediatric age group, as it is seen in only 1 person per 1 million younger than 20 years in the United States annually. These tumors can occur anywhere in the colon or rectum and are often associated with a family cancer syndrome. There is an increasing risk of colorectal carcinoma in members of families with a family history of intestinal polyposis, which can lead to the development of multiple adenomatous polyps *Juvenile polyps are not associated with an increased incidence or risk of cancer.*

Familial polyposis is inherited as a dominant trait, which confers a high degree of risk. Early diagnosis and surgical removal of the colon eliminate the risk of developing carcinomas of the large bowel. *Some colorectal carcinomas in young people, however, may be associated with a mutation of the adenomatous polyposis coli (APC) gene, which also is associated with an increased risk of brain tumors and hepatoblastoma.* The familial APC syndrome is caused by mutation of a gene on chromosome 5q, which normally suppresses proliferation of cells lining the intestine and later development of polyps. Another tumor suppressor gene on chromosome 18 is associated with progression of polyps to malignant form. Multiple colon carcinomas have also been associated with progression of polyps to a malignant form. Multiple colon carcinomas have been associated with neurofibromatosis type I (NF-1) and several other rarer syndromes.

The histologic types of colorectal cancer include adenocarcinoma, mucinous or colloid adenocarcinomas, signet ring adenocarcinoma, and scirrhous tumors. Most tumors in the pediatric age group are mucin-producing carcinomas, whereas only about 15% of adult lesions are of this histology. The tumors of younger patients with this histologic variant may be less responsive to chemotherapy. These tumors arise from the surface of the bowel, usually at the site of an adenomatous polyp. The tumor may extend into the muscle layer surrounding the bowel, or the tumor may perforate the bowel entirely and seed through the spaces around the bowel, including intra-abdominal fat, lymph nodes, liver, ovaries, and the surface of other loops of bowel. A high incidence of metastasis involving the pelvis, ovaries, or both may be present in girls.

Colorectal carcinoma usually presents with symptoms related to the site of the tumor. Changes in bowel habits are associated with tumors of the rectum or lower colon. Tumors of the right colon may cause more subtle symptoms, but are often associated with an abdominal mass, weight loss, decreased appetite, and blood in the stool. Any tumor that causes complete obstruction of the large bowel can cause bowel perforation and spread of the tumor cells within the abdominal cavity.

Because of its rarity, colorectal carcinoma is rarely diagnosed in a pediatric patient; however, vague gastrointestinal symptoms should alert the physician to investigate this possibility. Diagnostic studies that may be of value include examination of the stool for blood, studies of liver and kidney function, measurement of carcinoembryonic antigen, and various medical imaging studies, including direct examination using colonoscopy to detect polyps in the large bowel. Other conventional radiographic studies include barium enema followed by CT of the chest and bone scans.

Most patients present with evidence of metastatic disease, either as gross tumor or as microscopic deposits in lymph nodes, on the surface of the bowel, or on intra-abdominal organs. Complete surgical excision should be the primary aim of the surgeon, but in most instances this is impossible; removal of large portions of tumor provides little benefit for the individuals with extensive metastatic disease. Most patients with microscopic metastatic disease generally develop gross metastatic disease, and few individuals with metastatic disease at diagnosis become long-term survivors.

Current therapy includes the use of radiation for rectal and lower-colon tumors, in conjunction with chemotherapy using 5-fluorouracil with leucovorin. Other agents that may be of value include irinotecan and oxaliplatin. No significant benefit has been determined for interferon-alfa given in conjunction with 5-fluorouracil/ leucovorin.

Carcinoid Tumors

These tumors, like bronchial adenomas, may be benign or malignant and can involve the lining of the lung or the large or small bowel. Most lung lesions are benign; however, some metastasize. Most carcinoid tumors of the appendix are small, localized tumors and simple appendectomy is the therapy of choice. For larger (>2 cm) tumors or tumors that have spread to local nodes, cecectomy or rarely, right hemicolectomy, is the usual treatment. It has become accepted practice to remove the entire right colon in patients with large carcinoid tumors of the appendix (greater than 2 cm in diameter) or with tumors that have spred to the nodes. Treatment of metastatic carcinoid tumors of the large bowel or stomach becomes more complicated and requires treatment similar to that given for colorectal carcinoma. The carcinoid syndrome of excessive excretion of somatostatin is characterized by flushing, labile blood pressure, and metastatic spread of the tumor to the liver. Symptoms may be lessened by giving somatostatin analogues, which are available in short-acting and long-acting forms.

Genital/Urinary Tumors

Genital/urinary tumors include carcinoma of the bladder and ovarian cancer. The prognosis, diagnosis, classification, and treatment of these genital/urinary tumors are discussed below.

Carcinoma of the Bladder

Carcinoma of the bladder is extremely rare in children. The most common carcinoma to involve the bladder is transitional cell carcinoma, which generally presents with hematuria. The diagnosis and treatment of this tumor are the same for children, adolescents, and adults. Adolescents who develop this tumor are often prone to the development of other cancers, including other bladder cancers. Bladder cancer in adolescents may develop as a consequence of alkylating-agent chemotherapy given for other childhood tumors or leukemia. The association between cyclophosphamide and bladder cancer is the only established relationship between a specific anticancer drug and a solid tumor. One of the most important risk factors for bladder cancer in adults is cigarette smoking, which may be associated with up to 50% of these cancers in men and 33% in women.

Ovarian Cancer

Most cancers that affect the ovaries are of germ cell origin, which are more common in children than adults, in whom adenocarcinomas are more frequently encountered. Ovarian carcinomas of nongerm-cell origin include tumors derived from malignant epithelial elements, including adenocarcinoma, cystadenocarcinoma, endometrioid tumors, clear cell tumors, and undifferentiated carcinomas. Treatment is stage-related and may include radiation and chemotherapy with cisplatin, carboplatin, etoposide, topotecan, paclitaxel, and other agents.

Juvenile granulosa cell tumor (JGCT) of the ovary is one of the rare sex cord/stromal tumors of the ovary seen in girls under 18 years old (median age 7.6 years; range 6 months to 17.5 years in 1 study). They represent about 5% of ovarian tumors in children and adolescents and are distinct from the granulosa cell tumors seen in adults. Most patients present with precocious puberty. Other presenting symptoms include abdominal pain, abdominal mass, and ascites. JGCT has been reported in children with Ollier's disease and Maffuci syndrome Up to 90% of children will have low-stage disease (FIGO [International Federation of Gynecology and Obstetrics] stage I) and are usually curable with unilateral salpingo-oophorectomy alone. Patients with advanced disease (FIGO stage II-IV) and those with high mitotic activity tumors have a poorer prognosis. Use of a cisplatin-based chemotherapy regimen has been reported in both the adjuvant and recurrent disease settings with some success.

Other Rare Childhood Cancers

Other rare childhood cancers include multiple endocrine neoplasia syndrome, skin cancer, and cancer of unknown primary site. The prognosis, diagnosis, classification, and treatment of these other rare childhood cancers are discussed below.

Multiple Endocrine Neoplasia Syndrome

These syndromes are familial disorders that are characterized by neoplastic changes in more than 1 endocrine organ. Changes may include hyperplasia, benign adenomas, and carcinomas. There are distinct genetic disorders with characteristic clinical presentations referred to as MEN-1, MEN-2a, and MEN-2b. An additional complex is referred to as the Carney complex, which is an association of multiple endocrine neoplasia associated with heart and skin tumors.

The MEN-1 syndrome, also referred to as Werner's syndrome, may involve tumors of the pituitary gland, the parathyroid, adrenal, gastric, and pancreatic structures, which may secrete hormones such as insulin. The gene for this syndrome is located on chromosome 11q13. The MEN-2a syndrome (Sipple syndrome) is associated with medullary thyroid carcinoma, parathyroid hyperplasia, adenomas, and pheochromocytoma. The MEN-2b syndrome is associated with medullary thyroid carcinoma, parathyroid hyperplasia, adenomas, and pheochromocytoma, mucosal neuromas, and ganglioneuromas. Patients with the MEN-2b syndrome may have a slender body build, long and thin extremities, a high arch palate, and pectus excavatum or pes cavus. The face may be characterized by thick lips because of mucosal neuromas. Such patients can also be identified by performing a pentagastrin stimulation test or by genetic screening in families known to be affected.

A germ line mutation in the RET oncogene (tyrosine-kinase receptor) on chromosome 10q11.2 is responsible for the uncontrolled growth of cells in medullary thyroid carcinoma associated with MEN-2a and MEN-2b syndromes The current management of medullary thyroid cancer in children from families having the MEN-2 syndromes relies on presymptomatic detection of the RET proto-oncogene mutation responsible for the disease. Children with MEN-2a should undergo total thyroidectomy approximately at the age of 5 years old before the cancer spreads beyond the thyroid gland. Due to the increased virulence of medullary thyroid carcinoma in children with MEN-2b, it is recommended that these children undergo prophylactic thyroidectomy in infancy. Complete removal of the thyroid gland is the recommended procedure for surgical management of medullary thyroid cancer in children, since there is a high incidence of bilateral disease.

The Carney complex includes the association of primary pigmented nodular adrenocortical disease with blue nevi of the skin and mucosa and a variety of additional endocriné or nonendocrine tumors. There may be myxomas of the skin or breast and tumors of peripheral nerve sheath origin. The outcome of patients with the MEN-1 syndrome is generally good provided adequate treatment can be obtained for parathyroid, pancreatic, and pituitary tumors. The outcome for patients with the MEN-2a syndrome is also generally good, yet the possibility exists for recurrence of medullary thyroid carcinoma and pheochromocytoma. For patients with the Carney complex, prognosis depends on the frequency of recurrences of cardiac and skin myxomas and other tumors.

Skin Cancer (Melanoma, Basal Cell, and Squamous Cell Carcinoma)

Melanoma is thought to be the most common skin cancer in children, followed by basal cell and squamous cell carcinomas. The incidence of melanoma in children and adolescents represents approximately 1% of the new cases of melanoma that are diagnosed annually in this country. In all instances, melanoma in the pediatric population is similar to that of adults in relation to site of presentation, symptoms, description, spread, and prognosis.

The greatest cause of skin cancer of any type is exposure to the ultraviolet (UV) portion of sunlight. Other causes may be related to chemical carcinogenesis, radiation exposure, immunodeficiency, or immunosuppression. The person who is most likely to develop a melanoma is easily sunburned, has poor tanning ability, and generally has light hair, blue eyes, and pale skin. Worldwide, there is an increasing incidence of both melanoma and nonmelanoma skin cancers. Melanoma presents as a relatively flat, dark-colored lesion, which may enlarge, penetrate the skin, or metastasize.

Melanomas may be congenital. They are sometimes associated with large congenital black spots known as melanocytic nevi, which may cover the trunk and thigh. Melanomas can also develop in individuals with xeroderma pigmentosum, a rare recessive disorder characterized by extreme sensitivity to sunlight, keratosis, and various neurologic manifestations. Individuals with xeroderma pigmentosum may also develop other skin cancers, including squamous and basal cell carcinomas. Children with hereditary immunodeficiencies have an increased lifetime risk of developing melanoma.

Neurocutaneous melanosis is an unusual condition associated with large or multiple congenital nevi of the skin and melanin deposits within the central nervous system. These deposits may be detected by magnetic resonance imaging of the brain or spinal cord. Dysplastic nevi occur in about 5% of the U.S. population and are potential precursors of melanoma. Individuals with atypical moles, which include raised lesions (that may bleed) and various color hues (brown, tan, pink, black), are at an increased risk of having melanoma and of having children affected by these premalignant lesions.

Basal cell carcinomas generally appear as raised lumps or ulcerated lesions, usually in areas with previous sun exposure. These tumors may be multiple and exacerbated by radiation therapy as delivered for medulloblastoma. Squamous cell carcinomas are usually reddened lesions with varying degrees of scaling or crusting, and they have an appearance similar to eczema, infections, trauma, or psoriasis.

Biopsy or excision is necessary to determine the diagnosis of any skin cancer. Diagnosis is necessary for decisions regarding additional treatment. Basal and squamous cell carcinomas are generally curable with surgery alone, but the treatment of melanoma requires greater consideration because of its potential for metastasis. Surgery for melanoma depends on the size, site, level of invasion, and metastatic extent or stage of the tumor. Wide excision with skin grafting may become necessary. *It is currently recommended that surgical resection include a 2-cm-deep margin for melanoma lesions, with examination of the regional lymph nodes draining the site of the melanoma.* This procedure may require the injection of a radioisotope, following its distribution, and then performing excision of the associated regional lymph nodes (sentinel node biopsy technique). This requires injection of a vital blue stain and radioisotope into the skin to characterize the pattern of lymph node drainage. Lymph node dissection is necessary if sentinel nodes are involved with the tumor; however, if there is no spread of the disease beyond the lymph nodes, adjuvant therapy with interferon alfa-2b alone may be recommended for a period of 1 year. For individuals with metastatic disease, a combination of cisplatin, vinblastine, imidazole carboxamide, interleukin-2, and interferon alfa-2b has been proposed. Prognosis for melanoma in children and adolescents is similar to that for adults with similar stage disease, with the prognosis depending on the tumor thickness and the extent of spread at the time of diagnosis. Survival decreases with greater depth of invasion and with metastases to lymph nodes.

Cancer of Unknown Primary Site

These cancers present as a metastatic cancer for which a precise primary tumor site cannot be determined. As an example, lymph nodes at the base of the skull may enlarge in relationship to a tumor that may be on the face or the scalp but is not evident by physical examination or by radiographic imaging. Thus, modern imaging techniques may indicate the extent of the disease but not a primary site. Tumors such as adenocarcinoma, melanoma, and embryonal tumors such as rhabdomyosarcoma and neuroblastoma may have such a presentation.

For all patients who present with tumors from an unknown primary site, the treatment should be considered in relation to the pathology of the tumor and should be appropriate for the general type of cancer initiated, irrespective of the site or sites of involvement.[29] Chemotherapy and radiation therapy treatments appropriate and relevant for the general category of carcinoma or sarcoma (depending upon the histologic findings, symptoms, and extent of tumor) should be initiated as early as possible.

Wilms' Tumor and Other Childhood Kidney Tumors

General Information

Wilms' tumor is a curable disease in the majority of affected children. Approximately 500 cases are diagnosed in the United States annually. More than 90% of patients survive 4 years after diagnosis which is an improvement over the 80% survival observed from 1975 to 1984. The prognosis is related not only to the stage of disease at diagnosis, the histopathologic features of the tumor, patient age, and tumor size but also to the team approach to each patient by the pediatric surgeon, radiation oncologist, and pediatric oncologist. Previous clinical trials have, in part, evaluated whether reduced therapy is sufficient to control disease in patients with early-stage, favorable-histology Wilms' tumor with some success. Ongoing clinical trials are evaluating biologic factors in the development of Wilms' tumor, clear cell sarcoma, and rhabdoid tumor of the kidney.

Wilms' tumor normally develops in otherwise healthy children but just under 10% occur in individuals with recognized malformations. The phenotypes associated with Wilms' tumor can be classified as overgrowth or nonovergrowth syndromes. Overgrowth syndromes are the result of excessive prenatal and postnatal somatic growth, and result in macroglossia, nephromegaly, and hemihypertrophy. The two most common overgrowth disorders associated with Wilms' tumor are Beckwith-Wiedemann syndrome and isolated hemihypertrophy. Others include Perlman syndrome, Sotos syndrome, and Simpson-Golabi-Behemel syndrome. Nonovergrowth disorders associated with Wilms' tumor include isolated aniridia, trisomy 18, aniridia in combination with genitourinary malformations, and mental retardation (AGR) syndrome, Bloom syndrome, and Denys-Drash syndrome. Children with a predisposition to develop Wilms' tumor (e.g., Beckwith-Wiedemann, hemihypertrophy) should be screened with ultrasound every 3 months until they are at least 6 years of age.

Wilms' tumor (hereditary or sporadic) appears to result from changes in one or more of several genes. Specific germ-line mutations in one of these genes (Wilms' tumor gene-1, *WT1*) located on the short arm of chromosome 11 (band 11p13) are not only associated with Wilms' tumor but also cause a variety of genitourinary abnormalities such as cryptorchidism and hypospadias, and the rare Denys-Drash syndrome. A gene that causes aniridia is located near the WT1 gene on chromosome 11p13, and deletions encompassing the WT1 and aniridia genes may explain the association between aniridia and Wilms' tumor. Patients with aniridia or hemihypertrophy should be screened with ultrasound every 3 months until they are at least 6 years of age. Children with Wilms' Aniridia-Genitourinary abnormalities-(mental) Retardation (WAGR) syndrome are at increased risk of eventually developing renal failure and should be monitored. Patients with Wilms' tumor and aniridia without genitourinary abnormalities are at lesser risk but should be monitored. There appears to be a second Wilms' tumor gene at or near the Beckwith-Wiedemann gene locus on chromosome 11p15, and children with Beckwith-Wiedemann syndrome are at increased risk for developing Wilms' tumor. Approximately one fifth of patients with Beckwith-Wiedemann syndrome who develop Wilms' tumor present with bilateral disease, primarily at diagnosis, although metachronous recurrence is also observed.

Approximately one third of Wilms' tumors have loss of genetic material in the tumor cells from the short arm of chromosome 11, encompassing 1 or both of the Wilms' tumor gene regions on this chromosome. Genes on other chromosomes may also have an etiologic role in Wilms' tumor, and loss of genetic material from chromosome 16 and/or chromosome 1p occurs in some tumors. Many Wilms' tumors appear to arise from abnormally retained embryonic kidney precursor cells arranged in clusters termed nephrogenic rests. The different genetic lesions are associated with different subtypes of nephrogenic rests. Wilms' tumors that develop from intralobar nephrogenic rests generally contain heterologous elements such as smooth muscle, cartilage, and fat cells, and are associated with loss of DNA on the short arm of chromosome 11p and occasionally with *WT1* gene mutation. In contrast, Wilms' tumors that develop from perilobar nephrogenic rests, which appear to reflect a slightly later stage in renal embryonic development and are generally found in older children are associated with loss of imprinting of the *IGF2* gene, which stimulates cell proliferation. Usually the maternal copy of *IGF2* is imprinted, that is, not expressed in the embryo, and when it is expressed in the tumor, twice as much IGF2 RNA is made. Perilobar rests are also associated with Wilms' tumors in children with Beckwith-Wiedemann syndrome.

Despite the number of genes that appear to be involved in the development of Wilms' tumor, hereditary Wilms' tumor is uncommon, with 1 to 2% of patients having a positive family history for Wilms' tumor. The risk of Wilms' tumor among offspring of persons who have had unilateral (i.e., sporadic) tumors is quite low (<2%). Siblings of children with Wilms' tumor have a low likelihood of developing Wilms' tumor. About 4 to 5% of patients have bilateral Wilms' tumors, but these are not usually hereditary. Many bilateral tumors are present at the time Wilms' tumor is first diagnosed (i.e., synchronous), but a second Wilms' tumor may also develop later in the remaining kidney of 1 to 3% of children treated successfully for Wilms' tumor. The incidence of such metachronous bilateral Wilms' tumors is much higher in children whose original Wilms' tumor was diagnosed at less than 12 months of age and/or whose resected kidney contains nephrogenic rests. Periodic abdominal ultrasound is recommended for early detection of metachronous bilateral Wilms' tumor as follows: children with nephrogenic rests in the resected kidney (if <48 months of age at initial diagnosis)-every 3 months for 6 years; children with nephrogenic rests in the resected kidney (if > 48 months of age at initial diagnosis)-every 3 months for 4 years; other patients-every 6 months for 2 years, then yearly for an additional 1 to 3 years.

Although most patients with a histologic diagnosis of Wilms' tumor fare well with current treatment, approximately 10% of patients have histopathologic features that are associated with a poorer prognosis, and, in some types, with a high incidence of relapse and death. Wilms' tumor can be separated into 2 prognostic groups on the basis of histopathology:

- *Favorable histology:* Histologically mimics development of a normal kidney consisting of 3 components: blastema, epithelium (tubules) and stroma. There is no anaplasia.
- *Unfavorable histology:* Characterized by anaplasia (extreme cellular pleomorphism and atypia, diffuse). Focal anaplasia may not confer nearly as poor a prognosis as diffuse anaplasia. Anaplasia is associated with resistance to chemotherapy and may still be detected after preoperative chemotherapy.

Clear Cell Sarcoma

Clear cell sarcoma (CCSK) of the kidney is not a Wilms' tumor variant, but it is an important primary renal tumor associated with a significantly higher rate of relapse and death than favorable histology Wilms' tumor. In addition to pulmonary metastases, clear cell sarcoma also spreads to bone, brain and soft tissue. The classic pattern of CCSK is defined by nests or cords of cells separated by regularly spaced arborizing fibrovascular septa.

Rhabdoid Tumor of the Kidney

Initially thought to be a rhabdomyosarcomatoid variant of Wilms' tumor, it is a distinctive and highly malignant tumor type. A distinct clinical presentation with fever, hematuria, young age (mean 11 months), and high tumor stage at presentation suggests a diagnosis of rhabdoid tumor of the kidney. Rhabdoid tumor of the kidney (RTK) tends to metastasize not only to the lungs, but also to the brain. As many as 10 to 15% of patients with RTK also have central nervous system lesions, now designated atypical teratoid tumors. The most distinctive features of rhabdoid tumors of the kidney are rather large cells with large vesicular nuclei, a prominent single nucleolus, and in some cells, the presence of globular eosinophilic cytoplasmic inclusions.

The characteristic molecular lesion found in rhabdoid tumors of the kidney is loss-of-function mutations of the hSNF5/INI1 gene, which is located at chromosome band 22q11.2. This same molecular abnormality is found in tumors of the central nervous system termed atypical teratoid and rhabdoid tumors. Some patients with rhabdoid tumors have constitutional mutations of the hSNF5/INI1 gene, and these children are at increased risk for second primary brain tumors.

Stage Information

Wilms' Tumor

A clinicopathologic staging system has been devised by the National Wilms' Tumor Study Group. The clinical stage is determined by the pediatric surgeon in the operating room and is confirmed by the pathologist. Staging, which is based on the degree of gross and microscopic tumor extension, is the same for tumors with favorable or unfavorable histologic features. Thus, patients should be characterized by a statement of both criteria (for example, stage II, favorable histology or stage II, unfavorable histology).

A description of the staging system and incidence from the Third National Wilms' Tumor Study (NWTS-3) is given below.

Stage I (43% of patients): Stage I Wilms' tumor is defined as tumor limited to the kidney and completely excised. The surface of the renal capsule is intact. The tumor is not ruptured before or during removal. The vessels of the renal sinus are not involved. There is no residual tumor apparent beyond the margins of excision.

Stage II (23% of patients): Stage II Wilms' tumor is defined as tumor that extends beyond the kidney but is completely excised. No residual tumor is apparent at or beyond the margins of excision. Any of the following conditions may exist:

1. Regional extension of the tumor, i.e., penetration through the outer surface of the renal capsule into the perirenal soft tissue or more than 1 to 2 mm of tumor invasion into the renal sinus.
2. Vessels outside the kidney are infiltrated or contain tumor thrombus.
3. The tumor was biopsied or there was local spillage of tumor confined to the flank.
4. In the National Wilms' Tumor Study 5 (NWTS-5), tumors with evidence of invasion

of thc vessels in the renal sinus (without any other reason to classify as stage II) were classified as stage II versus the stage I classification they were given in NWTS-1 through 4.

Stage III (23% of patients): Stage III Wilms' is defined as residual tumor confined to the abdomen. One or more of the following conditions may exist:

1. Lymph nodes in the renal hilus, the periaortic chains, or beyond are found to contain tumor on biopsy. Lymph node involvement in the thorax or other extra-abdominal sites would be a criterion for stage IV.
2. There has been diffuse peritoneal contamination by the tumor, such as by spillage of tumor beyond the flank before or during surgery or by tumor growth that has penetrated through the peritoneal surface.
3. Implants are found on the peritoneal surfaces.
4. Tumor extends beyond the surgical margins either microscopically or grossly.
5. Tumor is not completely resectable because of local infiltration into vital structures.

Stage IV (10% of patients): Stage IV Wilms' tumor is defined as the presence of hematogenous metastases. There are metastatic deposits beyond stage III, e.g., to the lung, liver, bone, or brain or to a combination of these sites.

Stage V (5% of patients): Stage V Wilms' tumor is defined as bilateral renal involvement at the time of initial diagnosis.

For patients with bilateral involvement, an attempt should be made to stage each side according to the above criteria on the basis of extent of disease prior to biopsy. The 4-year survival was 94% for those patients whose most advanced lesion was stage I or stage II; 76% for those whose most advanced lesion was stage III.

Stage I-IV Anaplasia (unfavorable histology): Children with stage I anaplastic tumors have an excellent prognosis. They can be managed with the same regimen given to stage I favorable histology patients. Children with stage II through stage IV diffuse anaplasia, however, represent a higher-risk group. These tumors are more resistant to the chemotherapy traditionally used in children with Wilms' tumor (favorable histology).

Treatment Option Overview

Wilms' Tumor

Because of the relative rarity of this tumor, all patients with Wilms' tumor should be considered for entry into a clinical trial. Treatment planning by a multidisciplinary team of cancer specialists (pediatric surgeon or pediatric urologist, pediatric radiation oncologist, and pediatric oncologist) with experience treating Wilms' tumor is required to determine and implement optimum treatment.

The major treatment conclusions of the National Wilms Tumor Studies (NWTS 1-4) are:

1. Routine, postoperative radiation therapy of the flank is not necessary for children with stage I tumors or stage II tumors with favorable histology (FH) when postnephrectomy combination chemotherapy consisting of vincristine and dactinomycin is administered.
2. The prognosis for patients with stage III/FH is best when treatment includes: (a) dactinomycin, vincristine, doxorubicin, and 1,000 cGy of radiation therapy to the flank; or (b) dactinomycin, vincristine, and 2,000 cGy of radiation therapy to the flank.
3. The addition of cyclophosphamide to the combination of vincristine, dactinomycin, and doxorubicin does not improve prognosis for patients with stage IV/FH tumors.
4. Single-dose ("pulse-intensive") treatment with dactinomycin (stages I-II/FH, stage I anaplastic), and doxorubicin (stage III/FH, stages III-IV, or stages I-IV clear cell sarcoma of the

kidney) is equivalent to the divided-dose courses, and results in the same event-free survival, greater dose-intensity, and is associated with less toxicity and expense.

5. 18 weeks of therapy is adequate for patients with stage I/FH whereas other patients can be treated with 6 months of therapy instead of 15 months.

Operative principles have evolved from NWTS trials. The most important role for the surgeon is to ensure complete tumor removal without rupture and perform an assessment of the extent of disease. Radical nephrectomy-lymph node sampling via a transabdominal incision is the procedure of choice. Partial nephrectomy is currently not recommended, although it may be considered for very small tumors discovered by ultrasound screening. The contralateral kidney must be palpated and inspected through an opening in the fascia. Hilar, periaortic, iliac and celiac lymph node sampling is mandatory. Furthermore, any suspicious node basin should be sampled. Margins of resection, residual tumor, and any suspicious node basins should be marked with titanium clips. Liver wedge resection or partial duodenal or colonic resections are acceptable for complete en bloc excision. Wilms' tumor arising in a horseshoe kidney is rare and accurate preoperative diagnosis is important in planning the operative approach. Primary resection is possible in the majority of cases. In operable cases can usually be resected after chemotherapy. Patients with massive, nonresectable unilateral tumors, bilateral tumors, or venacaval tumor thrombus above the hepatic veins are candidates for preoperative chemotherapy because of the risk of initial surgical resection. Preoperative chemotherapy should follow a biopsy, which may be performed percutaneously. Preoperative chemotherapy makes the tumor removal easier and may reduce the frequency of surgical complications.

Newborns and all infants less than 12 months of age require a reduction in chemotherapy doses to 50% of those given to older children. This reduction diminishes toxic effects reported in children in this age group enrolled in NWTS studies while maintaining an excellent overall outcome. Liver function tests in children with Wilms' tumor should be monitored closely during the early course of therapy based on hepatic toxic effects (veno-occlusive disease) reported in those patients. Dactinomycin should not be administered during radiation therapy. Children treated for Wilms' tumor are at increased risk for developing second malignant neoplasms. This risk depends on the intensity of their therapy, including the use of radiation and doxorubicin, and on possible genetic factors. Congestive heart failure has been shown to be a risk in children treated with doxorubicin with the degree of risk influenced by cumulative doxorubicin dose, irradiation to the heart, and gender (females at increased risk). Efforts, therefore, have been aimed toward reducing the intensity of therapy when possible.

Stage I Wilms' Tumor

Regardless of histology, all stage I Wilms' tumor patients have an excellent prognosis with the same treatment.

Favorable histology (FH) tumors (94.9% 2-year relapse-free survival [RFS]; 98.7% 2-year survival):

- Nephrectomy with lymph node sampling and 18 weeks of chemotherapy with vincristine and pulse-intensive dactinomycin.

Focal or diffuse anaplasia (87.5% 2-year RFS, 85.5% 2-year survival):

- Nephrectomy with lymph node sampling and 18 weeks of chemotherapy with vincristine and pulse-intensive dactinomycin.

It may be possible to treat a subset of stage I Wilms' tumor patients with surgery alone without chemotherapy. The Children's Oncology Group (COG) is planning a large study to address this question. A pilot study was performed in National Wilms' Tumor Study Group-5 (NWTS-5) infants with stage I/FH Wilms' tumor who were less than 24 months of age and whose nephrectomy specimen weighed less than 550 grams. Even though there was 2 times the recurrence rate in this trial, it's possible that most of these patients may be successfully salvaged with chemotherapy.

Stage II Wilms' Tumor

Favorable histology tumors (85.9% 2-year relapse-free survival; 97% 2-year survival):

- Nephrectomy with lymph node sampling and 18 weeks of chemotherapy with vincristine and pulse-intensive dactinomycin.

Focal anaplasia:

- Nephrectomy with lymph node sampling, abdominal irradiation, and 24 weeks of chemotherapy with vincristine, doxorubicin, and pulse-intensive dactinomycin.

Diffuse anaplasia (70% 4-year survival):

- Nephrectomy with lymph node sampling, abdominal irradiation, and 24 weeks of chemotherapy with vincristine, doxorubicin, etoposide, cyclophosphamide, and mesna.

Stage III Wilms' Tumor

Favorable histology tumors (91.1% 2-year relapse-free survival; 98.2% 2-year survival):

- Nephrectomy with lymph node sampling, abdominal irradiation, and 24 weeks of chemotherapy with vincristine, doxorubicin, and pulse-intensive dactinomycin.

Focal anaplasia:

- Nephrectomy with lymph node sampling, abdominal irradiation, and 24 weeks of chemotherapy with vincristine, doxorubicin, and pulse-intensive dactinomycin.

Diffuse anaplasia (56% 4-year survival):

- Nephrectomy with lymph node sampling, abdominal irradiation, and 24 weeks of chemotherapy with vincristine, doxorubicin, etoposide, cyclophosphamide, and mesna.

Inoperable Tumors

Treatment Options

Patients who have tumors with caval extension above the hepatic veins or that are so massive that their surgeons consider the risk of initial surgical removal too great should be biopsied and treated with preoperative chemotherapy. If surgery is performed in a patient with caval or atrial extension, care should be taken to ensure that appropriate resources are available for pediatric cardiopulmonary bypass. On the National Wilms' Tumor Study-5 (NWTS-5), these patients are treated after biopsy by initial chemotherapy with vincristine and dactinomycin with or without doxorubicin. If no reduction in tumor size has occurred after using 3 drugs, then radiation therapy should be used. Surgery is performed as soon as sufficient tumor shrinkage has occurred, generally within 6 weeks of diagnosis. Patients are subsequently treated as for stage III tumors, which includes postoperative radiation therapy. Because of the 5% to 10% error rate in preoperative diagnosis of renal masses after radiographic assessment, confirmation of the diagnosis by biopsy (which may be performed percutaneously) should be obtained prior to chemotherapy.

Stage IV Wilms' Tumor

Favorable histology tumors (80.6% 2-year relapse-free survival; 89.5% 2-year survival):

- Nephrectomy with lymph node sampling, abdominal irradiation according to local stage of renal tumor, bilateral pulmonary irradiation for patients with chest X-ray evidence of pulmonary metastases, and 24 weeks of chemotherapy with vincristine, doxorubicin, and pulse-intensive dactinomycin.

Focal anaplasia

- Nephrectomy with lymph node sampling, abdominal irradiation according to local stage of renal tumor, bilateral pulmonary irradiation for patients with chest X-ray evidence of pulmonary metastases, and 24 weeks of chemotherapy with vincristine, doxorubicin, and pulse-intensive dactinomycin.

Diffuse anaplasia (17% 4-year survival):

- Nephrectomy with lymph node sampling, abdominal irradiation, whole-lung irradiation for patients with chest X-ray evidence of pulmonary metastases, and 24 weeks of chemotherapy with vincristine, doxorubicin, etoposide, cyclophosphamide, and mesna.

Stage V Wilms' Tumor

Previously, the surgical approach to bilateral Wilms' tumor was nephrectomy of the side with the larger lesion. However, initial unilateral nephrectomy may predispose patients with bilateral disease to late renal failure. Furthermore, studies demonstrate no difference in survival for children who undergo initial bilateral biopsy followed by chemotherapy and then surgical resection compared with patients who have initial resection followed by chemotherapy. Surgical strategy therefore attempts to preserve renal mass to minimize the risk of late renal failure. Surgical stage should be assigned to both kidneys. Thus, bilateral biopsies and lymph node sampling should be performed. Following 6 weeks of chemotherapy the patient is reassessed. If serial imaging studies show no further reduction in tumor, a second-look surgical procedure should be performed (partial nephrectomy or wedge excision) if negative margins can be obtained, otherwise another biopsy to confirm viable tumor. Chemotherapy and/or radiation therapy following the second-look operation is dependent on the response to initial therapy, with more aggressive therapy required for patients with inadequate response to initial therapy observed at the second procedure.

Approximately 10% of patients with bilateral tumors have unfavorable (anaplastic) histology and may benefit from more aggressive chemotherapy and radiation therapy and an aggressive surgical approach at the second-look operation.

Eighteen

Intraocular Melanoma

Melanoma of the uveal tract (iris, ciliary body, and choroid), although rare, is the most common primary intraocular malignancy in adults. The median age at diagnosis ranges from 55 to 62 years. Several factors likely play a role in the development of uveal melanoma. Host characteristics, such as light pigmentation (skin, hair, eye color) and genetic factors, as well as environmental exposures (sunlight, chemical), have been associated with increased risk.

Melanomas can arise in the anterior uveal tract (iris) or the posterior uveal tract (ciliary body or choroid). Iris melanomas have the best prognosis, whereas melanomas of the ciliary body have the worst. Most uveal tract melanomas originate in the choroid. The ciliary body is less commonly a site of origin, and the iris is the least common. The comparatively low incidence of this tumor in the iris has been attributed to the characteristic features of iris melanomas, i.e., they tend to be small, slow growing, and relatively dormant in comparison with their posterior counterparts. Iris melanomas rarely metastasize. Melanomas of the posterior uveal tract are cytologically more malignant, detected later, and metastasize more frequently than iris melanomas. The typical choroidal melanoma is a brown, elevated, dome-shaped subretinal mass. The degree of pigmentation ranges from dark brown to totally amelanotic.

Most melanomas of the iris, ciliary body, or choroid are initially completely asymptomatic. As the tumor enlarges, it may cause distortion of the pupil (iris melanoma), blurred vision (ciliary body melanoma), or markedly decreased visual acuity due to secondary retinal detachment (choroidal melanoma). Serous detachment of the retina frequently complicates tumor growth. If extensive retinal detachment occurs, secondary angle-closure glaucoma occasionally develops. Clinically, there are several lesions that simulate uveal melanoma, including metastatic carcinoma, posterior scleritis, and benign tumors such as nevi and hemangiomas.

A number of factors influence prognosis. The most important are cell type, tumor size, location of the anterior margin of the tumor, the degree of ciliary body involvement, and extraocular extension. Cell type, however, remains the most often used predictor of outcome. The selection of treatment depends on the site of origin (choroid, ciliary body, or iris), the size and location of the lesion, the age of the patient, and whether extraocular invasion, recurrence, or metastasis has occurred. Extraocular extension, recurrence, and metastasis are associated with an extremely poor prognosis, and long-term survival cannot be expected. The 5-year mortality rate due to metastasis from ciliary body or choroidal melanoma is approximately 30%, compared with a rate of 2 to 3% for iris melanomas. In a group of patients with large tumors of the choroid or choroid and ciliary body, the concurrent presence of abnormalities in chromosomes 3 and 8 was also associated with a poor outcome.

In the past, enucleation (eye removal) was the accepted standard treatment for primary choroidal melanoma, and it remains the most commonly used treatment for large tumors. Due to the effect of enucleation on the appearance of the patient, the diagnostic uncertainty encountered by the ophthalmologist (particularly in the case of smaller tumors), and the potential for tumor spread, alternative treatments, such as radiation therapy (brachytherapy or external-beam, charged-particle radiotherapy), transpupillary thermotherapy, photocoagulation, and cryotherapy have been developed in an attempt to spare the affected eye and possibly retain useful vision. Initial results from the randomized Collaborative Ocular Melanoma Study have demonstrated comparable 5-year survival rates for patients with medium-size tumors treated primarily with brachytherapy (I^{125} plaque irradiation) or enucleation.

Primary intraocular melanomas originate from melanocytes in the uveal tract. Four distinct cellular types are recognized in intraocular melanoma (revised Callendar classification):

1. *Spindle A cells* (spindle-shaped cells with slender nuclei and lacking visible nucleoli).
2. *Spindle B cells* (spindle-shaped cells with larger nuclei and distinct nucleoli).
3. *Epithelioid cells* (larger polygonal cells with 1 or more prominent nucleoli).
4. *Intermediate cells* (similar to but smaller than epithelioid cells).

Most primary intraocular melanomas contain variable numbers of epithelioid, spindle A, and spindle B cells (mixed-cell melanomas). Pure epithelioid-cell primary melanomas are infrequent (approximately 3% of cases).

Several microscopic features can affect the prognosis of intraocular melanoma, including cell type, mitotic activity, lymphocytic infiltration, and, possibly, fibrovascular loops. Cell type remains the most often used predictor of outcome following enucleation, with spindle A cell melanomas carrying the best prognosis and epithelioid cell melanomas carrying the worst.

Metastatic Disease

Because the uveal tract is a vascular structure without lymphatic channels, tumor spread occurs principally by local extension and by dissemination through the blood stream. If regional preauricular, submandibular, or cervical lymph node involvement is seen, subconjunctival extension of the primary tumor has occurred. Systemic metastases are generally hematogenous in origin and the first site identified is usually the liver. Lung, bone, and subcutaneous sites are also common]. In approximately two thirds of patients, the liver is the only site of detectable metastasis. At the time of death, however, other sites of metastasis have been detected in patients for whom the liver was the only known location of tumor spread. In patients with a history of ocular melanoma who present with hepatic metastases of unknown origin, metastatic melanoma should be considered in the differential diagnosis.

It is particularly unusual for choroidal melanomas of any size to invade the optic nerve or its meninges. Metastasis of choroidal melanoma to the contralateral choroid is also rare. Other unusual cases of melanoma metastasis have been reported in the literature, including cardiac, pancreatic, spleen, and stomach metastasis.

Iris Melanoma

Melanocytic stromal proliferations of the iris are the most common tumors of the iris. Clinical differentiation between an iris nevus and a melanoma might sometimes be difficult and at times impossible. Melanomas of the iris are usually small discrete lesions, although, occasionally, they may be diffuse, infiltrative, multiple, and may result in heterochromia, chronic uveitis, or spontaneous hyphema. Iris melanomas that involve more than two thirds of the angle circumference are associated with secondary glaucoma.

Routine evaluation of iris melanomas includes gonioscopy, transillumination of the globe, and indirect ophthalmoscopy with 360 degrees of scleral depression. Photographic documentation is essential to document progression in size or growth of the tumor. Anterior segment fluorescein angiography may be helpful in demonstrating the vascularity of the lesion, but is not diagnostic. High-resolution ultrasound biomicroscopy can be used to measure small lesions (basal dimensions and thickness) and assess tumor involvement of the anterior ciliary body, angle, and overlying sclera. The main disadvantage with this technology is its limited penetration of large lesions. In these cases, conventional ultrasonography is more accurate.

In general, iris melanomas have relatively good outcomes, with a 5-year survival rate of more than 95%. Iris melanomas are predominantly of the spindle cell type and are usually smaller in size than posterior melanomas due to earlier detection. Clinical features, including prominent tumor vascularity, rapid growth, and heterogeneous pigmentation, are associated with an epithelioid cell component. Involvement of the iridocorneal angles is frequently associated with ciliary body invasion.

Conservative management is generally advocated whenever possible, but surgical intervention may be justified with unequivocal tumor growth and with extensive disease at initial examination.

Standard Treatment Options

1. *Observation with careful follow-up:* In asymptomatic patients with stable lesions; follow-up includes serial photography.
2. *Local resection:* When progressive and pronounced growth is documented.
3. *Enucleation:* If the tumor is not amenable to local resection (diffuse involvement of the iris, involvement of more than one half of the iris and anterior chamber angle, intractable glaucoma, and extraocular extension).
4. *Plaque radiotherapy:* Offered as an alternative for large, diffuse, surgically-nonresectable lesions of the iris.

Choroidal Melanoma

The natural history of small choroidal melanoma remains poorly understood. Small, pigmented choroidal lesions cannot always be differentiated reliably on examination. Growth is a presumed indicator of malignant potential.

Although patients diagnosed with small choroidal tumors were not eligible for participation in the Collaborative Ocular Melanoma Study, these patients were offered participation in a prospective follow-up study to evaluate the natural history of small lesions. Clinical risk factors associated with tumor growth included increased tumor thickness, presence of subretinal fluid, orange pigmentation, absence of drusen, absence of retinal pigment, margin at the optic disc, and epithelial changes surrounding the tumor.

The 5-year melanoma-related mortality rate in patients treated for small choroidal melanomas has been reported as high as 12%. Several studies indicate the 2 most important clinical factors predictive of mortality are larger tumor size (at the time of treatment) and documentation of tumor growth. Typical features of the tumor on ophthalmoscopy, fluorescein angiography, and ultrasound examination of the eye contribute to the clinical diagnosis. Accuracy of the tumor thickness measurement by echography is an important issue with very small tumors. Wide-field photography is helpful in detecting the rate of choroidal tumor growth. Although these techniques have improved the diagnostic differentiation of larger size melanomas, the accuracy of diagnosis for small melanomas is more uncertain. Furthermore, smaller tumors may not produce symptoms, depending on their location with respect to the macula, and may go undetected unless discovered during the course of a routine eye examination.

The management of small choroidal melanomas is controversial. The likelihood of progression from the time of diagnosis to growth warranting treatment has not been well characterized. In the past, many ophthalmologists advocated observation. This was justified on several grounds, including the difficulty in establishing a correct diagnosis, the lack of any documented efficacy for globe-conserving treatments, and concerns for severe treatment-related morbidity. Some investigators have advocated earlier therapeutic intervention, since smaller tumor size at the time of treatment appears to be associated with lower mortality rates.

The management of choroidal melanomas depends on many factors; most important are tumor size and location. In otherwise healthy patients, a small choroidal melanoma in the posterior fundus is amenable to several treatment options, including radiotherapy, laser photocoagulation, transpupillary thermotherapy, a combination of these methods, or even enucleation.

Standard Treatment Options

1. *Observation:* In patients for whom the diagnosis is uncertain or in whom tumor growth is not documented; also prudent in asymptomatic patients with stable lesions, particularly in elderly or debilitated patients, or in patients with tumor growth in their only useful eye.
2. *Plaque radiotherapy:* Used for small or medium-sized uveal melanomas, amelanotic tumors, or tumors that touch the optic disc for greater than 3 O'clock-hours of optic disk circumference.
3. *External-beam, charged-particle radiotherapy:* Provides precisely focused radiation with a homogeneous dose distribution pattern and little lateral spread; requires sophisticated equipment available only at selected centers; patient cooperation during treatment (voluntarily fixating the eye on a particular point so the tumor is positioned properly in the radiation beam) is important; in eyes with tumors less than 6 mm in thickness and located more than 3 mm distant from the optic disc or fovea, clinically significant visual loss can usually be avoided.
4. *Gamma knife radiosurgery:* A newer method of radiotherapy; preliminary experience suggests this treatment may be a feasible option for small-size to medium-size melanomas.
5. *Laser photocoagulation:* Can be used in very selected cases of small posterior choroidal melanoma; indirect ophthalmoscope laser therapy may be combined with plaque radiotherapy.
6. *Transpupillary thermotherapy:* Causes substantial tumor necrosis in choroidal melanomas up to 3.5 mm in thickness; currently used in selected cases with deeply pigmented small choroidal melanomas in the posterior pole with minimal or no contact with the optic nerve; can be used as a primary treatment or as an adjunctive method to plaque radiotherapy.
7. *Local tumor resection:* Used mainly for selected ciliary body or anterior choroidal tumors with smaller basal dimension and greater thickness.
8. *Enucleation:* Severe intraocular pressure elevation is a factor favoring enucleation; may also be considered in small and medium-size

melanomas that are invading the tissues of the optic nerve; an eye-sparing procedure rather than enucleation should be considered if there is hope for useful vision.

Enucleation remains the standard therapy for most large choroidal melanomas and melanomas causing severe glaucoma or invading the optic nerve. Some reports have suggested that enucleation may not help improve survival and may actually result in tumor metastasis. Episcleral radionuclide plaque therapy (brachytherapy) and external-beam, charged-particle radiotherapy offer patients eye-sparing and vision-sparing alternatives to enucleation. Episcleral plaque brachytherapy is the most frequently used eye-sparing treatment for choroidal melanoma. Iodine-125 (I^{125}), gold-198 (^{198}Au), palladium-103 (^{103}Pd), and other ophthalmic plaques can be effective in the treatment of medium-size melanomas.

Retinoblastoma

Retinoblastoma is a relatively uncommon tumor of childhood that arises in the retina and accounts for about 3% of the cancers occurring in children younger than 15 years. The estimated annual incidence is approximately 4 per million children. Although it may occur at any age, it most often occurs in younger children, usually before the age of 2 years. Ninety-five percent of cases are diagnosed before the age of 5 years. The tumor may be either unilateral (75%) or bilateral (25%). Retinoblastoma is usually confined to the eye, and as a result, more than 90% of children with retinoblastoma will be cured. The present challenge for those who treat retinoblastoma is to prevent blindness and other serious effects of treatment that reduce the life span or the quality of survival.

Retinoblastoma is a tumor that occurs in germline (40%) and sporadic (60%) forms. Germline disease includes those patients with a positive family history (hereditary disease) and those patients who have sustained a new germline mutation. The genetic locus responsible for a predisposition to retinoblastoma is located within the q14 band of chromosome 13.

The germline form of retinoblastoma may manifest as unilateral or bilateral disease. Most unilateral disease is sporadic or nongermline, whereas all children with bilateral disease have the germline form. Germline tumors tend to occur at a younger age than sporadic tumors. Unilateral tumors in infants are more likely to have germline mutations, whereas older children with unilateral tumors are more likely to have sporadic tumors. Unilateral tumors in younger children have fewer genetic abnormalities than those in older children. Children with the germline form (positive family history and/or bilateral retinoblastoma or mutations in the *RB* gene) who have a normal examination in at least 1 eye on initial presentation need to be examined frequently for the development of new retinoblastoma tumors. It is recommended that they be examined every 2 to 4 months for at least 28 months. Following treatment, patients require careful surveillance until 7 years of age.

Trilateral retinoblastoma is a well recognized syndrome that consists of unilateral or bilateral germline retinoblastoma associated with an intracranial neuroblastic tumor. It has been observed that 5 to 15% of children with either familial, multifocal, or bilateral retinoblastoma may develop an intracranial neuroblastic tumor as well.

All siblings of patients with retinoblastoma should be examined, and studies suggest that DNA polymorphism analysis may help predict which persons are at risk and warrant close follow-up. Cytogenetic abnormalities (e.g., deletion on the long arm of chromosome 13) are sometimes observed. Clinical laboratory service is now becoming available in some centers for performing genetic testing of relatives of retinoblastoma patients to determine risk of hereditary susceptibility to the disease. Although confined to use in research, "exon by exon" sequencing of the RB1 gene demonstrates germline mutation in 90% of patients with germline retinoblastoma. Although a positive finding confirms susceptibility with current technology, a negative finding cannot absolutely rule it out.

Most patients with retinoblastoma have extensive disease within the eye at diagnosis, with either massive tumors involving more than one half of the retina, multiple tumors diffusely involving the retina, or obvious seeding of the vitreous. The goals of therapy are 2-fold: eradicate the disease and preserve as much vision as possible.

Although there are several staging systems currently available for retinoblastoma, for the purposes of treatment retinoblastoma is categorized into intraocular and extraocular disease.

Intraocular

5-year Disease-free Survival: >90%

Intraocular retinoblastoma is localized to the eye and may be confined to the retina or may extend to involve the globe; however, it does not extend beyond the eye into the tissues around the eye or to other parts of the body.

Extraocular

5-year Disease-free Survival: <10%

Extraocular retinoblastoma has extended beyond the eye. It may be confined to the tissues around the eye, or it may have spread, typically to the central nervous system (CNS) or to other parts of the body.

Reese-Ellsworth Classification for Intraocular Tumors

Reese and Ellsworth have developed a generally adopted classification for intraocular retinoblastoma that has been shown to have prognostic significance for maintenance of sight and control of local disease. The system is relevant to decisions regarding the use of local treatment modalities.

Group I: very favorable for maintenance of sight:

A. Solitary tumor, smaller than 4 disc diameters at or behind the equator.
B. Multiple tumors, none larger than 4 disc diameters all at or behind the equator.

Group II: favorable for maintenance of sight:

A. Solitary tumor, 4-10 disc diameters at or behind the equator.
B. Multiple tumors, 4-10 disc diameters behind the equator.

Group III: possible for maintenance of sight:

A. Any lesion anterior to the equator.
B. Solitary tumor, larger than 10 disc diameters behind the equator.

Group IV: unfavorable for maintenance of sight:

A. Multiple tumors, some larger than 10 disc diameters.
B. Any lesion extending anteriorly to the ora serrata.

Group V: very unfavorable for maintenance of sight:

A. Massive tumors involving more than one half the retina.
B. Vitreous seeding.

Intraocular Retinoblastoma

Treatment of retinoblastoma should be planned after the extent of the tumor within and outside the eye is known. Treatment options consider both cure and preservation of sight.

Treatment options for the involved eye include the following:

1. Enucleation, if the tumor is massive or if there is little expectation for useful vision.
2. External-beam radiation with doses ranging from 3,500 to 4,600 cGy. Because of the need to sedate young children and the intricacies of field planning, special expertise in pediatric radiation therapy is important.
3. Cryotherapy, used in addition to radiation or in place of photocoagulation for lesions

smaller than 4 disc diameters in the anterior portion of the retina.

4. Light coagulation (photocoagulation) is occasionally used alone with small tumors. In patients with early stages of disease, light coagulation is usually used in addition to radiation therapy or when there is limited recurrence following radiation therapy. Photocoagulation is used for posteriorly located tumors that are smaller than 4 disc diameters, distinct from the optic nerve head and macula, and without involvement of large nutrient vessels or choroid involvement. Thermotherapy delivered via infrared radiation is an alternative to laser photocoagulation.
5. Brachytherapy with radioactive plaques for either focal unilateral presentations or recurrent disease following previous external-beam irradiation.
6. During the past 10 years, systemic chemotherapy to reduce tumor volume (chemoreduction) and to avoid the long-term effects of radiation therapy for patients with intraocular tumors has succeeded in rendering many eyes amenable to treatment with cryotherapy or photocoagulation. Chemotherapy may also be continued or initiated with concurrent local control interventions. Factors, such as tumor location (macula), patient age (patient older than 2 months), and tumor size, correlate with responsiveness to chemotherapy. Most tumors treated with vincristine and carboplatin require additional local therapy; the addition of etoposide to the chemotherapy regimen may improve outcome, but may increase the risk of developing acute leukemia.

Unilateral Disease

Treatment Options

Since most unilateral disease is usually massive and there is often no expectation that useful vision can be preserved, surgery (enucleation) is usually undertaken and radiation therapy is not given to the tumor bed. However, even this is being tested, as patients with unilateral disease have been treated with chemotherapy in an attempt to save a potentially seeing eye.

When there is potential for preservation of sight because the tumors are smaller, treatment with other modalities (radiation therapy, photocoagulation, cryotherapy, thermotherapy, chemoreduction, and brachytherapy) instead of surgery should be considered. In selected children with unilateral disease, chemoreduction reduced the need for enucleation or external-beam radiation to 68% within 5 years of treatment. Reese-Ellsworth (RE) group correlated with successful chemoreduction: 11% of children classified as having RE group II or III disease, 60% of children having RE group IV disease, and 100% of children having RE group V disease required enucleation or external-beam radiation within 5 years of treatment.

Since a proportion of children who present with unilateral retinoblastoma will eventually develop disease in the opposite eye, it is very important that children with unilateral retinoblastoma receive periodic examinations of the unaffected eye. Asynchronous bilateral disease occurs most frequently in families with affected parents.

Careful examination of the enucleated specimen by an experienced pathologist is necessary to determine if high-risk features for metastatic disease are present. These include anterior chamber seeding, choroidal involvement, tumor beyond the lamina cribrosa, intraocular hemorrhage, or scleral and extrascleral extension. Systemic adjuvant therapy with vincristine, doxorubicin, and cyclophosphamide, or vincristine, carboplatin, and etoposide, has been used in patients with certain high-risk features assessed by pathologic review after enucleation to prevent the development of metastatic disease. Clinical trials are needed to determine precisely what features are truly high risk.

Bilateral Disease

The management of bilateral disease depends on the extent of the disease in each eye.

Treatment Options

Usually the disease is more advanced in 1 eye, with less involvement in the other eye. The standard of care in the past has been to enucleate the more involved eye; however, if there is potential for vision in both eyes, bilateral irradiation or chemotherapy with close follow-up for response and focal treatment (e.g., cryotherapy or laser therapy) is indicated.

A number of large centers in Europe and North America have published the trial results of using systemic chemotherapy for patients whose intraocular tumors are not initially amenable to local management. Examples of such tumors are those that are too large to be treated with either cryotherapy, laser photocoagulation, or plaque radiation therapy (brachytherapy). Another example is the newborn with a tumor over the optic nerve head. All these situations have in common the likelihood that local therapy would so limit vision as to offer little improvement over enucleation. Most centers have limited this approach to patients with bilateral disease, reasoning that for patients with unilateral disease the morbidity of enucleation is modest. When disease is massive and there is no expectation that useful vision can be preserved, surgery is usually undertaken and radiation therapy is not given.

All the institutional pilot protocols have in common the use of carboplatin and etoposide. Most centers add vincristine and one has advocated the use of cyclosporin A as a modulator of the p-glycoprotein. In all cases, the goal of chemotherapy is the reduction (hence the term "chemoreduction") of tumor volume, making possible the use of local therapy (cryotherapy, photocoagulation, thermotherapy, plaque radiation therapy) and avoiding the use of enucleation or external-beam irradiation. Chemotherapy has been combined with diode laser hyperthermic local therapy.

Extraocular Retinoblastoma

Few patients with retinoblastoma present with extraocular disease. Extraocular disease may be localized to the soft tissues surrounding the eye or to the optic nerve beyond the margin of resection. However, further extension may occur into the brain and meninges with subsequent seeding of the spinal fluid, as well as distant metastatic disease involving the lungs, bones, and bone marrow. In patients with the genetic form of retinoblastoma, central nervous system (CNS) disease is less likely the result of metastatic or regional spread than a primary intracranial focus, such as a pineal tumor. Early diagnosis may be helpful and it has been recommended that cranial computerized tomography or magnetic resonance imaging be done twice a year until age 5 years for those who carry the gene (bilateral and unilateral germline cases).

Standard Treatment Options

There is no clearly proven effective therapy for the treatment of extraocular retinoblastoma, although orbital irradiation and chemotherapy have been used. In general, palliative therapy with radiation (including craniospinal irradiation when there is meningeal involvement) and/or intrathecal chemotherapy with methotrexate, cytarabine, and hydrocortisone, and supportive care has been used.

Index